CLARK'S
POSITIONING IN
RADIOGRAPHY

TENTH EDITION
Volume One

Edited by Louis Kreel MD FRCP FRCR
with the assistance of Ann Paris FCR TE DMU

A WILLIAM HEINEMANN MEDICAL BOOKS
PUBLICATION

Distributed by
YEAR BOOK MEDICAL PUBLISHERS, INC.
35 East Wacker Drive, Chicago

First edition published in January 1939
Second edition published in January 1941
Third edition published in June 1942
Fourth edition published in April 1945
Fifth edition published in October 1949
Sixth edition published in February 1951
Seventh edition published in December 1956
Eighth edition published in July 1964
Eighth edition (revised) published in May 1967
Ninth edition (Volume 1) published in 1973
Tenth edition (Volume 1) published in 1979

(ISBN 0–8151–5190–X)

Library of Congress Catalog Card Number: 79–56325

INTRODUCTION
to the TENTH EDITION

The last ten years have seen considerable advances in radiography, radiology departments and hospital practice. Rare-earth screens are now widely used with a marked reduction in radiation exposure making slow exposure times possible without recourse to high kilovoltage or high output generators.

Many old procedures have been modified and new procedures introduced, now being an integral part of normal practice. Angiography is available in all but the smallest departments, double contrast barium meals and enemas performed routinely as well as arthography, renal cyst puncture, antegrade pyelography, mammography and endoscopic retrograde cholangio-pancreotography (ERCP).

Automatic processing is currently so widespread that 'wet processing' is not only unknown in many departments but can hardly be remembered while radiographic equipment with automatic exposure control is gaining wider acceptance. Radiography has consequently become easier and pleasanter with cleaner and more efficient dark rooms, fewer repeat examinations and a saving in cost and radiation.

Fluoroscopy has also become simpler and pleasanter with the universal introduction of image intensification and television viewing. Gone are the old days of red goggles, dark adaptation and barium examinations in the dark. Moreover, the new caesium iodide intensifier tubes produce images of very high quality. Even the films are in the process of change with the acceptance of 70 and 100 mm films, storage by miniaturisation and the use of Xerography.

Central sterilisation departments provide sterile angiographic, aspiration, myelographic and hystersalpingography packs. Emergency examinations are now readily organized with a minimum of fuss and bother, and have consequently become safer and more tolerable for the patient. A more important reason for the increased safety is that the newer contrast agents for these invasive procedures are less toxic and more easily managed.

Intensive Care and Coronary Care units (ITU/CCU) are an accepted part of general hospital practice and many more hospitals move patients to radiology departments in their beds. Mobile examinations are therefore more confined and are of much better quality especially with the new higher output units.

There has also been a greater awareness of the potential hazard from radiation in the early months of pregnancy and the almost universal implementation of the 10 day rule is especially gratifying. The most dramatic change however is the introduction of ultrasonography in obstetrics which has completely displaced conventional radiography. But it is not only in obstetrics that the new scanning methods are revolutionizing diagnostic radiology. Non-invasive methods including isotope imaging, computed tomography and nuclear magnetic resonance scanning are being applied to all areas of the body and every organ. The new generation of radiographers are likely to be as familiar and unimpressed by these innovations as the present generation are with automatic processors and image intensifiers.

Thus radiology departments have changed radically in the last decade, making exact diagnoses more readily available to larger numbers with less discomfort to the patient and easier for the radiographer. However, radiographers now need a far greater knowledge to cover the increasing scope of the subject. With the new scanning methods being introduced computers and computer technology may yet also find a place in radiographic practice. However, there can be no progress in radiography without the basic skills in patient positioning based on an accurate knowledge of basic anatomy. "Positioning in Radiography" will therefore continue as an essential guide to good radiographic practice.

ACKNOWLEDGEMENTS

We gratefully acknowledge the rôle of the Clinical Research Centre and Northwick Park Hospital. In producing a new Edition to "Kitty" Clark's book; a modern department is obviously essential. The farsighted policy of the Department of Health and Social Security (DHSS) in combining with the Medical Research Council (MRC) under the auspices of the North West Regional Board, helped to conceive and build the institution. Modern equipment and adequate staffing is obviously needed for good radiography.

Our thanks are therefore due to the Staff of the Radiology Department who have developed and maintained high standards since its opening in 1970.

ACKNOWLEDGEMENTS
to the NINTH EDITION

Miss K C Clark was principal of the ILFORD Department of Radiography and Medical Photography, Tavistock House, from 1935 to 1958. Her intense interest in teaching and radiographic projections led to an invitation by Ilford Limited to produce 'Positioning in Radiography' which has now reached its 10th edition. Her infectious enthusiasm was most gratifying to all visitors. She was ably assisted by her colleagues, leading to many innovations in radiography, especially in developing mass miniature radiography.

She accepted Honorary Fellowship of the British Society of Radiographers after being President of the Society and in 1959 was made an Honorary member of the Faculty of Radiologists and an Honorary Fellow of the Australian Institute of Radiography.

Miss Clark died in 1968 and the Kathleen Clark Memorial Library established by the Society of Radiographers at Upper Wimpole Street in fitting respect of her contribution.

The ninth edition was produced in two volumes being edited and revised by James McInnes FSR, TE, FRPS, having been involved with Positioning in Radiography from 1946 when he joined the team at Tavistock House. He originated many aspects in radiography and contributed numerous articles to radiographic journals, becoming Principal of Lecture and Technical Services at Tavistock House and lecturing widely to X-ray Societies in Britain, Canada, America, South and West Africa.

Over two hundred new photographic illustrations have been incorporated in this new edition. Renewal of considerable previous illustrations has taken place, to both up-date and improve the accuracy of presentation. Photographic illustration of all additional techniques has also been included.

In the production of these we are indebted to the photographic artistry and skill of Mr Michael Barrington-Martin.

Acknowledgement is also made to the considerable assistance given by GEC Medical Equipment Limited (Wembley) who, on two occasions, installed the necessary X-ray equipment in the photographic studios and to Sierex Limited and Philips Medical Systems Ltd on further occasions. The accuracy and convenience required, to present photographs of radiographic positioning technique, is largely a function of having good X-ray equipment, and on each occasion We were well served in this respect.

In connection with the above we are also indebted to Leslies Limited (Polyfoam Division) for the use of their Polyfoam positioning aids and foam table mattress, these proved a major factor in comfort, convenience and positional accuracy.

Thanks are also due to Miss H M Fowles MSR, Westminster Hospital X-ray Department for providing the facilities for photographing the tomographic positioning techniques. Thanks are also due to Miss D M Chesney, Hon FSR, TE, Coventry and Warwickshire Hospital for permission to adapt her article, "Acute Abdomen Emergency" within the format of Positioning In Radiography.

Consultation is a very necessary feature in the preparation of descriptive and accurate text, in this respect we are indebted to the following:
Miss S J Smith FSR and Mr J Causton FSR, Salford College of Technology. Mr E Higginbottom MSR, Lodge Moor Hospital, Sheffield. Mr W J Stripp, Royal National Orthopaedic Hospital, London. Miss M England FSR, and Mr Norman Baldock FSR, Royal Northern Hospital, London. Thanks are due to Mr J Coote for making available the X-ray room facilities at Tavistock House, in order to clarify many of the problems associated with positioning technique.
Mr Kenneth Lawley and Mr Michael Smith have been responsible for the design and production of the 9th edition in the new two volume form. We are most grateful for their valued co-operation.

Our thanks are due to the directors of CIBA-GEIGY Limited for making this edition possible and allowing us to be associated with this acknowledged world-wide authoritative work on radiographic positioning.

In preparing the ninth edition of Positioning In Radiography we wish to acknowledge the radiographic illustration content from the following sources:

Albert Einstein Medical Center, Philadelphia, USA
Dr J Gershon-Cohen and Miss Barbara M Curcio

Bradford Royal Infirmary, Yorkshire
Dr R J Carr

Bristol Royal Hospital, Royal Infirmary Branch
Dr J H Middlemiss

Brompton Hospital, London
Dr L G Blair and Miss V G Jones

Child Study Centre, University of London, Institute of Education and Child Health
Dr J M Tanner, group investigations

Children's Hospital Medical Center, Boston, USA
Dr E B D Neuhauser and Dr M H Wittenborg, Mr Eric Hammond

Chorley and District Hospital, Lancashire
Dr G Sullivan

Cuckfield Hospital, Sussex
Miss H E M Noller

Dublin
Dr T Garratt Hardman

Halifax, Yorkshire
Dr R I Lewis

Harefield Hospital, Middlesex
Dr L G Blair, Mr V C Snell and Mr A W Holder

Hospital for Sick Children, London
Dr L G Blair, Dr G N Weber, also Miss H Nicol and Miss M Riocreux

Hospital for Sick Children, Toronto, Canada
Dr J D Munn, Mr Richard Harmes, Mr Walter Johns, also Mr L J Cartwright

Ipswich and East Suffolk Hospital
Miss S M Stockley

Johnson and Johnson (Great Britain) Limited, Slough, Buckinghamshire

Lodge Moor Hospital, Sheffield, Yorkshire
Dr T Lodge and Mr E Higginbottom

London Hospital
Dr J J Rae and Miss F M A Vaughan

Department for Research in Industrial Medicine
Dr L J Rae, Dr A I G McLaughlin and Miss F M A Vaughan

Maidenhead Hospital, Berkshire
Dr A W Simmins, Mr David W Bain and Miss A Crofton

Manchester Royal Infirmary, Lancashire
Dr E D Gray, Dr R G Reid

Medical Arts X-ray Department, Niagra Falls, Canada
Mr Lewis Edwards

Melrose-Wakefield Hospital, Massachusetts, USA
Dr William E Davis and Mr Clarence W Coupe

Memorial Hospital, Cirencester, Gloucestershire
Dr G C Griffiths

Memorial Hospital, New York City, USA
Dr Robert S Sherman and Dr George Schwarz

Middlesex Hospital, London
Dr F Campbell Golding and Miss H J Weller, Dr M J McLoughlin and Miss Marion Frank

Mulago Hospital, Kampala, Uganda
Dr A G M Davies

National Hospital, Queen Square, London
Dr Hugh W Davies, Dr J W D Bull, Mr Harvey Jackson and Mr Peter Gortvai, Dr J Marryat, Mr A M Hastin Bennett, Mr A E Prickett, Miss A M Hamilton, Mr L S Walsh

National Heart Hospital, London
Dr Peter Kerley, CVO, CBE and Miss K M A Pritchard

New Britain Hospital, Connecticut, USA
Dr John C Larkin and Mr Nicholas R Barraco

Newcastle General Hospital, Newcastle-Upon-Tyne
Dr S Josephs

New England Center Hospital, Pratt Diagnostic Clinic, Boston, USA
Dr Alice Ettinger

Nuffield Orthopaedic Centre, Oxford (Wingfield Morris Orthopaedic Hospital)
Dr F H Kemp, Dr J L Boldero, Mr J Agerholm, Miss B Robbins

NV Optische Industrie 'De Oude Delft', Holland

Prince of Wales's General Hospital, London
Dr A Elkeles

Queen Victoria Hospital, Plastic Surgery and Jaw Injuries Centre, East Grinstead, Sussex
Dr William Campbell

Radcliffe Infirmary, Oxford
Dr F H Kemp

Robert Jones and Agnes Hunt Orthopaedic Hospital, Oswestry, Shropshire
Dr J W Foy, Mr J Rowland Hughes, Mr F B Thomas, Mr R Roaf and Mr W G Davies

Royal Cornwall Infirmary, Truro
Dr H S Bennett, Mr J G Kendall, Mrs V Wheaton

Royal Dental Hospital, London
Dr Sydney Blackman, Miss D O Gibb and Mrs D White

Royal Hospital, Sheffield, Yorkshire
Dr T Lodge and Mr G W Delahaye

Royal Marsden Hospital, London
Dr J J Stevenson, Dr J S McDonald, Dr E J Pick

Royal National Orthopaedic Hospital, London
Dr F Campbell Golding, Mr J N Wilson, Mr C W S F Manning, Mr J I P James, Mr W J Stripp

Royal National Orthopaedic Hospital, Brockley Hill, Stanmore, Middlesex
Dr F Campbell Golding, Mr J N Wilson, Mr C V S F Manning

Royal Northern Hospital, London
Dr L S Carstairs, Mr A M Hastin Bennett, and Miss M J England, Mr N Baldock

Royal Portsmouth Hospital, Hampshire
Dr R S MacHardy

St Anthony's Hospital, Cheam, Surrey
Mr Aubrey York Mason

St Mary's Hospitals for Women and Children, Manchester
Dr J Blair Hartley and Miss A Stirling Fisher

St Thomas's Hospital, London
Dr J W McLaren

St Vincent's Hospital, New York City, USA
Dr Francis F Ruzicka Jnr, and Dr M M Schechter

St Vincent's Orthopaedic Hospital, Eastcote, Pinner, Middlesex
Dr L G Blair, Mr V C Snell and Sister Francis

Salford Royal Hospital, Lancashire
Dr A H McCallum

Stuttgart, Germany
Dr Georg Thieme Verlag

Sydney, Australia
Dr Majorie Dalgarno

Temple University Hospital, Philadelphia, USA
Professor Herbert M Stauffer and Miss Margaret J McGann

The Hague, Holland
Dr V Fiorani

Universiteit Van Amsterdam, Holland
Professor Dr B G Ziedses des Plantes

University College Hospital, London
Dr David Edwards, Dr M E Grossmann, Dr M E Sidaway and Mrs S Gordon and Sister H Quirke

War Memorial Children's Hospital, London Ontario, Canada
Dr D S Rajic and Mr Bryan Fisher

Westminster Hospital, London
Dr B Strickland, Dr Roger Pyle and Dr S Holesh

Weston-Super-Mare General Hospital, Somerset
Dr H B Howell and Mr E J Quick, Mrs S S Duncan

Women's College Hospital, Toronto, Canada
Dr M E Forbes, Dr Jean Toews and Mrs Elizabeth Mills

PREFACE

The object of this book is to present in as practical a form as possible, the essentials of radiographic technique and to provide students, radiographers and radiologists with a reference book on the more widely used radiographic techniques and procedures. The last ten years have seen profound changes in radiographic practice and the next ten years will see further progress. However, basic radiographic techniques will continue to form the major part of the work of radiology departments.

Correct positioning for routine examinations is illustrated photographically together with resulting radiographs and occasional explanatory line diagrams and photographs of dry bones as well. There are a limited number of abnormal radiographs, mostly of fractures, which are described in the text to show how positioning and exposure require modification. Suitable exposure factors are shown for each position.

Radiographers must know basic anatomy, particularly as shown on radiographs in various projections. The anatomical appearances will obviously change as the position of the patient changes, but also with changes in tube angulation. However, it is not just the change in position but in radiographic density with variation of the overlying soft tissues and bone.

Radiographic anatomy is therefore not just a simple translation of named parts from one view to another but an imaginative step in projection to allow for changed tissue density. Similarly physiological changes must also be taken into account. Not only must respiratory, cardiac and gastro-intestinal movements be recognized, understood and their effects circumvented, but on occasion even used to good effect in radiographic examinations.

The development of new techniques often introduces new factors which previously may have been irrelevant. Contrast agents and various drugs are now commonly used in X-ray diagnosis and radiographers must familiarize themselves with these as well. But above all radiography is about radiation which must be used efficiently. Radiation dose to patients must be kept at its lowest consistent with accurate diagnosis which can only be done with correct location, positioning and exposure to avoid repeat examinations.

While radiographers are not expected to be responsible for the interpretation of radiographs, their expert opinions, when requested, can be most helpful. However, a familiarity with clinical conditions given on request forms is essential for the translation of very brief instructions into high quality radiographs.

The care and comfort of the patient is paramount not only for the sake of the patient but also to ensure an adequate examination. General comfortable relaxation in the correct position for a particular projection, encourages local relaxation and immobility. Radiographic rooms must be warm, and the parts of the patient not being examined, well covered. Apprehensive patients must be reassured and asked to co-operate. A clear explanation of what the examination entails will help to gain the patient's confidence and co-operation.

Every radiograph must be clearly labelled with the patient's name, date and X-ray or hospital number. It is also absolutely essential that the labels as to right or left must be clearly visible on the film and correspond with the request as shown on the request form. When relevant the position of the patient must also be indicated on the film, particularly whether erect, supine, right or left side up or head or feet down. Without this information it may be impossible to interpret the films correctly.

Radiographic Appearances

Living anatomy is portrayed on each film taken but is limited by the physical properties of X-rays and current technology. Good radiographic practice tries to avoid any further downgrading of the anatomical image by a meticulous attention to detail especially in using the correct projection for the part of the body or particular organ being examined. But internal organs change their position with regard to each other and to their surface relationships with changes of patient position. A knowledge of these changes is absolutely essential in radiographic practice. The most marked changes in the position of internal organs occurs with a change from the supine to erect.

There are also significant differences between supine and prone and right and left decubitus positions and quite marked changes in position of organs also occurs with respiration. A three dimensional appreciation of anatomy is therefore extremely important in radiography.

Radiographic appearance is the term used in this book for what is seen on the resulting film and takes into account the many factors which contribute to the result. For a better appreciation of technique required to produce these films many radiographs are annotated, especially those of bones and joints and projections are further illustrated by line drawings and photographs.

The radiographic illustrations have been reproduced from negative prints to keep their appearances as close as possible to that of the actual radiographs, except of course in size.

A high speed Bucky grid with a ratio of 10:1 is used for all areas of the body other than arms, hands and feet to eliminate scattered radiation and yet keep short exposure times. Fine-lined stationary grids (100 lines to the inch) have also been used but cross hatched grids tend to increase exposures by a factor of ×2 or ×3.

Technical Factors

Exposure factors are given for each projection shown, namely kilovolts (peak) milliampere-seconds and focus-film distance (FFD) as well as the type of intensifying screens, film and type of grid when relevant and assumes that all films will be developed under recognized standard conditions for automatic or manual processing. These factors will be suitable for a patient of average physique.

Each factor associated with exposure technique is a variable because of the wide range of radiological equipment in use and the various combinations of film and intensifying screen possible. The exposure factors given are for a full wave rectified X-ray unit. However for any particular unit the factors will need to be increased or decreased due to unit output difference but the same percentage difference can be applied to all exposure throughout the book.

The focus-film distance may vary according to the type of examination but should wherever possible be kept constant and at 120 cm (48 ins). For Bucky exposures it ranges from 100 cm (40 ins) to 120 cm (48 ins), however when using a Bucky the FFD must be within the limits specified for the grid in use. For teleradiography it ranges from 150 cm (60 ins) to 180 cm (72 ins) except for high kV chest radiography using an air gap when it may be increased considerably. Radiation must be restricted to the smallest possible area of the region being examined, and the genital organs must be protected by lead shields of suitable size and shape. The conventional 2 mm aluminium filter at the tube aperture reduces radiation exposure to the patient and extra filters should be added when kilovoltages over 150 kV are used. Every possible care must be taken to minimize radiation hazards both to the patient and to the operator.

Kilovoltage and Radiographic Appearances

Increasing the kilovoltage increases the energy of the X-rays, decreases their wavelengths and increases their penetration. There is however a loss of contrast on the more penetrated films taken at higher kV exposures. Some simple rules can therefore be used to obtain good quality films.

For good bone detail the kV should not be increased above 100 and a kV of 60–70 is preferred. However, for very thick parts such as the pelvis, higher kV's may be needed.

For soft tissue detail particularly in mammography, very low kV's in the order of 20–30 kV are used requiring a special X-ray tube, screens and film.

For opaque contrast agents high kV is needed for penetration. However, most contrast examinations have now been so profoundly modified that kV's in the range of 60–80 give the best results. Fine detail in double contrast barium examinations are most easily shown in this range which is also recommended for the demonstration of small vessels on arteriography.

However, exposure times must be kept wherever possible within the 0·04–0·06 range to avoid movement blurring.

Qualities Desirable in a Radiograph

A good image requires good definition which is a function of both contrast and sharpness of the image. Contrast is determined by the radiographic density of adjacent areas and is adequate when the different radiographic densities between adjacent areas are visible. Increasing the film contrast makes these differences in radiographic densities more readily visible. Sharpness on the other hand depends on (a) eliminating 'subject movement' (μm) by keeping the patient still and using the shortest possible times for an adequate exposure; (b) using the smallest focal spot size, longest focal film distance and shortest object-film distance (μg) consistent with an adequate exposure and (c) choosing a film screen combination compatible with the X-ray unit which minimizes movement unsharpness (μm) and equipment unsharpness (μg).

Positioning terminology usually describes the projection from the tube towards the film but also still occasionally from the film towards the tube. The latter is still used because radiologists describe projections from fluoroscopic examinations which are accepted by long standing tradition especially the oblique views of the heart and aorta.

POSITIONING TERMINOLOGY

Patient Aspect

Anterior aspect, is the view of the patient from the front and posterior aspect, the view of the patient from the back.

Antero-posterior (AP) and postero-anterior (PA) describe the direction of the central ray from the portal of entry towards the exit. In the antero-posterior (AP) position the front of the body faces the X-ray tube, and in the postero-anterior (PA) position the X-ray tube is closest to the back of the body.

In projections for the upper and lower limbs, AP, PA and oblique views are described from the tube side as well as for skull projections. The AP and PA terminology also applies to all prone, supine and erect positions, e.g. chest postero-anterior or lumbar spine antero-posterior.

In examinations of the abdomen, vertebral column and pelvis, oblique positions are described from the patient's aspect (anterior or posterior) nearest to the film, together with the side (left or right) of the subject nearest the film.

Thus, if the patient is supine with the right side raised and left side toward the film, it is called a left posterior oblique.

Oblique Positioning

Right Anterior Oblique—anterior aspect of patient is towards the film, right side of the patient in contact, left side raised. **Left Anterior Oblique**—anterior aspect of patient is towards the film, left side of patient in contact, right side raised. **Right Posterior Oblique**—posterior aspect of patient is towards the film, right side of patient in contact, left side raised. **Left Posterior Oblique**—posterior aspect of patient is towards the film, left side of patient in contact, right side raised.

Lateral Positioning

Right lateral indicates the right side of patient in contact with film. Left lateral indicates the left side of patient in contact with film.

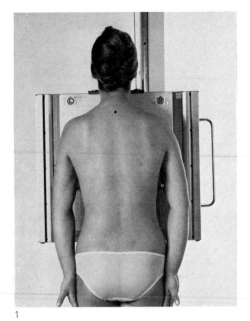

1

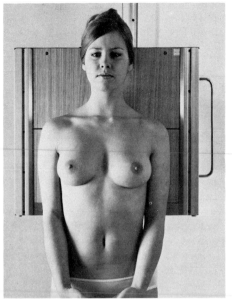

2

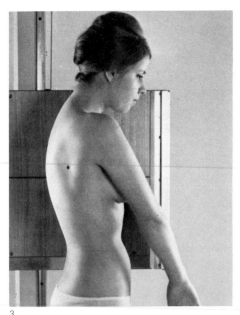

3

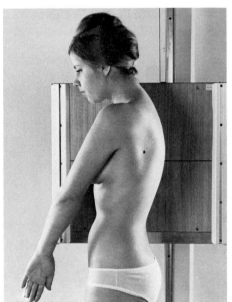

4

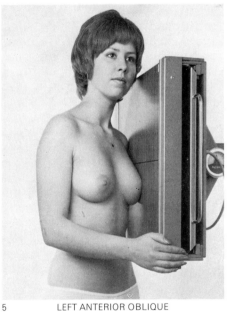

5   LEFT ANTERIOR OBLIQUE

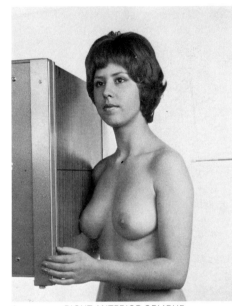

6   RIGHT ANTERIOR OBLIQUE

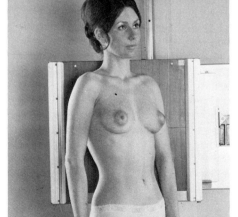

7   LEFT POSTERIOR OBLIQUE

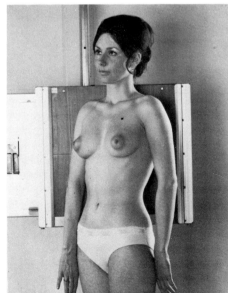

8   RIGHT POSTERIOR OBLIQUE

Erect Positioning
1   Postero-Anterior
2   Antero-Posterior
3   Left Lateral
4   Right Lateral
5   Left Anterior Oblique
6   Right Anterior Oblique
7   Left Anterior Oblique
8   Right Posterior Oblique

Horizontal Positioning
1   Supine
2   Prone
3   Right Lateral
4   Left Lateral
5   Left Posterior Oblique
6   Right Posterior Oblique
7   Right Anterior Oblique
8   Left Anterior Oblique

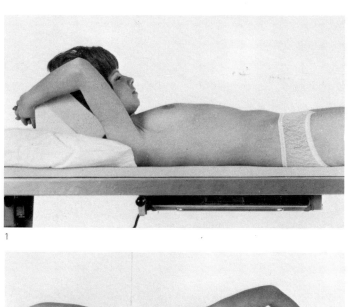

1

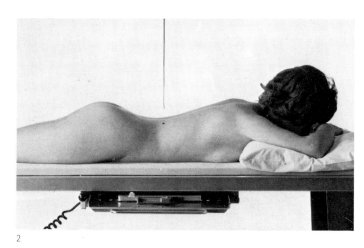

2

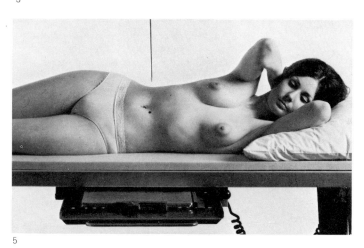

3

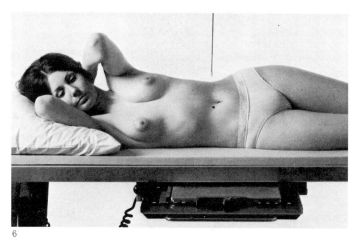

4

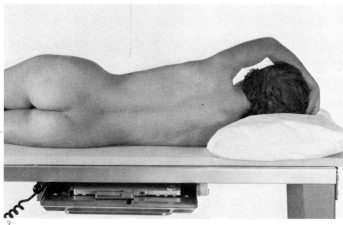

5

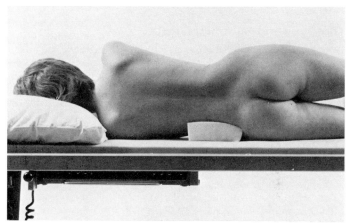

6

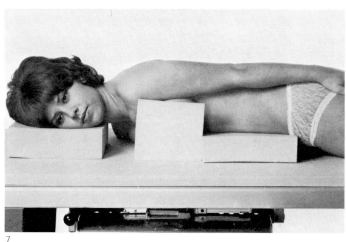

7

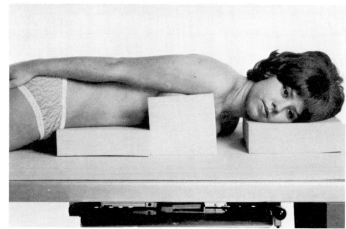

8

CONTENTS
VOLUME ONE

The Tenth Edition of
Positioning in Radiography
has been produced in two volumes.
An outline of the contents
of volume two is shown below:

CONTENTS
VOLUME TWO

1

UPPER LIMB

1 SECTION 1

UPPER LIMB

General and Technical

Because examinations of the upper limb are elementary and routine the standards of any department can immediately be judged by the quality of films of this region. But more importantly the best possible radiographs are essential as decisions about injuries in the upper limb especially of the elbow and wrist affect the future dexterity, employment and earnings of patient.

When examining the upper limb, the whole of the arm should rest on the X-ray couch to bring the adjacent joints level with the area to be radiographed.

(1) In the antero-posterior (AP) position the arm is supine lying with the palm of the hand facing upward, the elbow extended and the shoulder well down, the tube being centred from above the couch.

(2) In the lateral position the elbow is flexed to a right angle and the arm and forearm rest on the table top with the palm of the hand at right angles to the couch.

(3) When a postero-anterior projection is taken for the hand and wrist the elbow is flexed and the hand rotated into the prone position.

(4) Where the arm and forearm of the patient are in Plaster of Paris the examination may be done in the postero-anterior position; for accurate centring use a tape measure to compare affected and unaffected limb lengths. (3)

(5) The AP view to show the long bones of the forearm should be taken with the hand supinated as the radius and ulna are super-imposed when the hand is pronated.

■ Centring points for wrist, forearm and elbow are indicated by black spots (1,2).

The patient must be relaxed and the arm must be immobilized by the use of non-opaque supports of plastic sponge around the area to be radiographed. Remember the limb will only remain stationary if it is in a comfortable position.

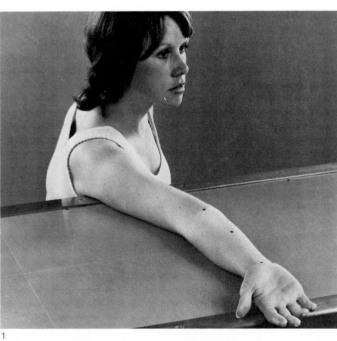

1

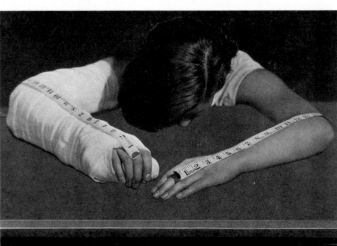

2

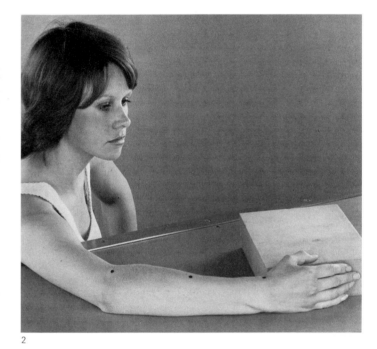

2

Radiation is kept to a minimum by collimating the beam with a light beam diaphragm or by the use of an extension cone. Unless otherwise stated the tube is straight, at right angles to the table top and the central ray at 90° to the film. The carpus, metacarpus, phalanges and their interarticulation at the wrist joint are shown in the three positions of the hand (6,8,10)

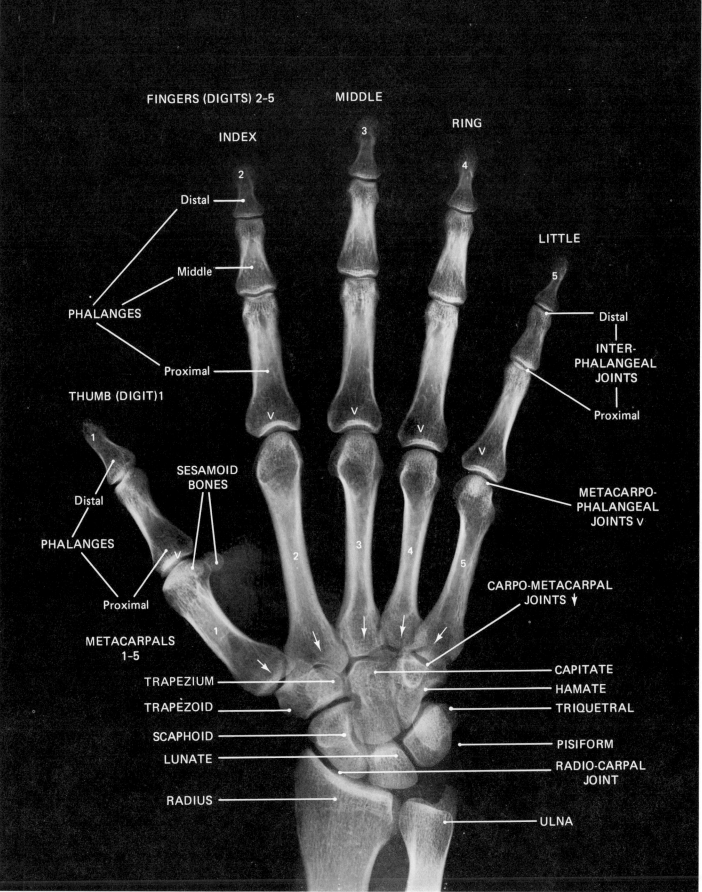

FINGERS (DIGITS) 2-5   MIDDLE

INDEX   RING

2   3   4

Distal

LITTLE

Middle   5

PHALANGES   Distal

INTER-
PHALANGEAL
JOINTS

Proximal   Proximal

THUMB (DIGIT)1

1

SESAMOID
BONES

Distal

PHALANGES   V

METACARPO-
PHALANGEAL
JOINTS V

Proximal

CARPO-METACARPAL
JOINTS ↓

METACARPALS
1-5

1   CAPITATE

TRAPEZIUM   HAMATE

TRAPEZOID   TRIQUETRAL

SCAPHOID   PISIFORM

LUNATE   RADIO-CARPAL
JOINT

RADIUS   ULNA

RIGHT HAND   POSTERO-ANTERIOR

Postero-anterior (basic)

The forearm is placed on the table in pronation, with the fingers extended, but relaxed and separated to bring them into close contact with with film.

■ Centre over the head of the third metacarpal bone (5,6)

Lateral (basic)

From the prone position the hand and forearm are turned into the lateral position so that the palm of the hand is at 90° to the film with the fingers overlapping and the thumb resting on a nonopaque support. (7,8)

■ Centre over the head of the second metacarpal bone.

Note—Although the metacarpal bones overlap, this projection does show forward or backward displacement at the fracture site; it also shows whether a foreign body is on the palmar or dorsal aspect of the hand.

Oblique—postero-anterior (basic)

From the lateral position the hand is rotated forward to midway between the postero-anterior and the true lateral. At an angle of approximately 45° to the film, the fingers are separated and rest on a 45° non-opaque pad for immobilization.

■ Centre over the head of the fifth metacarpal bone or angle the tube towards the head of the third metacarpal to reduce the area of irradiation by 50% (9,10).

Note—This projection avoids superimposition of the bones, being used in the diagnosis of crack fractures and in pathological conditions.

Hand

kVp			mAS				Film	Screens	
PA	Lat	Obl	PA	Lat	Obl	FFD	ILFORD	ILFORD	Grid
50	50	50	8	12	10	100 cm (40")	RAPID R	SUPER HD	—

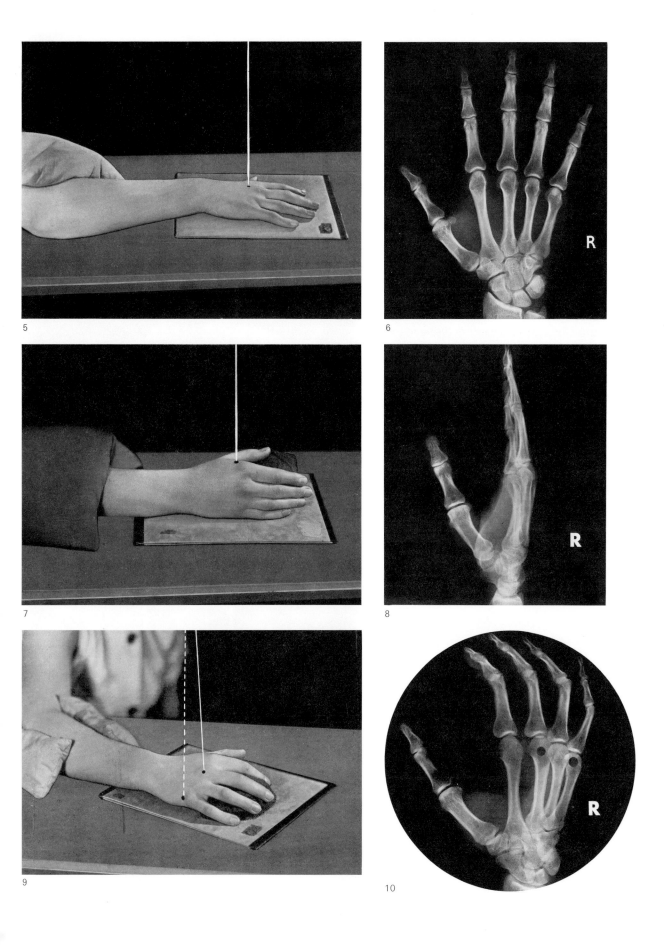

5

6

7

8

9

10

Metacarpus

When required the antero-posterior projection using the horizontal beam (11) may replace the basic postero-anterior position previously shown (5,6).

Antero-posterior—horizontal beam

The injured hand is placed laterally on a non-opaque sponge block on the couch in a relaxed position; the back of the hand is rested against the vertically placed film which is supported by a wooden block or sandbag (11).

■ The horizontal beam is centred to the middle of the third metacarpal in the palm of the hand (11)

Lateral—localized

Without moving the limb a film is inserted beneath the hand (on the surface of the non-opaque sponge support) and the tube is returned to the vertical position (12); the beam is collimated.

■ Centre to the middle of the second metacarpal bone (12)
For **Exposure Factors** see page 4.

Radiographs

A series of radiographs (13) show the initial radiographs of the hand following an injury (13).

■ This is a typical subject for the technique shown in (11, 12) but the third basic projection (the oblique) is also an essential part of the examination.

In (14) frontal and lateral views of the wrist showing ununited epiphyses of the radius and ulna.

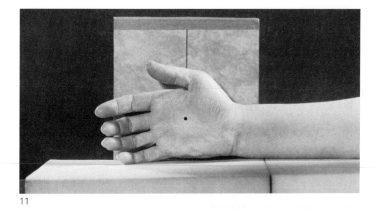

11

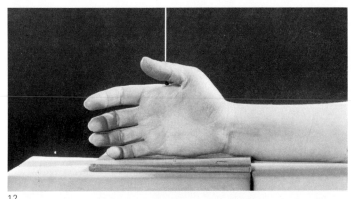

12

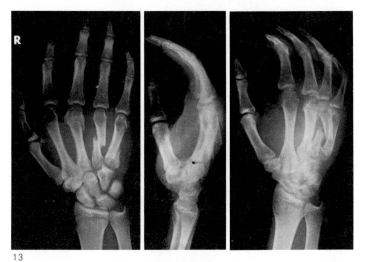

13

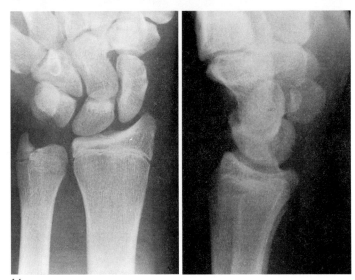

14

Pathology
Radiograph (15) shows the right and left hands exposed side by side as is the usual practice in all such pathological conditions; oblique view comparison of both hands is also recommended.

Foreign bodies
Postero-Anterior and Lateral
(16) To show Presence, Palmar or Dorsal aspect of Foreign Body.

Fracture radiographs
It is important to take both lateral and oblique projections of such injuries, as shown in (17, 18, 19).

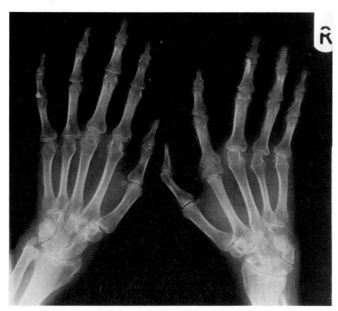

15

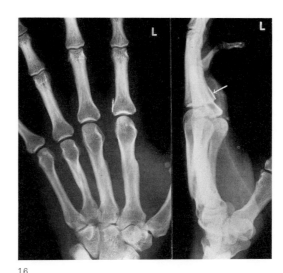

16

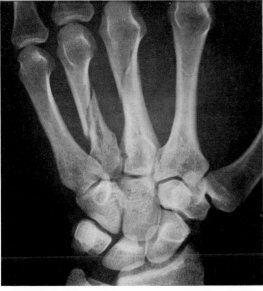

POSTERO-ANTERIOR
17

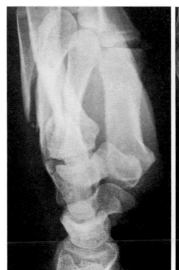 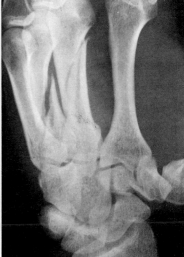

LATERAL   OBLIQUE   7
18   19

Fingers

Postero-anterior
The hand is placed in position as for the general projection of the hand (5) but using a smaller film and centring over the proximal interphalangeal joint.

Lateral
Place the hand so that the finger is either on the film (index, little) or parallel to the film (middle, ring) and support the raised fingers on a non-opaque pad. The other fingers must be flexed to get them away from the finger being radiographed.

Index and Middle Fingers
Index and middle fingers are examined in pronation with the lateral aspect of the index finger in contact with the film. The middle finger is supported on a non-opaque pad and the remaining fingers flexed to the palm of the hand. The forearm is raised and supported on sandbags.

■ Centre over the proximal interphalangeal joint of the index finger (20, 21)

Ring and Little Finger
Ring and little finger are examined with the hand in the true lateral position and the medial aspect of the little finger in contact with the film. The ring finger is supported on a non-opaque pad and the remaining fingers flexed to the palm of the hand.

■ Centre over the proximal interphalangeal joint of the little finger (22, 23)

Fingers							
kVp		mAS			Film	Screens	
PA	Lat	PA	Lat	FFD	ILFORD	ILFORD	Grid
50	50	6	6	100 cm (40″)	RAPID R	SUPER HD	—

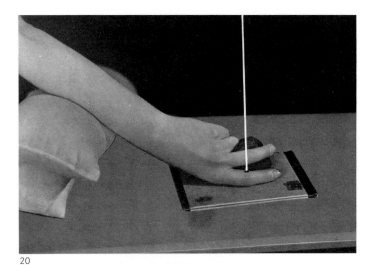

20

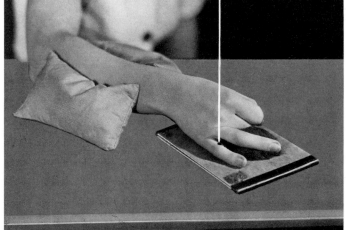

22

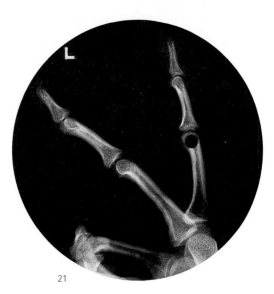

21

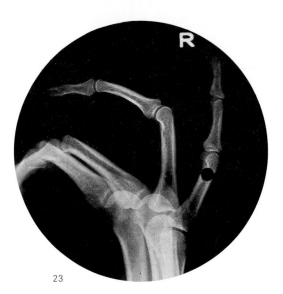

23

Distal and Middle Phalanges
Postero-anterior

For examination of individual fingers the palm of the hand is supported on a non-opaque pad and the fingers rest on the film which is raised to the same level (24, 25).

■ Centre over the middle phalanx.

Lateral

For the examination of individual fingers, a small film is placed between the finger being examined and the one below it. The finger above is flexed to the palm of the hand.

Remember to use a lead film divider to enable the PA and lateral views to be radiographed on one film.

■ Centre over the middle phalanx.

Fracture radiographs

Radiograph (26) shows a fracture of the terminal phalanx of the middle finger and (27) a dislocation at the proximal interphalangeal joint of the middle finger.

When metal splints are used, it is difficult to obtain satisfactory postero-anterior and lateral projections. It may be necessary to angle both hand and X-ray tube to obtain sufficient separation of splint and finger to show the region being treated.

In radiographs (28) overlapping of the bone and splint shadows has been avoided to show the injury to the head of the middle phalanx.

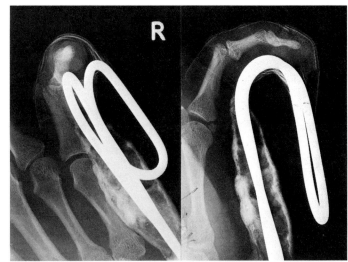

28

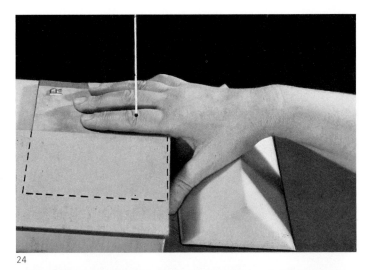

24

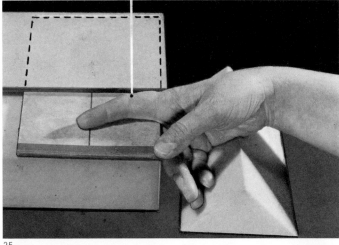

25

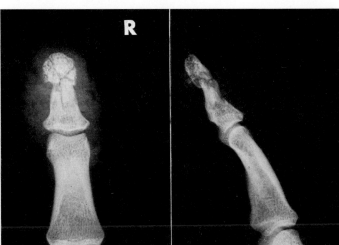

26

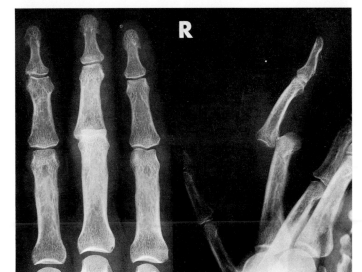

27

Thumb

The carpo-metacarpal joint must be included in both projections to cover the possibility of a fracture to the base of the first metacarpal. (29, 30, 44) The choice of antero-posterior or postero-anterior projections for the thumb depends upon the injury sustained and on the mobility of the upper limb.

Lateral (basic)
The forearm is pronated and the palm of the hand raised on a non-opaque pad to bring the lateral aspect of the slightly flexed thumb in contact with the film.
■ Centre over the metacarpo-phalangeal joint (29, 31(a), 32(a)).

Postero-anterior (basic)
The hand is placed in the lateral position with the thumb supported in abduction on a non-opaque pad (30)

Note—The loss of definition due to increased subject-film distance is negligible. This is the most suitable technique in the case of a badly injured thumb.

These two projections are shown from the tube position in Fig. 32.

Thumb									
kVp			mAS			Film	Screens		
Lat	PA	AP	Lat	PA	AP	FFD	ILFORD	ILFORD	Grid
50	50	50	10	10	10	100 cm (40″)	RAPID R	SUPER HD	—

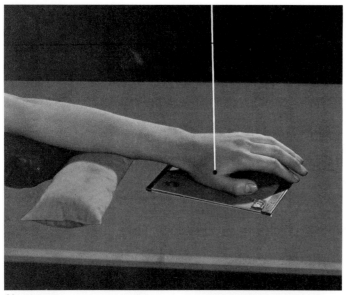

29

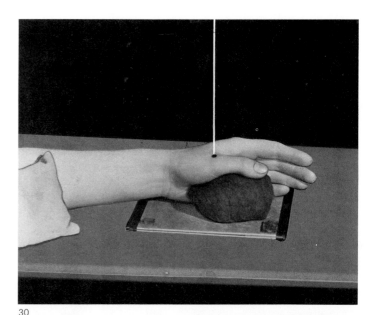

30

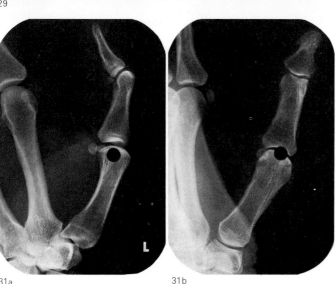

31a   31b

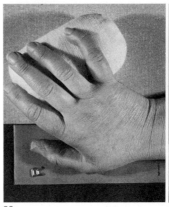 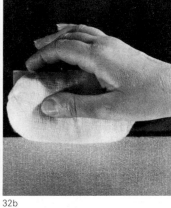

32a   32b

Antero-posterior (1)

The arm is rotated internally until the lateral margin of the index finger is in contact with the couch and the posterior aspect of the thumb is in contact with the film. A non-opaque pad is placed under the index finger and the elbow supported on sandbags. (33)

■ Centre over the metacarpophalangeal joint (33, 34)

Note—In this position, the carpo-metacarpal joint is frequently obscured.

Antero-posterior (2)

The hand is rotated externally until the posterior aspect of the thumb is in contact with the film, the fingers being supported on a non-opaque pad. (35)

■ Centre over the metacarpo-phalangeal joint (35, 36)

Note The carpo-metacarpal joint and adjacent structures are now clearly shown.

The Exposure Factors, (see page 10) are the same for postero-anterior (basic).

The two projections of the thumb are done on a single film using a lead divider to protect each half of the film in turn (33, 35). In each position the thumb is placed lengthwise on the film and correctly aligned to the long axis of the film with the carpo-metacarpal joint included. In changing the position of the lead divider between exposures avoid reversing the film position or the image will be reversed, for example, thumb up in one projection and thumb down in the other (37a).

Figure 37a shows a fracture at the base of the thumb.

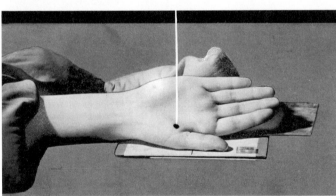

33

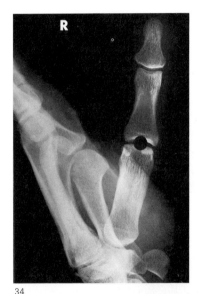

34

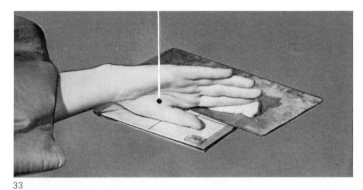

35

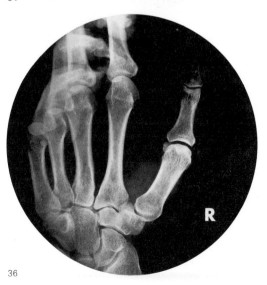

36

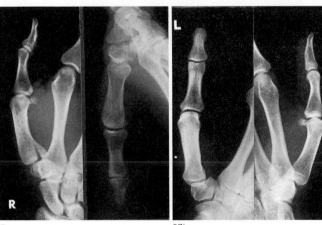

37a 37b

Foreign Body in Thenar Eminence

It is difficult to show whether a foreign body is on the dorsal or palmar aspect of the thumb, because in postero-anterior (basic) and lateral (basic) positions of the hand, the thumb is oblique in position whereas in the lateral (29) and postero-anterior (39) projections for the thumb, its true relationship with the hand is not shown.

When radiographing the thumb for suspected foreign bodies, the thumb must not be allowed to move in relation to the hand until the examination is finished.

Lateral

The hand is placed in the true lateral position as for lateral hand (basic) (7), the outer third of the length of the thumb is then positioned over the index finger.
■ Centre to the middle of the first metacarpal bone (38, 39)

Lateral-tilted (1)

From (38) tilt the hand forward 10°–15°.
■ Centre to the middle of the first metacarpal.

Lateral—tilted (2)

From (38) tilt the hand backwards 10–15°.
■ Centre to the middle of the first metacarpal (40)

Note—The tilted lateral projections help to localize the position of a foreign body by showing how it moves in relation to the first metacarpal (41)

Postero-anterior

Leave the hand in the lateral position (38). Rotate the X-ray tube until it is in position for a horizontal ray view.

Support the film perpendicular to the central ray against the dorsal aspect of the hand.
■ Centre to the middle of the first metacarpal.

Thenar eminence							
kVp		mAS			Film	Screens	
Lat	PA	Lat	PA	FFD	ILFORD	ILFORD	Grid
50	50	10	10	100 cm (40″)	RAPID R	SUPER HD	—

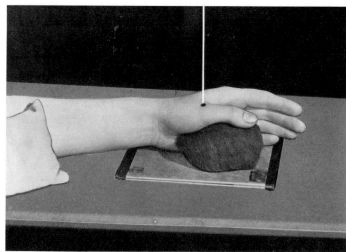

38

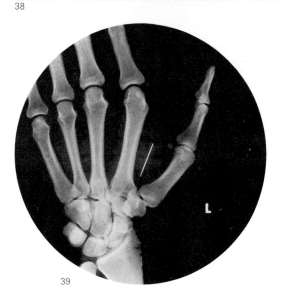

39

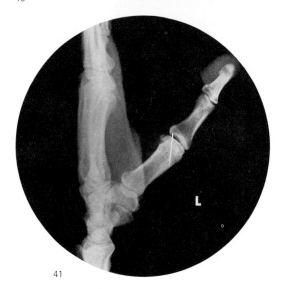

40

41

Fracture Radiographs

Two projections of a fractured base of thumb are shown in (42), and post reduction films with splinting in (43a, 43b)

Note—The adequate demonstration of the fractured metacarpal in spite of the metallic splint.

A fracture through the base of the thumb is shown in Fig. 44.

A comminuted fracture of the terminal phalanx is shown in Fig. 45, using the modified technique (postero-anterior view) as described on p. 8.

Sesamoid bones

Sesamoid bones develop in the palmar and plantar tendons at the metacarpo-phalangeal and metatarso-phalangeal joints and are seen as small rounded opacities lying on their anterior aspects. Sesamoid bones also occur in other regions of the body. The patella is a large sesamoid bone lying in the tendon of quadriceps femoris muscle of the thigh.

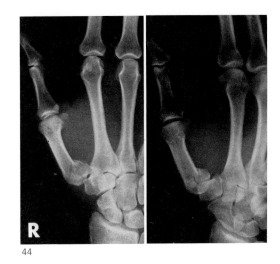

44

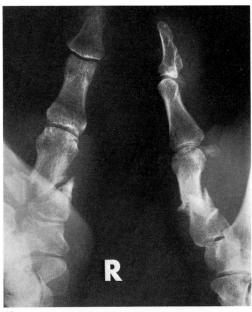

42

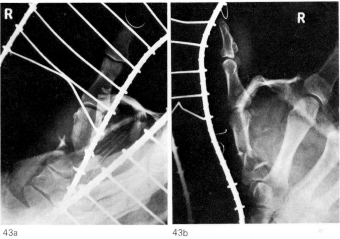

43a   43b

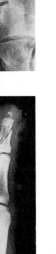

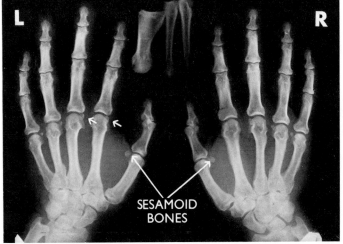

45   46

SESAMOID BONES

Note—In (46) the dry metacarpal bones have been included to show a method of checking the consistent quality of radiographs for pathological conditions examined at intervals over a considerable period of time.

Wrist Joint

Radiographic appearances

Radiographs of the five basic positions, postero-anterior, lateral, postero-anterior oblique, antero-posterior oblique and axial indicate the relative positions of the carpal bones in the different projections. The carpal bones are also shown on the tunnel (axial) view (51b) together with a line diagram (51a).

The carpal bones are arranged in a distal and a proximal group as follows:

(Thumb)			(Little Finger)
Distal			
Trapezium	Trapezoid	Capitate	Hamate
Proximal			
Scaphoid	Lunate	Triquetral	Pisiform
(Radius)		(Ulna)	

The more commonly used basic projections are the postero-anterior straight (52) or with ulna flexion (62), lateral (54) and oblique (66).

Radiographs of the wrist joint must include the distal ends of the radius and ulna, the carpus and the bases of the metacarpal bones. X-ray examination is most frequently carried out for a diagnosis of a Scaphoid or Colles' fracture. For a Colles' fracture the maximum area of radius and ulna should be included in preference to the upper third of the metacarpus. When using a small film it is advisable to place the centre of the film one inch distal to the tube centring point as shown in (52).

Exposure Factors

When suitable, the exposure factors are given in the one table, postero-anterior (PA, lateral (Lat.) and oblique (Obl.).

As for the hand, after deciding on the exposure for the antero-posterior or postero-anterior position, the milliampere seconds may be doubled for the lateral projection and increased by one half for the oblique projection (see page 16).

Complimentary exposures such as postero-anterior and lateral (53, 55) are usually made on one film as shown in (56). For the scaphoid, all four views, postero-anterior (65), lateral (55), postero-anterior oblique (67) and antero-posterior oblique (69) are usually done on one film.

Recommended views

Colles' Fracture	Postero-anterior
	Lateral
Scaphoid	Postero-anterior (Ulna deviation)
	PA Oblique
	AP Oblique
	Additional Obliques
Lunate	Postero-anterior
	Lateral
Trapezoid	PA Oblique with Ulna deviation
Pisiform	AP Oblique
Radial Carpal Joints	PA—25° angulation
Carpal Tunnel	Axial View

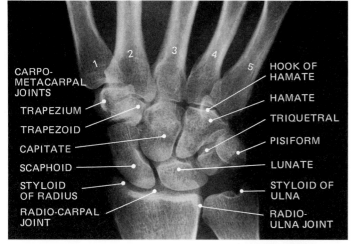

CARPO-
METACARPAL
JOINTS

TRAPEZIUM

TRAPEZOID

CAPITATE

SCAPHOID

STYLOID
OF RADIUS

RADIO-CARPAL
JOINT

1 2 3 4 5

HOOK OF
HAMATE

HAMATE

TRIQUETRAL

PISIFORM

LUNATE

STYLOID OF
ULNA

RADIO-
ULNA JOINT

RIGHT WRIST   POSTERO-ANTERIOR
47

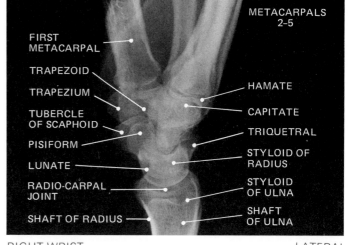

METACARPALS
2-5

FIRST
METACARPAL

TRAPEZOID

TRAPEZIUM

TUBERCLE
OF SCAPHOID

PISIFORM

LUNATE

RADIO-CARPAL
JOINT

SHAFT OF RADIUS

HAMATE

CAPITATE

TRIQUETRAL

STYLOID OF
RADIUS

STYLOID
OF ULNA

SHAFT
OF ULNA

RIGHT WRIST   LATERAL
48

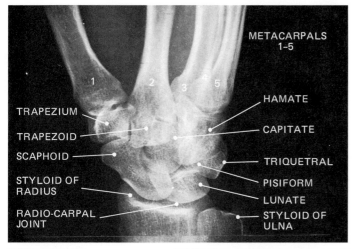

METACARPALS
1-5

TRAPEZIUM

TRAPEZOID

SCAPHOID

STYLOID OF
RADIUS

RADIO-CARPAL
JOINT

1 2 3 4 5

HAMATE

CAPITATE

TRIQUETRAL

PISIFORM

LUNATE

STYLOID OF
ULNA

RIGHT WRIST   POSTERO-ANTERIOR OBLIQUE
49

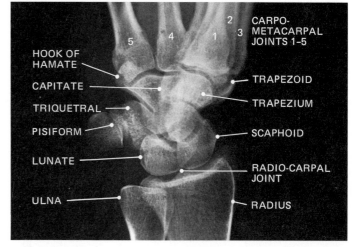

2 3
CARPO-
METACARPAL
JOINTS 1-5

HOOK OF
HAMATE

CAPITATE

TRIQUETRAL

PISIFORM

LUNATE

ULNA

5 4 1

TRAPEZOID

TRAPEZIUM

SCAPHOID

RADIO-CARPAL
JOINT

RADIUS

RIGHT WRIST   ANTERO-POSTERIOR OBLIQUE
50

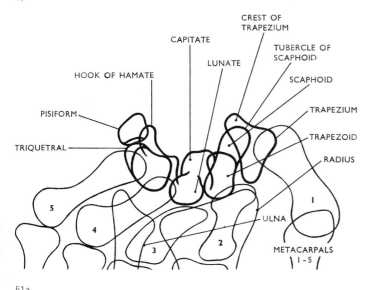

CREST OF
TRAPEZIUM

CAPITATE

LUNATE

TUBERCLE OF
SCAPHOID

SCAPHOID

HOOK OF HAMATE

TRAPEZIUM

PISIFORM

TRAPEZOID

TRIQUETRAL

RADIUS

5

4

3 2

ULNA

1

METACARPALS
1-5

51a

CARPAL TUNNEL   AXIAL
51b

Postero-anterior (basic)

The forearm is placed on the couch with the elbow flexed and the hand pronated, i.e. palm to couch. The wrist and the hand should be relaxed with the digits slightly flexed and a non-opaque pad placed under the metacarpo-phalangeal joints for stability. Anything more than minimal extension raises the wrist from the film and is to be discouraged.

■ Centre midway between the radial and ulnar styloid processes (52, 53)

Lateral (basic)

With the elbow flexed to 90° supinate the forearm so that the medial margin of the little finger lies on the table top. An additional backward tilt is then given to the wrist to superimpose the radius on the ulna (54). As the hand is inclined to fall forward into a naturally more relaxed and comfortable position, the position is maintained with sandbags, and with support for the thumb.

■ Centre to the radial styloid processes (54, 55)

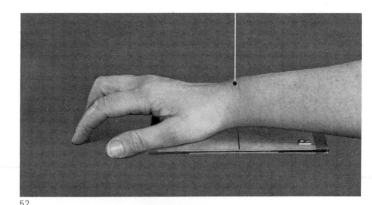

52

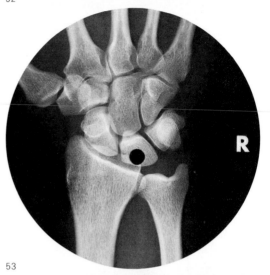

53

Wrist									
kVp			mAS				Film	Screens	
PA	Lat	Obl	PA	Lat	Obl	FFD	ILFORD	ILFORD	Grid
50	50	50	10	12	10	100 cm (40″)	RAPID R	SUPER HD	—

Slipped epiphysis (child)

Radiographs (56) showing a slipped epiphysis and separation of a small fragment of bone posteriorily emphasizing careful positioning and good quality radiographs.

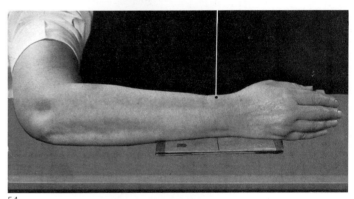

54

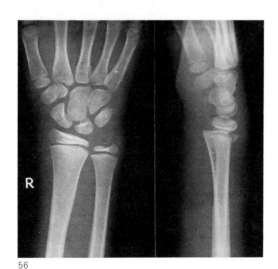

56

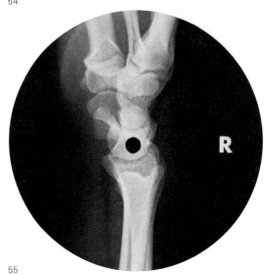

55

Injuries

True postero-anterior and lateral projections are essential for comparison throughout manipulation and healing of a fracture. When the wrist cannot be positioned correctly due to pain or presence of splint or plaster, the tube is angled to compensate for any rotation of the wrist, as shown in (57) for the postero-anterior projection. Similarly the cross-sectional diagram (57a) shows compensation by tube angulation for the lateral projection or as required with horizontal tube projection (60).

Fracture Radiographs

Radiographs of an injured wrist (58, 59), exposed twice from postero-anterior and lateral aspects, indicate the possible variations due to positioning which could be very misleading to the surgeon manipulating the fragments, and stress the importance of taking true postero-anterior and lateral projections. In radiographs (58, 59) the correct position is that shown on the right.

Radiographs (61) show the original injury in (a, b) and in a plaster splint after reduction of the fracture in (c, d). To obtain comparable results with a plaster splint, the exposure should be increased.

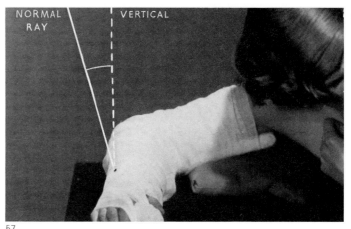

57

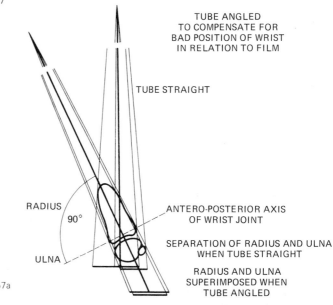

TUBE ANGLED
TO COMPENSATE FOR
BAD POSITION OF WRIST
IN RELATION TO FILM

TUBE STRAIGHT

RADIUS

90°

ULNA

ANTERO-POSTERIOR AXIS
OF WRIST JOINT

SEPARATION OF RADIUS AND ULNA
WHEN TUBE STRAIGHT

RADIUS AND ULNA
SUPERIMPOSED WHEN
TUBE ANGLED

57a

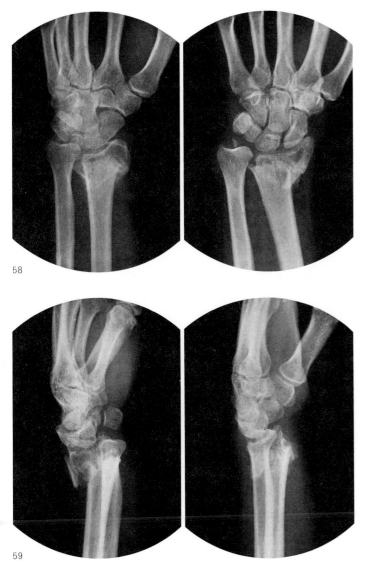

58

59

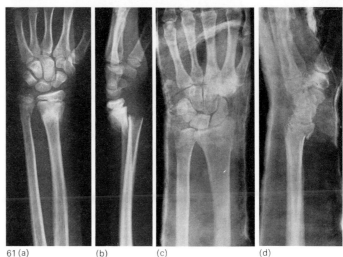

60

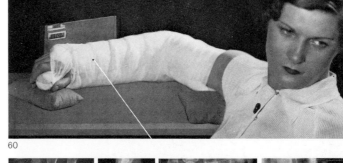

61 (a)   (b)   (c)   (d)

Scaphoid

Postero-anterior with Flexion to Ulna (basic)

The forearm is pronated and the hand is moved gently but firmly in adduction toward the ulnar side (62). In this position the proximal row of carpal bones moves simultaneously in the opposite direction towards the radial side (65).

■ Centre midway between the radial and ulnar styloid processes (62, 63, 64, 65(a))

Note—This view shows good separation of the carpal bones, especially the scaphoid. It is not always possible to apply ulnar flexion to an injured wrist, in which case the straight position must be used (52).

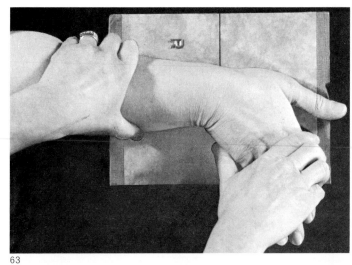

63

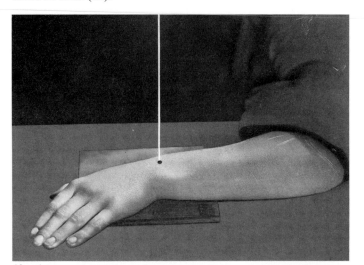

62

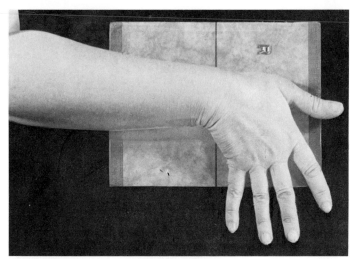

64

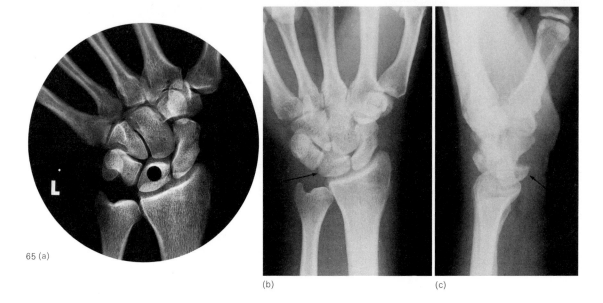

65 (a)

(b)

(c)

Radiographs 65(b) (c) show the appearance of a dislocation of the lunate which is barely recognizable on the frontal view but obvious on the lateral.

Oblique—postero-anterior (basic)

From the lateral position the wrist is rotated forward to a position midway between the postero-anterior and the true lateral as for the oblique projection of the hand with the ulnar side immediately adjacent to the border of the unexposed film. A small wedge of plastic sponge under the raised side supports the hand and wrist in position (83). With the type of lead divider shown in (66) two or more projections may be included on a single film (87).

■ Centre over the ulnar styloid process (66,67)

Note—This is a necessary additional projection and may demonstrate a minor injury which is obscured in other exposures. Both wrists may be taken for comparison on the one film (85,86).

1

Oblique—antero-posterior

From the postero-anterior oblique position the forearm is rotated backward through approximately 90°, again with the small wedge of plastic sponge under the raised side. The position is maintained by loosely-filled sandbags about the hand.

■ Centre to the ulnar styloid process (68,69)

The exposure factors are shown in the above table.

Note—This second oblique position (68) provides a projection through the long axis of the scaphoid in addition to showing the pisiform with its antero-posterior relationship to the triquetral (69). See also reference to pinning for scaphoid on page 20. These two views are essential for examination of the wrist especially for demonstration of a scaphoid fracture.

Scaphoid									
kVp			mAS				Film	Screens	
PA	Lat	Obl	PA	Lat	Obl	FFD	ILFORD	ILFORD	Grid
50	50	50	10	12	10	100 cm (40″)	RAPID R	SUPER HD	—

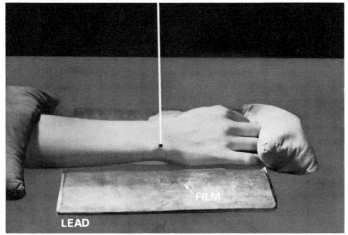

66

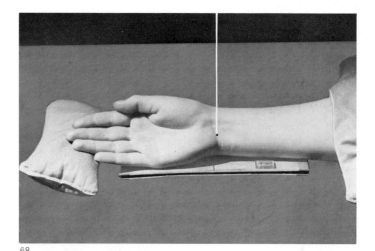

68

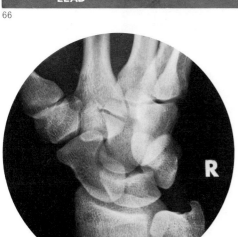

67

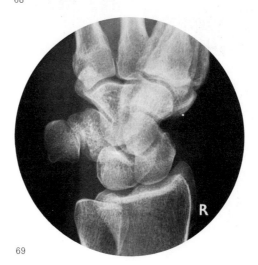

69

The two general oblique positions of the carpus are mandatory to show the axial and lateral views of the scaphoid itself (66,68). A variation of the technique (70,72) produces similar results. The postero-anterior oblique position (66,70) provides the postero-anterior view of the scaphoid (67,71), whilst antero-posterior oblique position (68,72) provides the lateral view of the scaphoid (69,73). These two projections enable the surgeon to estimate the direction for insertion of a pin into fracture fragments.

A support may be used for taking the radiographs and for pinning operations (70,72). This support is a right-angled trough with the sides inclined at an angle of 45° to the horizontal and a slot for the film cassette immediately below. Half the length is backed with lead foil to allow two projections on a 12 × 25 cm (6 × 12″) film.

The wrist is exposed in turn in the standard oblique postero-anterior, and oblique antero-posterior positions (70,72), the cassette being moved in the slot, between exposures, to give each section in turn the protection of the lead backing.

Owing to the angle at which the trough supports the limb the first exposure gives a true postero-anterior projection of scaphoid and the second a true lateral.

■ Centre to the angle of the trough (70,71,72,73) 1 cm distal to the radial styloid.

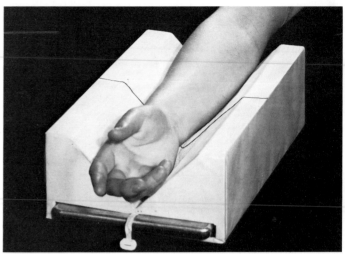

72

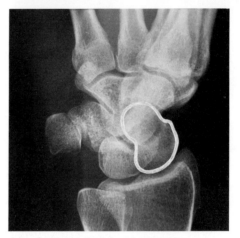

OBLIQUE (ANTERO-POSTERIOR)
73

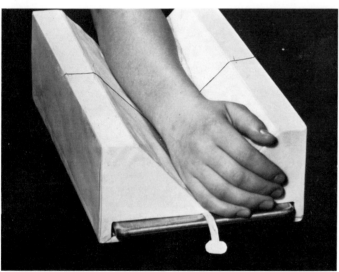

70

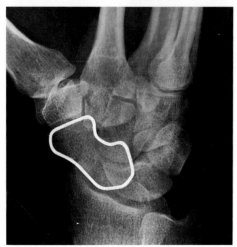

OBLIQUE (POSTERO-ANTERIOR)
71

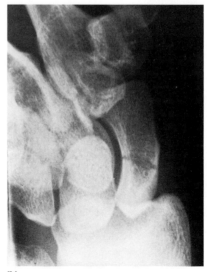

74

Complementary obliques
Scaphoid

Small fissure cracks may not be shown where the X-ray beam is not in line with the fracture through the waist of the scaphoid in the 45° oblique positions. Three modifications may then prove successful.

(a) 30° modified oblique—Postero-anterior
From the postero-anterior position, raise the radial aspect of the wrist 30° to the film.
■ Centre with the tube perpendicular to the styloid process of the Ulna (75)

(b) 60° extended oblique—Postero-anterior
From the previous position the radial aspect is raised through a further 30° to be at 60° to the film.
■ Centre with the tube perpendicular to the styloid process of the Ulna (76, 74).

(c) Elongated oblique
From the postero-anterior position, raise the radial aspect of the wrist 20° to the film.
■ With the tube angle 35° towards the elbow centre over the radial styloid.

Radial-Carpal Joint

Postero-anterior with tube angled

The wrist is placed in the postero-anterior position; raise the palm of the hand on a plastic sponge pad to produce an angle of approximately 25° at the wrist joint.
■ Centre in the midline between the styloid processes.
   The resulting radiograph shows a clear joint space between the radial surface and the carpal bones. The carpo-metacarpal joint tends to be obscured (78).

Radiograph (74) shows a 60° extended oblique—Postero-anterior view of the scaphoid with a fracture clearly visible but not seen on the other routine scaphoid films.

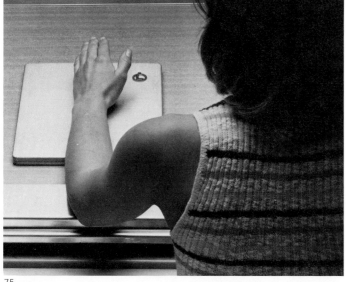

75

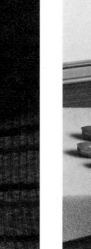

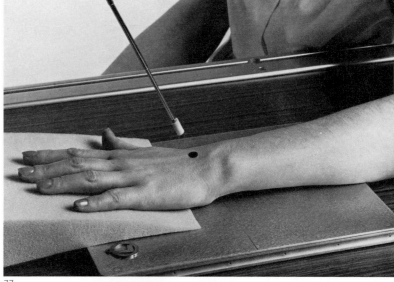

77

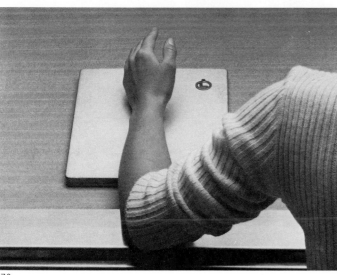

76

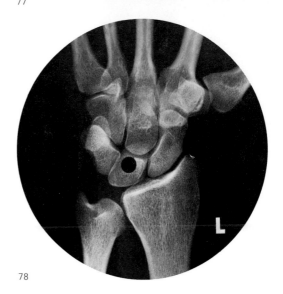

78

Lunate

Both postero-anterior and lateral projections are required to show a dislocation of the lunate (82). The dislocation produces an abnormal position of the lunate on the postero-anterior view but is particularly well demonstrated on the lateral projection.

Lateral—right and left for comparison

Comparative projections of sound and injured limbs may be needed to show a minor injury. It is best to radiograph each limb separately as previously described (55) and each wrist should be exposed on a separate film.

When comparative radiographs or multiple projections are taken on one film it is good practice to have the area of interest at the same level on the film, so that they are viewed in a straight line, and is obtained by marking the position of the film on the patient's forearm.

The value of comparison between sound and injured sides is shown in a postero-anterior projection (81).

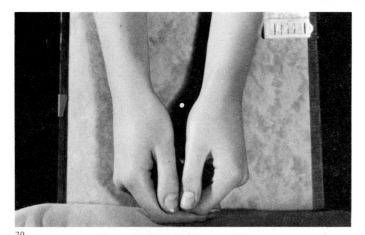

79

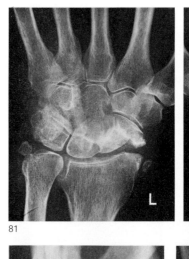

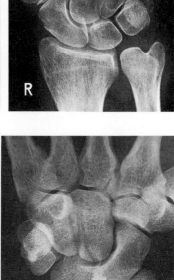

81

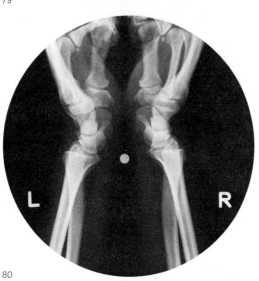

80

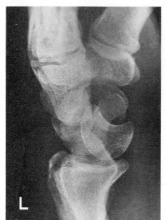

82

Injuries to Trapezium

After placing the hand in the oblique position over a small wedge-shaped support, the hand is deviated toward the ulnar side taking particular care in the alignment of the wrist with the border of the film.

■ Centre to the ulnar styloid process (83)

Oblique with flexion to ulna both wrists

Both wrists may be exposed in this position on one film, with the thumbs in contact and the hands in ulnar deviation away from each other (85).

■ Centre between the wrists, at the level of the styloid processes for a simultaneous projection (85,86)

Radiograph (87) showing a fracture of the right trapezium as well as the left scaphoid illustrating the value of a comparison of the sound side with the injured in the oblique projection with ulna flexion (83,84).

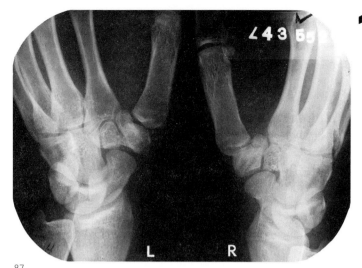

87

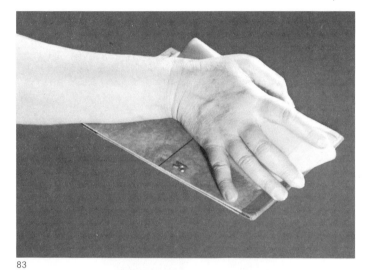

83

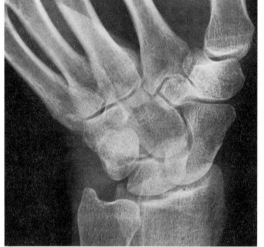

84

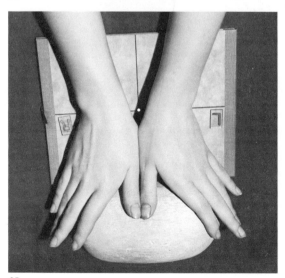

85

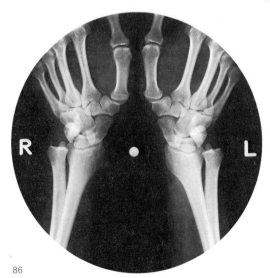

86

Carpal tunnel

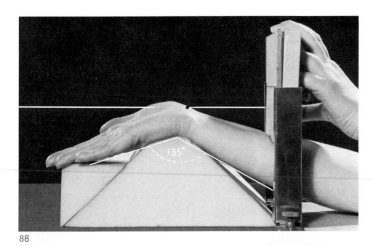

88

The carpal tunnel is the area bounded by the carpal bones and the transverse carpal ligament (the annular ligament). The carpal bones form a shallow concavity anteriorly, and the transverse carpal ligament completes the tunnel by its attachment medially to the pisiform and the hook of the hamate, and laterally to the tubercle of the scaphoid and the ridge of the trapezium (see page 15, 51a,b). The median nerve and the flexor tendons of the fingers pass through the tunnel.

The carpal tunnel is shown by axial projection of the wrist joint; three methods are described.

Axial

(1) The forearm is extended, and the wrist dorsi-flexed at an angle of approximately 135° with ulnar deviation, over a wedge-shaped plastic sponge block; the film is held vertically in position proximal to the wrist joint (88,91).

(2) The film is placed on the surface of a plastic sponge block against which the forearm is supported; dorsi-flexion at the wrist joint at an angle of approximately 135°, with ulnar deviation, is maintained by traction on a bandage round the palm of the hand (89,91).

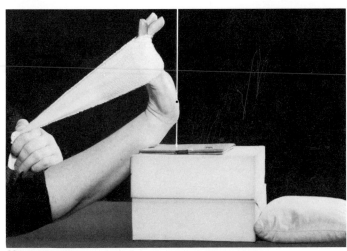

89

(3) The patient stands back to the table, with the palm of the hand pressing on the film supported on the table surface (90, 91).
■ Centre along the line of the forearm to between the pisiform and the hook of the hamate medially, and the tubercle of the scaphoid and the ridge of the trapezium laterally (bony projections which are readily palpable) with the tube directed either horizontally or vertically, as appropriate, toward the tunnel and at right-angles to the film (88,89,90,91).

Note—(92) is included as an unsatisfactory projection compared with (91).

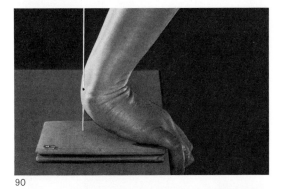

90

Carpal Tunnel

kVp	mAS	FFD	Film ILFORD	Screens ILFORD	Grid
60	20	100 cm (40")	RAPID R	SUPER HD	

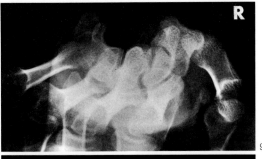

91

Radial Deviation
Ulnar and Radial Flexion
Although flexion of the hand toward the ulna (95) is the more commonly used and more readily achieved, flexion toward the radius (97) may also be required. This series of photographs and radiographs—ulnar flexion (95,96) radial flexion (97,98) and the routine straight position (93,94) is included for comparison and guidance.

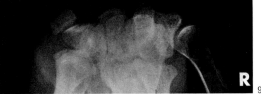

92

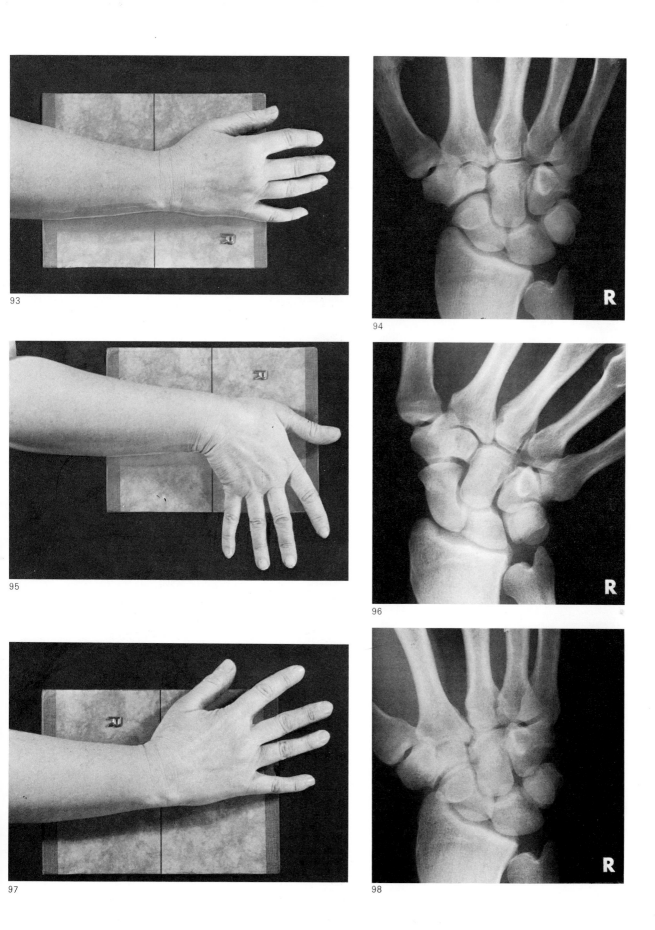

93

94

95

96

97

98

Lateral on Flexion and Extension

Although it is the usual practice to expose the wrist joint in the straight lateral position (100, 101), it is sometimes necessary to obtain radiographs showing flexion or extension at the joint. This series of illustrations shows the three positions with the resulting radiographs for comparison—straight (100, 101), flexed (102, 103) and extended (104, 105). The additional photograph (99) shows the actual placing of the wrist and the necessary backward tilt to achieve a true lateral projection. It should be noted that gentle, smooth, but firm movement is required in making these adjustments at the wrist joint.

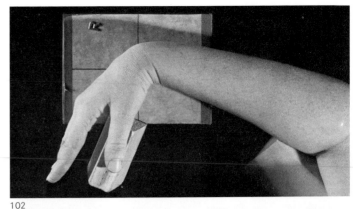

102

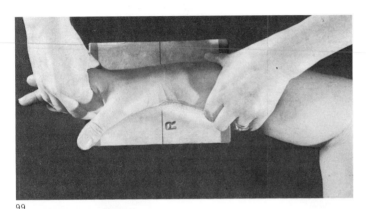

99

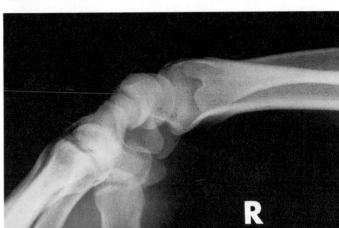

103

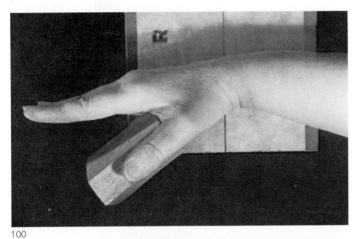

100

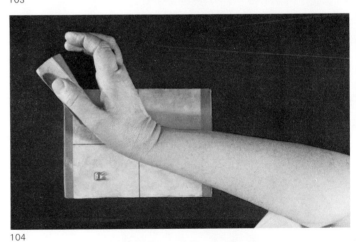

104

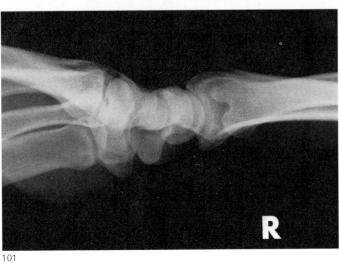

101

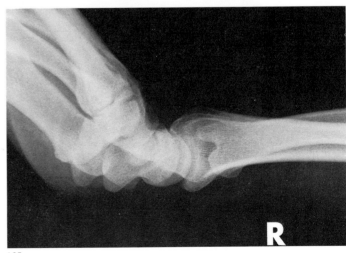

105

Forearm

Positioning for the forearm is quite different from positioning for the wrist joint.

To obtain two views of the ulna, at right angles to each other, either the elbow must be extended between the lateral (106) and antero-posterior views (108) or, if the forearm has to remain flexed at the elbow, the tube should be moved through ninety degrees (110,112) between the two projections.

Note—For a general exploratory view of the forearm both the wrist and the elbow joint must be included.

Lateral (basic)
The limb is placed in the lateral position with the elbow flexed; the hand is also in the lateral position with the ulnar border of the hand and forearm on the cassette.
■ Centre to the middle of the forearm (106,107)

Antero-posterior (basic)
The arm is extended at the elbow so that the shoulder, elbow and wrist are on the same level. Place the dorsum of the forearm on the cassette. The extended arm is now in full supination with the wrist slightly extended.
■ Centre to the middle of the forearm (108,109).

Forearm							
kVp		mAS			Film	Screens	
Lat	AP	Lat	AP	FFD	ILFORD	ILFORD	Grid
60	60	8	8	100 cm (40″)	RAPID R	SUPER HD	—

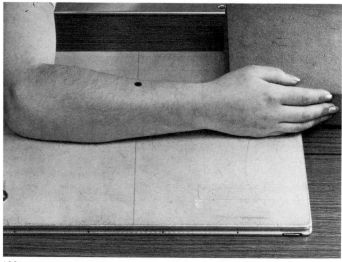

106

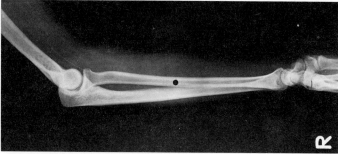

107

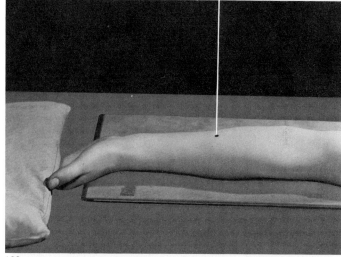

108

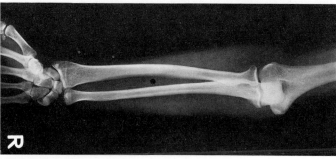

109

Injuries

A splint or plaster immobilizing the elbow and wrist joints will complicate the previous projections. After taking the arm in the prone position (110) without moving the patient the film is placed vertically on the posterior aspect of the forearm. The X-ray beam is projected horizontally from the trunk aspect of the forearm (112).

■ Centre to the middle of the forearm (110, 111, 112, 113)

Note—Always use a film large enough to include both the wrist and elbow joints. As it is sometimes impossible to place the injured arm on the table, the necessary projections are obtained by bandaging the films to the arm and by directing the beam horizontally for the postero-anterior position and from above the shoulder for the lateral position (114). Thus, two near routine projections are obtained (115). Radiograph (115) shows a dislocation of the radio-ulnar joint at the elbow and a

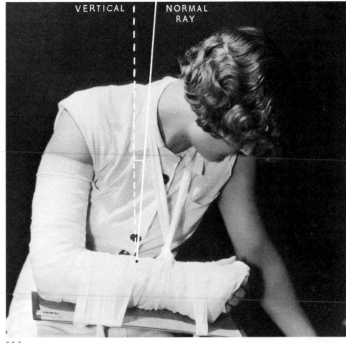

114

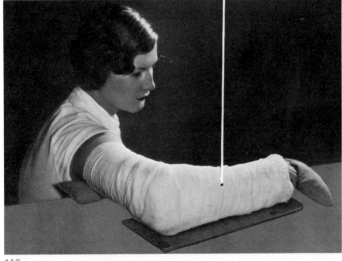

110

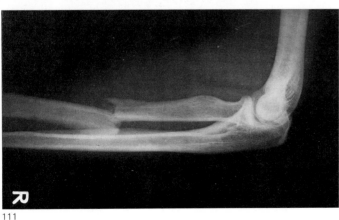

111

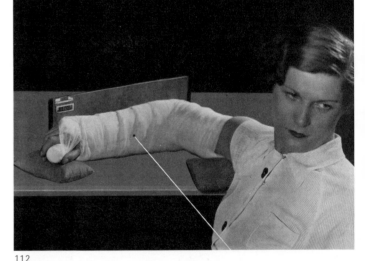

112

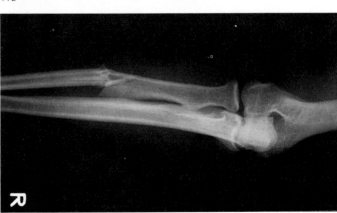

113

greenstick fracture of the ulna. A greenstick fracture is common in children where the bone is bent and only partially broken as occurs when trying to break a piece of green wood. The importance of including the full length of the bone to show alignment, both before and after reduction, will be appreciated, particularly in the lateral projection.

A serious injury suffered by an adult patient is shown in (117) where there is a fracture of the wrist joint and of the shaft of the ulna. In this case the arm could not be moved into the general antero-posterior and lateral positions and the radiographs were taken as shown in (110,112), producing an antero-posterior projection of the elbow joint and lateral of the wrist joint, (116) and a postero-anterior projection of the wrist joint and lateral of the elbow joint (117).

Foreign Bodies in Forearm
When examining the forearm for foreign bodies, the succeeding projection must be taken without moving the limb. The forearm should be placed with the palm of the hand in contact with the couch, the elbow should be flexed, as shown in (110).

After this exposure (118) without moving the limb the second film is placed against the outer aspect of the forearm and at right angles to the couch, the X-ray beam being projected horizontally as shown in (112) giving a view at right angles to the one previously described (119).

1

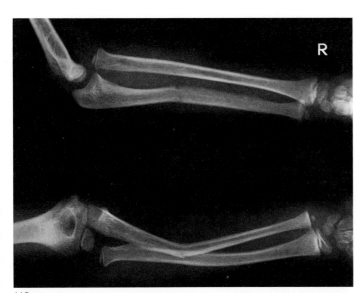

115

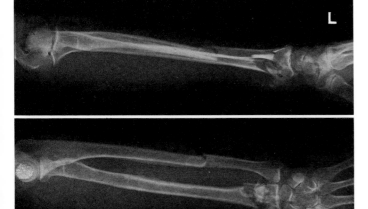

116(top) 117(above)

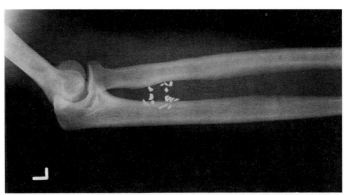

118

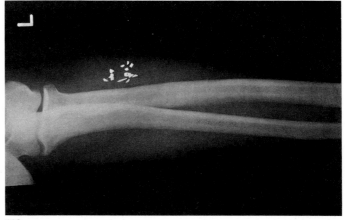

119

Elbow joint

Radiographic appearances

Annotated radiographs of the elbow joint, antero-posterior (120), lateral (121), oblique (122) and extreme flexion (123), will help the student understand the anatomical references in the text.

The most satisfactory projections of the elbow joint are obtained when the upper arm is on the same plane as the forearm, and in order to gain the patient's confidence, the more readily placed lateral position is exposed before adjusting the arm to the antero-posterior position.

The text initially describes the basic antero-posterior and lateral projections. Frequently, however, the antero-posterior position will cause the patient too much discomfort. Alternative views are given to overcome this difficulty.

Arthrography

Arthrography is the examination for the internal structures of a joint and can be carried out either with a gas (negative contrast medium) or with a positive contrast medium. Where air or oxygen is used it is known as pneumo-arthrography; where a water-soluble organic iodine compound is used, it is referred to as arthrography.

The elbow joint is injected from the lateral side into the space between the head of the radius and capitulum, with 3 ml of a 35% water soluble non-ionic organic iodide contrast medium. Following injection the elbow is flexed and extended many times to disperse the contrast medium throughout the joint. The proprietary names of the contrast agents are given in supplement 1.

The injections are made with the patient on the X-ray couch so that exposures can follow immediately, antero-posterior (120), lateral (121) and oblique (122).

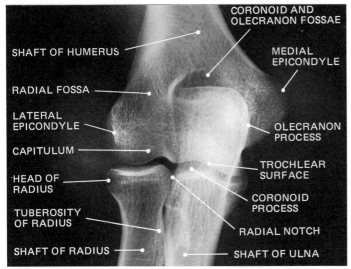

SHAFT OF HUMERUS

CORONOID AND
OLECRANON FOSSAE

RADIAL FOSSA

MEDIAL
EPICONDYLE

LATERAL
EPICONDYLE

OLECRANON
PROCESS

CAPITULUM

HEAD OF
RADIUS

TROCHLEAR
SURFACE

CORONOID
PROCESS

TUBEROSITY
OF RADIUS

RADIAL NOTCH

SHAFT OF RADIUS

SHAFT OF ULNA

RIGHT ELBOW   ANTERO-POSTERIOR
120

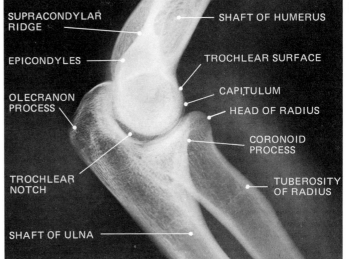

SUPRACONDYLAR
RIDGE

SHAFT OF HUMERUS

EPICONDYLES

TROCHLEAR SURFACE

OLECRANON
PROCESS

CAPITULUM

HEAD OF RADIUS

CORONOID
PROCESS

TROCHLEAR
NOTCH

TUBEROSITY
OF RADIUS

SHAFT OF ULNA

RIGHT ELBOW   LATERAL
121

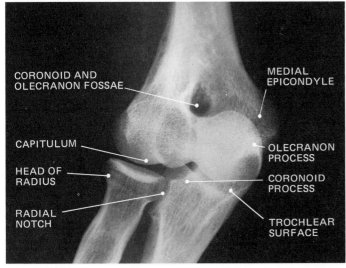

CORONOID AND
OLECRANON FOSSAE

MEDIAL
EPICONDYLE

CAPITULUM

OLECRANON
PROCESS

HEAD OF
RADIUS

CORONOID
PROCESS

RADIAL
NOTCH

TROCHLEAR
SURFACE

RIGHT RADIO-ULNAR JOINT   OBLIQUE
122

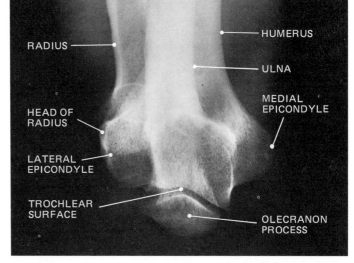

RADIUS

HUMERUS

ULNA

HEAD OF
RADIUS

MEDIAL
EPICONDYLE

LATERAL
EPICONDYLE

TROCHLEAR
SURFACE

OLECRANON
PROCESS

RIGHT ELBOW   EXTREME FLEXION
123

Lateral (1) (basic)

The arm and forearm are placed in the usual lateral position with the elbow joint flexed to an angle of approximately 90°. The hand and forearm are supported and immobilized.

■ Centre to the lateral epicondyle of the humerus (124, 125)

This position gives a true lateral projection of all bones of the elbow joint.

Note—If the arm cannot be raised to the level of the shoulder joint then a lateral view may be obtained by keeping the elbow in the lateral position but placing the film between the elbow and the body and adjusting the tube to a 90° angle to the long axis of the arm.

Antero-posterior (1) (basic)

From the lateral position the arm is rotated and extended outward to the fully supinated position with the palm facing the tube. The shoulder must be well down so that the arm and forearm are in one plane and the elbow joint is in the true antero-posterior position.

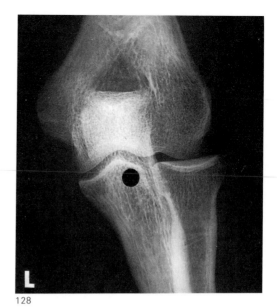

128

■ Centre through the joint space 2·5 cm (1 inch) below the midpoint between the epicondyles (126, 127)

The radiograph (128) shows the effect of allowing the hand to rotate into the prone position so that the shaft of the radius crosses that of the ulna.

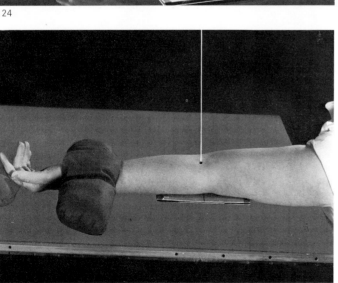

124

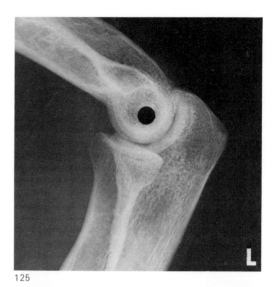

125

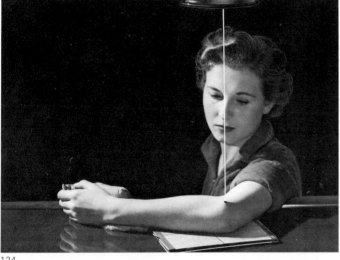

126

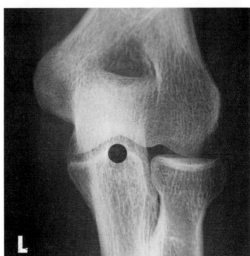

127

32

Lateral (2)

From the previous lateral position the hand is allowed to rotate forward until the palm is in contact with the couch.
■ Centre to the lateral epicondyle of the humerus (129, 130)

Note—The lateral (1, basic) gives a true lateral projection of the radius (124), however, it is usually easier for the patient to adopt the lateral (2) position (129).

Lateral (3)

With the elbow flexed, the hand rotates forward until the radial aspect is in contact with the couch, and the palm of the hand faces away from the trunk (131, 132).

The third lateral position (131) is included to show a further variation in the appearance of the head of the radius. In each of the three positions the only movement at the elbow is the rotation of the radial head, when each part of the head is in turn projected clear of the shadow of the coronoid process. The additional lateral projections may help in the detection of a poorly visible fracture to the head of the radius.

By comparing lateral radiographs with the articulated dry bones of the skeleton, the almost complete rotation of the radial head in the three projections (125, 130, 132) will be appreciated.

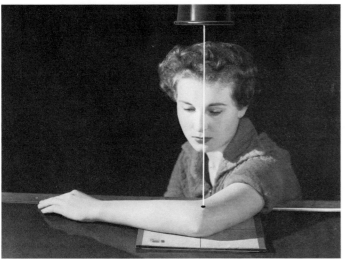

129

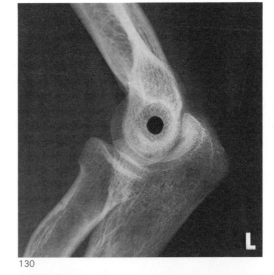

130

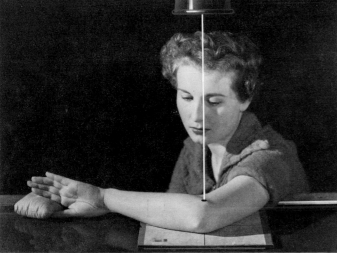

131

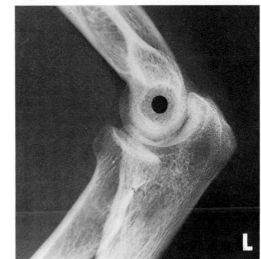

132

Note—This position gives a general projection of the joint, with equal distortion of upper and lower aspects. Its chief value is in showing the upper surface of the head of the radius.

Antero-posterior (2)

When the joint cannot be fully extended and there is no alternative but to examine the elbow in partial flexion, the most satisfactory result is obtained when the forearm is placed in contact with the film and the humerus supported.

■ Centre to the mid-point 2·5 cm (1 inch) below the crease of the joint (133, 134)

Antero-posterior (3)

It is common practice, when it is necessary to examine the elbow in partial flexion, to position the limb so that both angles between limb and film, above and below the joint, are equal. To keep the elbow in the partially flexed position, support for both the arm and forearm will be needed, thus avoiding pressure on the olecranon process.

■ Centre to the crease of the elbow (135, 136)

					Elbow		
kVp		mAS			Film	Screens	
Lat	AP	Lat	AP	FFD	ILFORD	ILFORD	Grid
60	60	10	10	100 cm (40″)	RAPID R	SUPER HD	—

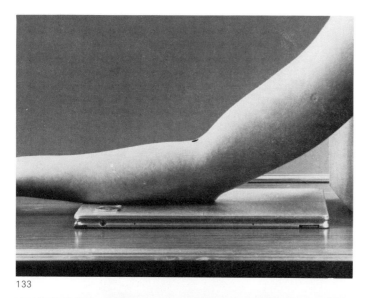

133

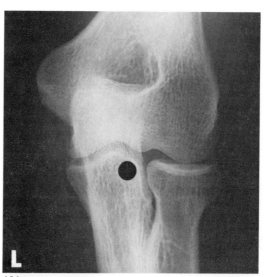

134

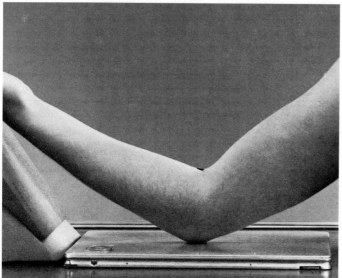

135

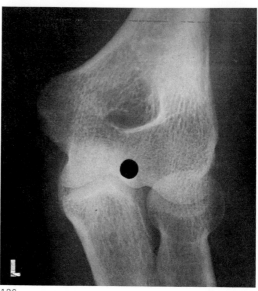

136

Antero-posterior (4)

When the elbow cannot be fully extended and a supracondylar fracture is suspected, then the projection must be made with the upper arm in contact with the film and the forearm supported.
■ Centre midway between the epicondyles (137,138)

It is necessary to increase the exposure by 5 kVp for this view of the lower humerus.

Note—Compare the radiographs of the elbow joint (127,134,136,138) with similarly positioned articulated skeletal bones.

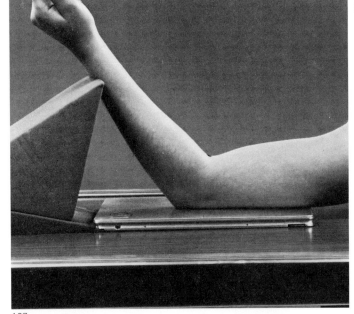

137

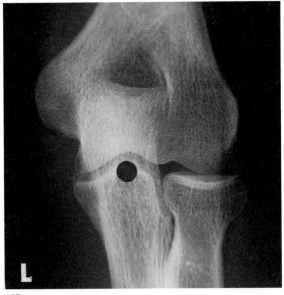

Antero-posterior (1)

127

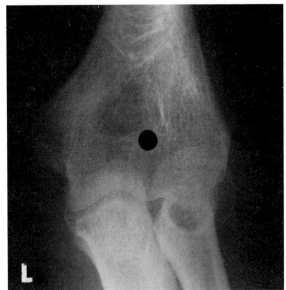

Antero-posterior (4)

138

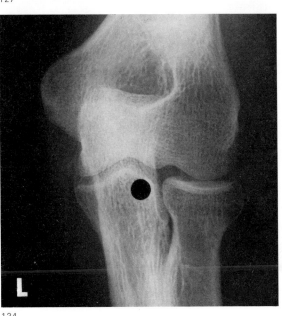

Antero-posterior (2)

134

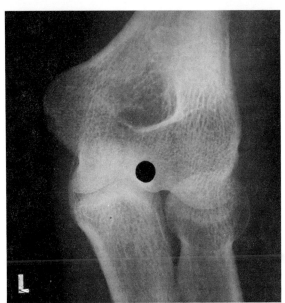

Antero-posterior (3)

136

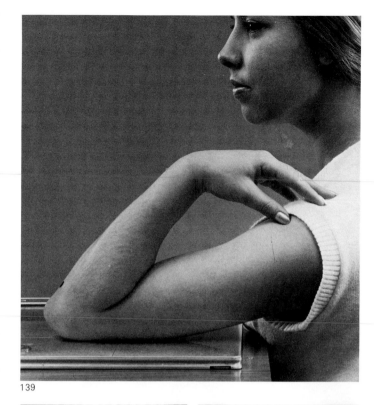
139

Axial—infero-superior

The axial view is obtained when the hand is in contact with the shoulder, the upper arm is in contact with the film, and the beam directed axially through both forearm and humerus.

■ Centre 5 cm (2 ins) distal to the olecranon process with the tube straight (139), or with the tube angled 30° toward the shoulder (140).

Note—This projection shows the bones of the forearm superimposed upon the humerus. The olecranon process and its articulation are shown when the tube is straight, and also the circumference of the radial head. The radio-humeral joint space is shown when the tube is tilted. Compare (140) with annotated radiograph (123), page 31.

Elbow Axial

kVp	mAS	FFD	Film ILFORD	Screens ILFORD	Grid
70	8	100 cms (40″)	RAPID R	SUPER HD	—

Exposure factors

The value of taking the axial projection of the elbow (139) is shown in the radiograph of a child with a supracondylar fracture (141).

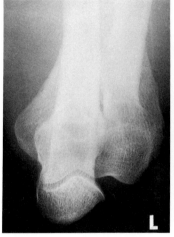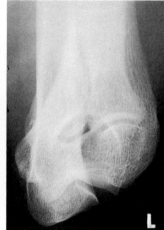

(a) TUBE STRAIGHT   (b) TUBE TILTED
140

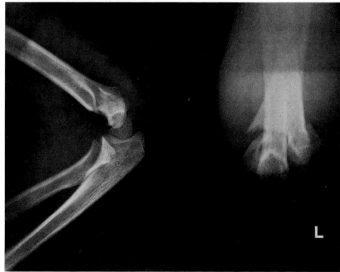

141

Axial—supero-inferior

On occasion it is desirable and more suitable to examine the arm from the reverse aspect. Rotation at the shoulder joint enables the forearm to be in contact with the film as in (142).

■ Centre to just above the level of the humeral epicondyles (142) with the tube straight (a) or angled (b) (142, 143)

Note—Compare the axial radiographs (140) and (143).

Ulnar Groove

The ulnar groove or sulcus at the distal end of the humerus transmits the ulnar nerve from the upper to lower arm and is a depression between the trochlea (lying laterally), and the medial epicondyle (lying medially). This region is superficial and the condyle and groove are readily palpable. The supero-inferior projection is used to show the ulnar groove and adjacent soft tissues.

Supero-inferior

With the patient sitting back to the couch, extend the limb from the shoulder joint so that the elbow, which is flexed to an angle of approximately 35°, rests on the film holder which is on the couch surface.

■ Centre to the groove immediately lateral to the medial epicondyle, with the tube vertical using a small aperture cone (144, 145, 146)

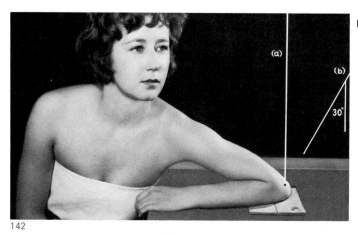

142

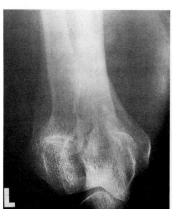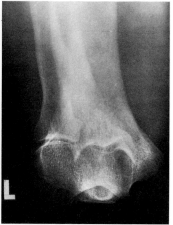

143

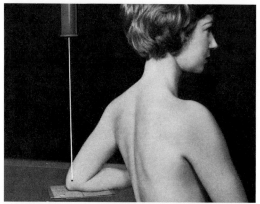

144

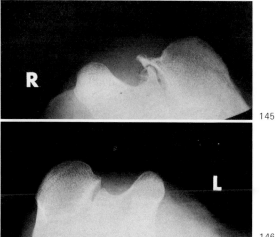

145

146

Ulnar Groove

kVp	mAS	FFD	Film ILFORD	Screens ILFORD	Grid
70	10	100 cm (40″)	RAPID R	SUPER HD	—

Proximal Radio-Ulnar Joint
For the demonstration of poorly-visible fractures of the head of the radius further views may be required.

Antero-posterior (5)
From the basic antero-posterior position for the elbow joint (126), the arm is rotated slightly outward to separate the proximal radius and ulna.
■ Centre over the head of the radius (147, 148)

Exposure factors

			Radio Ulnar Jt.			
kVp	mAS	FFD	Film ILFORD	Screens ILFORD	Grid
60	10	100 cm (40″)	RAPID R	SUPER HD	—

Fracture Radiographs
Two radiographs of the elbow (149), using the position shown (147) disclose a fracture, through the head of the radius (149).

Horizontal Ray View
With patients on a splint or in plaster of Paris, a horizontal ray view may be required. Raise the arm and forearm to the level of the shoulder joint and centre to the crease of the elbow with the film at right angles to central ray (150).

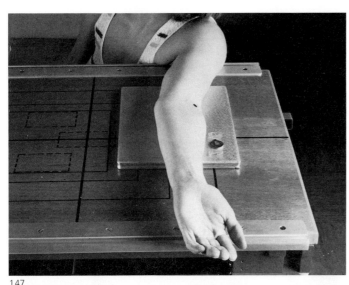

147

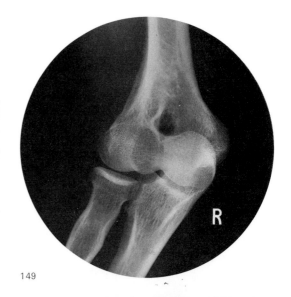

149

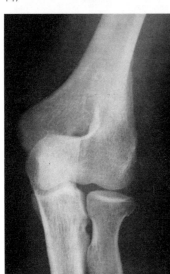
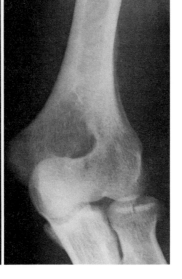

148

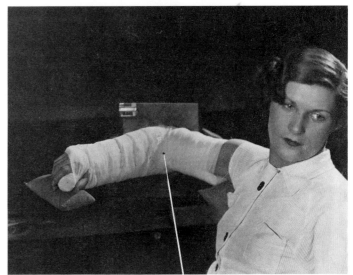

150

Elbow Immobilized to Trunk

When an injured elbow is immobilized and cannot be moved away from the trunk, it can be radiographed either by positioning a film between the elbow and the trunk, or by an exposure through the trunk. The latter projection will mean more radiation to the patient.

Erect—Lateral (A)

Film between trunk and body.

A cassette is slipped between the elbow and the patient's trunk with lead rubber behind the cassette to minimize radiation to the patient.
■ The horizontal ray is centred on the lateral epicondyle

Erect—Lateral (B)

With the patient in the erect position the lateral aspect of the elbow joint is in contact with the vertical Bucky. The trunk must be positioned in such a way that the vertebral column appears anterior to the elbow joint but overlying the distal radius and ulna (151).

■ Centre through the trunk directly over the elbow joint, covering only the small localized area required to include the joint (152)

Note—In view of the increased tissue thickness, a Bucky or stationary grid must be used, otherwise the film will be too grey from scattered radiation.

Elbow Immobilized to Trunk

kVp	mAS		Film	Screens	
Lat	Lat	FFD	ILFORD	ILFORD	Grid
80	20	100 cm (40")	RAPID R	SUPER HD	Grid

Horizontal or Lying

This view is particularly useful when the patient is unable to stand or sit; then, with the patient lying in the lateral position, so that the injured elbow is uppermost, the cassette is slipped in between the elbow and the trunk as previously described.

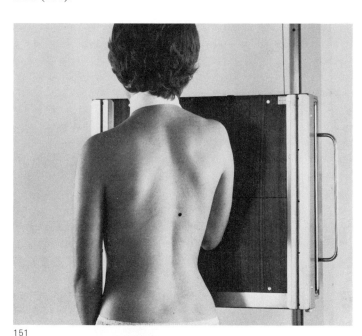

151

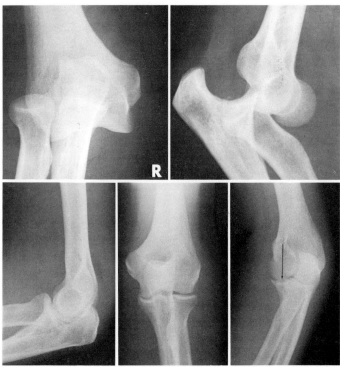

153(top) 154(above)

■ Centre directly over the elbow joint with the central ray perpendicular to the film

Radiographs

Radiograph (153) shows a frontal and lateral view of a dislocation at the elbow.

In (154) there is a large effusion in the elbow joint but no fracture visible on lateral and frontal views but shown on an oblique view (arrow) on the Coracoid process.

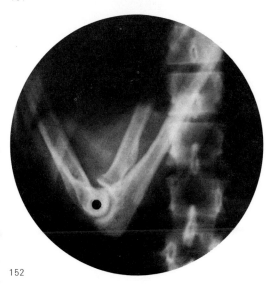

152

39

Children

In children, because the epiphyses are still developing, there is often difficulty in interpreting radiographic anatomy. A comparison film of the normal side is used to assess the presence of an abnormality in the injured limb.

It was previously recommended that the two exposures be done on a single film (155) but this means that mirror image views are compared. However, if the views are taken on separate films then the radiograph of the normal side can be turned round to make comparison easier. If the two exposures are made on one film, a lead divider must be used to cover the portion of the film not being exposed.

In the antero-posterior projection (156) the effect of incomplete supination of the forearm causes the radius to be superimposed on the ulna, but being similarly positioned for right and left sides, the radiographs are comparable.

					Elbow (Child)		
kVp		mAS			Film	Screens	
Lat	AP	Lat	AP	FFD	ILFORD	ILFORD	Grid
50	50	8	8	100 cm (40″)	RAPID R	SUPER HD	—

Injuries

Radiographs (157) of a child show a supracondylar fracture of the humerus. The post-reduction film (158) in a plaster splint is in a comparable position.

A good quality film can be obtained by increasing the exposure.

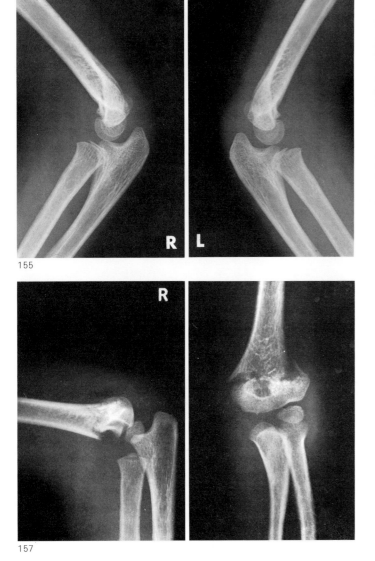

155

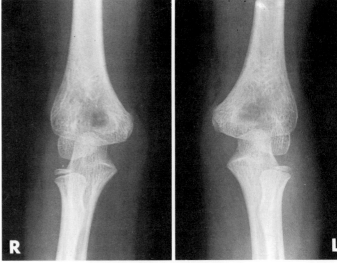

156

157

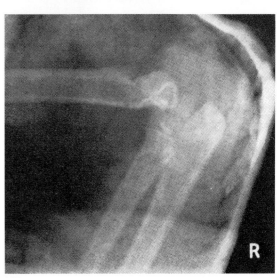

158

2

HUMERUS AND
SHOULDER GIRDLE

HUMERUS AND SHOULDER GIRDLE

Radiographic Appearances

Lettered radiographs showing five projections of the shoulder will assist the student in following the anatomical references in the text. Additionally, a diagram (226) showing various muscle attachments is included on page 60.

(159) Shows the standard antero-posterior position of the shoulder and humerus, with the arm slightly abducted and extended at the elbow joint, with the palm of the hand facing the tube, as in (201), page 54.

(160) Shows the antero-posterior position of the shoulder, with the arm raised above shoulder level and rotated medially with flexion at the elbow joint, as in (256), page 67.

(161) Shows the scapula in lateral projection with medial and lateral borders superimposed. The trunk is in the oblique position with some abduction of the arm and the elbow flexed to obtain separation of the humeral shaft and scapula, as in (251), page 66.

(162) Shows an axial, infero-superior projection of the shoulder, with the arm extended and abducted to shoulder level with the palm of the hand facing away from the tube (palm up) as in (186a), page 50.

(163) In the same general axial position as (162), but the arm is rotated medially with the palm of the hand facing toward the tube (palm down) as in (186b), page 50.

Note—(162) and **(163)** are axial projections providing a general plan of the shoulder in the third dimension. The scapula and clavicle form a 'V'-shape above the lung fields.

General and Technical

Because of movement during respiration the patient's breath must be held while the radiograph is being taken and a short exposure time is required. Exposures are made in expiration as there is then less tension with the body at rest. In children, elderly people and in other patients where respiratory movements cannot be controlled, exposure times should be reduced to a minimum. A maximum exposure time of 0·1 second should be used but 0·05 second is preferred. For walking or chair patients, especially when elderly or obese, it is less disturbing to be examined in the erect position, and when distressed as a result of an accident should be allowed to remain seated in the casualty chair. A wheelchair has been designed to enable all such examinations to be made without disturbing the patient.

With a little ingenuity, even when the patient is in an ordinary wheelchair cassettes can be placed and supported in position for the X-ray tube to be angled from any direction to obtain the necessary projections.

Intensifying screens are used and a grid, either stationary or moving type is advised for many of the projections in this section, particularly when high kilovoltages are employed and is essential for all projections through the trunk. The exposure factors given for each position refer to an adult of average physique.

Radiographic quality should ensure that the soft tissues are seen in addition to bony structures. The various projections given in the text allow each part of a bone such as the tuberosities of the humerus as well as soft tissues such as ligaments and muscles to be shown in profile. Changes in outline and in density can then be demonstrated.

Note—To avoid confusion from the many alternative techniques included in the text, the basic projections for each region are indicated accordingly as (BASIC).

The section is presented in the following order with appropriate positioning.

Humerus (General)
Humerus (Head) fracture
Shoulder (General)
Humerus (Head) pathology
Shoulder Joint (dislocation)
Positioning and Identification of Tendons
Acromio-Clavicular Joint (subluxation)
Scapula
Acromion Process
Clavicle
Sterno-Clavicular Joints

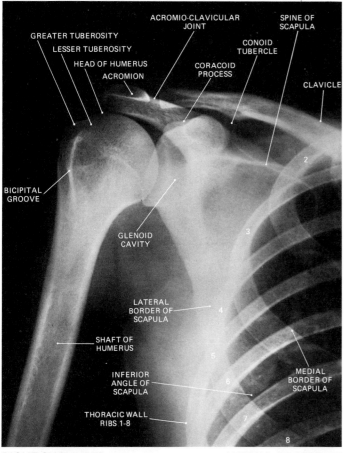

GREATER TUBEROSITY
LESSER TUBEROSITY
HEAD OF HUMERUS
ACROMION
ACROMIO-CLAVICULAR JOINT
CONOID TUBERCLE
CORACOID PROCESS
SPINE OF SCAPULA
CLAVICLE
BICIPITAL GROOVE
GLENOID CAVITY
LATERAL BORDER OF SCAPULA
SHAFT OF HUMERUS
INFERIOR ANGLE OF SCAPULA
THORACIC WALL RIBS 1-8
MEDIAL BORDER OF SCAPULA

RIGHT SHOULDER · ANTERO-POSTERIOR
159

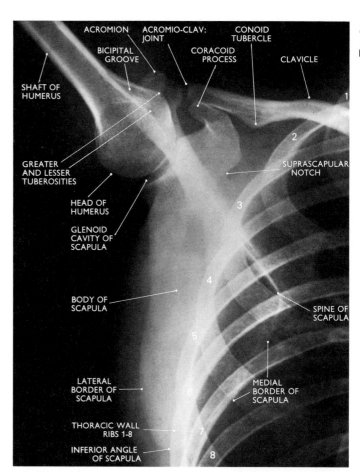

ACROMION
ACROMIO-CLAV: JOINT
CONOID TUBERCLE
BICIPITAL GROOVE
CORACOID PROCESS
CLAVICLE
SHAFT OF HUMERUS
GREATER AND LESSER TUBEROSITIES
HEAD OF HUMERUS
GLENOID CAVITY OF SCAPULA
SUPRASCAPULAR NOTCH
BODY OF SCAPULA
SPINE OF SCAPULA
LATERAL BORDER OF SCAPULA
MEDIAL BORDER OF SCAPULA
THORACIC WALL RIBS 1-8
INFERIOR ANGLE OF SCAPULA

RIGHT SHOULDER · ANTERO-POSTERIOR
160

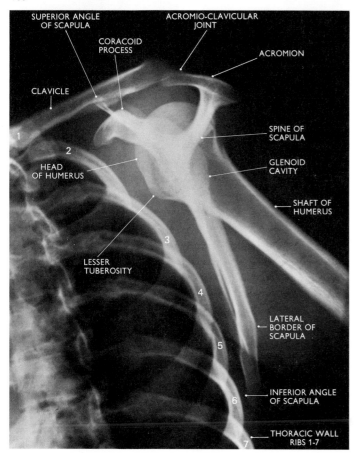

SUPERIOR ANGLE OF SCAPULA
ACROMIO-CLAVICULAR JOINT
CORACOID PROCESS
ACROMION
CLAVICLE
HEAD OF HUMERUS
SPINE OF SCAPULA
GLENOID CAVITY
SHAFT OF HUMERUS
LESSER TUBEROSITY
LATERAL BORDER OF SCAPULA
INFERIOR ANGLE OF SCAPULA
THORACIC WALL RIBS 1-7

RIGHT SCAPULA · LATERAL
161

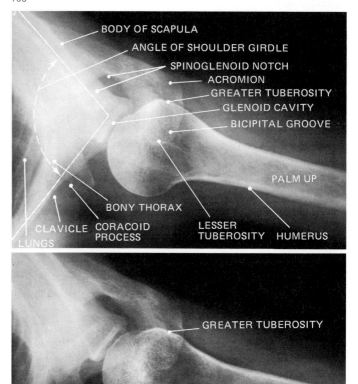

BODY OF SCAPULA
ANGLE OF SHOULDER GIRDLE
SPINOGLENOID NOTCH
ACROMION
GREATER TUBEROSITY
GLENOID CAVITY
BICIPITAL GROOVE
PALM UP
CLAVICLE
LUNGS
CORACOID PROCESS
BONY THORAX
LESSER TUBEROSITY
HUMERUS

GREATER TUBEROSITY
PALM DOWN
BICIPITAL GROOVE
LESSER TUBEROSITY

INFERO-SUPERIOR · LEFT SHOULDER
162(top) 163(above)

43

Humerus

Antero-posterior (basic)

With the patient supine and facing the tube, the trunk is rotated toward the affected side and the opposite shoulder raised on sandbags to bring the injured arm into contact with the cassette. The arm is supinated with full extension at the elbow and slight abduction at the shoulder. A sandbag is placed on the hand for immobilization. Adjustments in positioning of an injured arm should be done by moving the trunk in relation to the arm wherever possible.

■ Centre midway between the shoulder and elbow joint (164,165)

Lateral (basic)

From the previous position flex the forearm at the elbow to 90° abduct the arm to 45° and rest the forearm on the table in the lateral position with the thumb uppermost.

■ Centre midway between the shoulder and elbow joint (166,167)

The basic antero-posterior and lateral views are only possible when there is full movement of the limb. Alternative positions are necessary in injured subjects. The whole of the humerus is included when there is a fracture in the middle third but for fractures at the upper and lower ends the views are for the shoulder and elbow respectively.

Note—In both antero-posterior and lateral positions the film is placed well up under the shoulder joint because in centring to the middle of the humerus, the oblique ray tends to project the shoulder joint which is not in close contact with the film, to a much higher level than is generally anticipated. The positioning for antero-posterior (basic) and lateral (basic) can also be done with the patient erect (205,206) page 55.

To emphasize the difference in the two positions on rotating the humerus from antero-posterior to lateral (164,167), the shoulder section of radiographs (165,166) is shown in larger size (168,169).

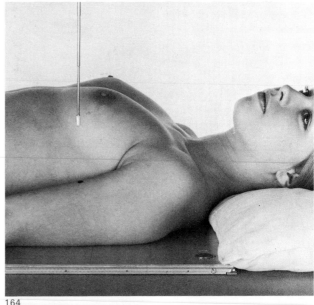

164

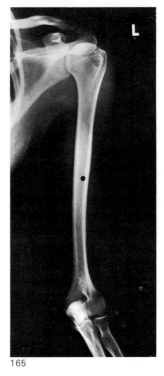

165

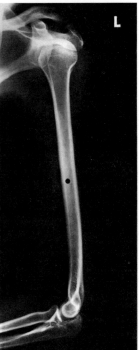

166

Exposure conditions are shown for each region, but when both joints are to be included in a single exposure a mean average of the two sets of factors should be used.

Humerus

kVp		mAS			Film	Screens	
AP	Lat	AP	Lat	FFD	ILFORD	ILFORD	Grid
60	60	30	30	100 cm (40")	RAPID R	SUPER HD	—

Fracture Radiographs

Antero-posterior view (170) of the shoulder showing a fracture of the neck and great tuberosity of the humerus. The axial view (171) also shows a fracture of the Coracoid process.

It is usually necessary to increase the exposure by 50–70% to compensate for a plaster splint.

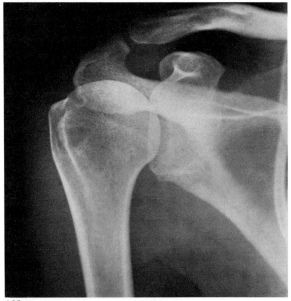

168

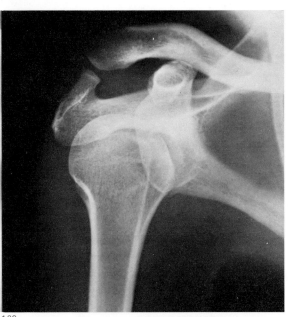

169

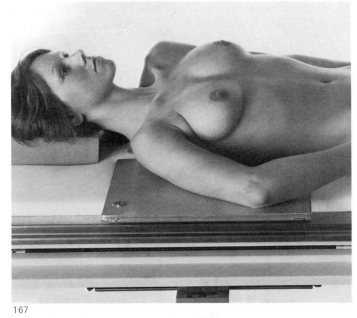

167

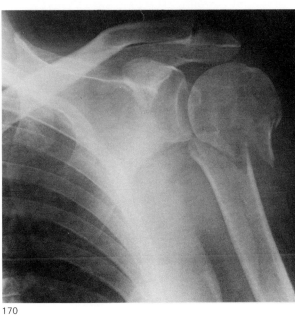

170

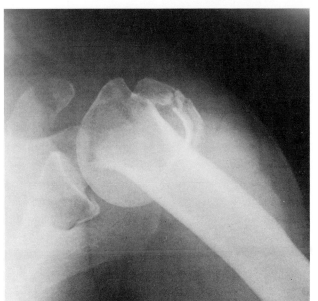

171

2 Humerus and shoulder girdle
Humerus (after injury)

(1) When the arm is restricted in movement relative to the trunk, the patient may sit or stand. Ignoring the trunk, the films should be placed to the anterior or posterior and lateral aspects of the humerus (172, 173), with the beam directed through the thorax when necessary (174). It is usually possible to obtain either antero-posterior or postero-anterior, and lateral projections of a fracture, with the alignment of the fragments being clearly shown.

The following exposure factors apply to (172) and (173)

Humerus (after injury)

kVp	mAS	FFD	Film ILFORD	Screens ILFORD	Grid
65	40	100 cm (40")	RAPID R	Super HD	Grid

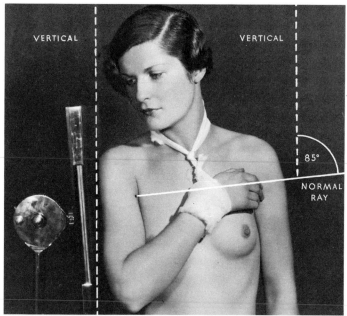

172

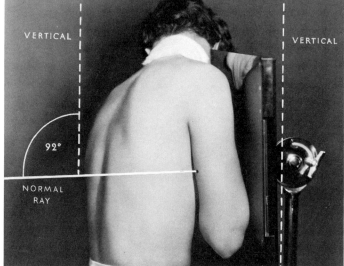

173

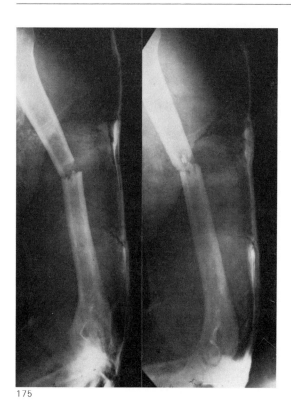

175

Fracture Radiographs

Radiographs of the arm in a plaster splint (175) show how two satisfactory projections can be made by using similar positioning to that shown in (172, 173). In view of the plaster splint the exposure was increased by 40%.

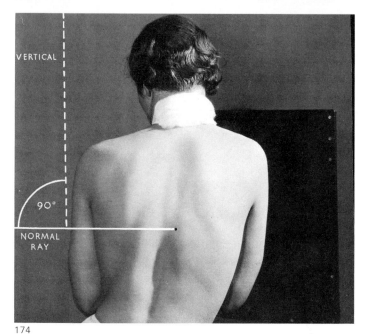

174

(2) When the injured arm is suspended freely beside the trunk and cannot be moved without causing considerable discomfort, the patient is again examined in an erect or sitting position. After the exposure for the antero-posterior projection with the patient facing the tube, the patient is moved to the lateral position with the injured arm against the vertical stand. The sound arm is raised and folded over the head, the trunk leaning toward the film so that the injured shoulder assumes a lower level than the uninjured side. This position (176) is an alternative to (174).

■ Centre through the axilla, to the upper third of the injured arm (176, 177, 178)

Exposure factors

Humerus thro' Trunk					
kVp	mAS		Film	Screens	
Lat	Lat	FFD	ILFORD	ILFORD	Grid
85	100	100 cm (40″)	RAPID R	STANDARD	Grid

Note—The outline of the humerus is well shown, (177). Slight rotation of the trunk backward or forward to position the spine away from the humerus is necessary.

Although unnecessary irradiation of the trunk is to be avoided whenever possible there are occasions such as this, when the small additional exposure (176, 177) is justified.

Greater clarity of the humerus can be obtained if the patient continues to breathe quietly during a long exposure. The arm must remain quite still while the ribs move during breathing. By doing this, the overlying rib shadows are blurred out. Similar clarity on a lateral thoracic spine radiograph can be obtained by a long exposure in quiet breathing.

The four photographs (172, 173, 174, 176) illustrate some of the positions used in examining the humerus when the arm is immobilized. Radiographs (178) are of a fracture of the surgical neck of the humerus. In (b) the upper end of the humerus is projected through the thorax for the lateral projection. The erect or possibly the sitting position is more readily acceptable to the patient.

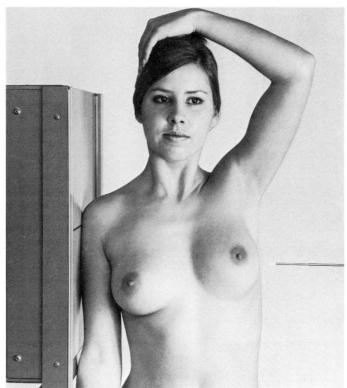

176

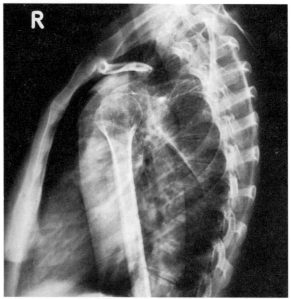

177

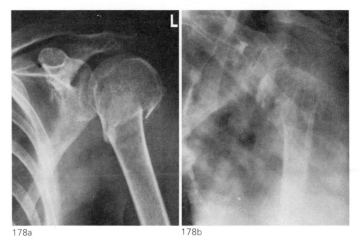

178a   178b

Abduction

(3) When the arm is fixed by splint or plaster in abduction at an angle of from 70° to 90° with the trunk, the patient is usually examined in the supine position.

Antero-posterior

With the injured arm supported in abduction, the cassette is placed well up under the shoulder to include the shoulder joint and the upper one-third of the humerus.

■ Centre over the head of the humerus (179, 180a)

Humerus Abduction

kVp		mAS			Film	Screens	
AP	Axial	AP	Axial	FFD	ILFORD	ILFORD	Grid
60	60	30	40	100 cm (40″)	RAPID R	SUPER HD	—

Lateral—Infero-superior

Again the arm is supported in abduction and the shoulder slightly raised on a non-opaque pad, the head is turned and the neck inclined towards the sound side, allowing the cassette, supported vertically above the shoulder, to be pressed against the neck, thus ensuring the inclusion of the essential parts of the shoulder joint. This applies particularly when considerable tube angulation is required (183).

■ Centre toward the axilla using horizontal tube projection and with the angulation away from the trunk at a minimum according to the conditions prevailing (181, 180b, 182, 183)

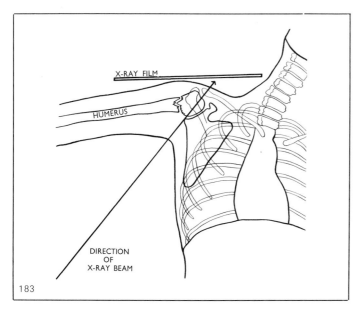

183

A frontal view diagram shows the importance of placing the cassette well into the neck to accommodate the oblique projection of the head of the humerus on to the film (183), particularly with an oblique tube projection as shown on the tracing from a radiograph.

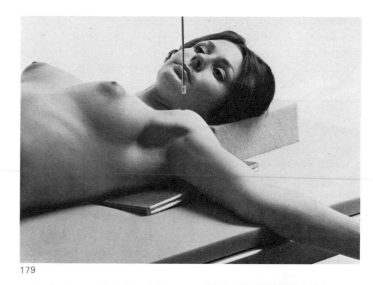

179

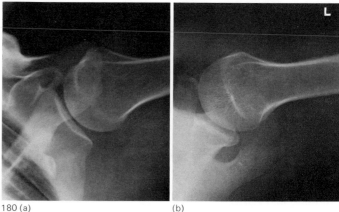

180 (a)   (b)

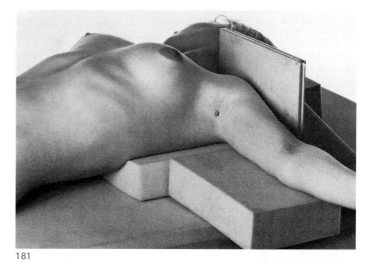

181

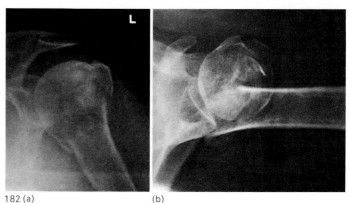

182 (a)   (b)

Fracture Radiographs

This method gives an undistorted lateral projection in all circumstances. Metal splints and heavy plaster may partially obscure the bone, but the general alignment of the fragments can be seen. Radiographs (184) are examples of satisfactory technique in the two positions, to show a fracture of the humerus—After reduction film with the arm abducted and in a heavy plaster splint.

It is difficult to see the fracture of the lesser tuberosity in (a) the antero-posterior, is shown in profile in the lateral position (b) but best seen in the infero-superior position (c) with the tube directed through the axilla (181) page 48.

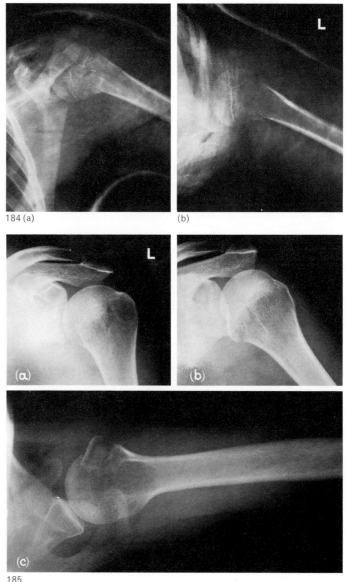

184 (a) (b)

185

Lateral—Infero-superior

(4) As an alternative the patient may be examined in the erect position.

Two projections in the axial lateral position show the difference in appearance of the head of the abducted humerus with the arm extended (186a) palm upward, away from the tube, and (186b) palm downward facing the tube.

Note—the change in position of the lesser and greater tuberosities. Reference should be made to (162, 163) page 43.

PALM UP

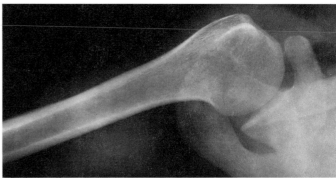

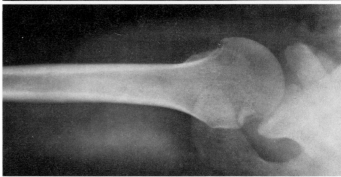

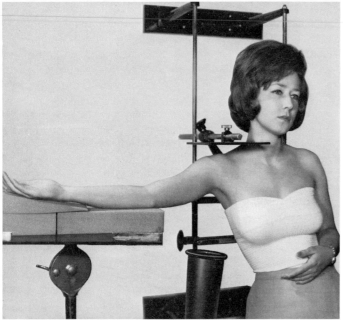

186a

PALM DOWN
187a(top)   187b(above)

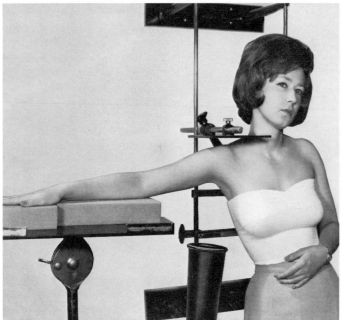

186b

(5) (a) The patient may stand, or sit on the end of the couch. The tube, with a small extension cone attached, is lowered and directed upward to bring the cone aperture between the arm and trunk. The cassette rests above the shoulder on a long-handled support which may be clamped to the vertical stand (188, 189).

■ Centre through the axilla toward the acromion

When an injury is being treated with a large pad in the axilla and the arm strapped to the trunk, the patient should be seated on the end of the table with the injured arm supported by the sound limb. The cassette is placed above the shoulder joint and held in position on the long-handled support. The tube is projected upwards (189).

■ Centre through the axilla posteriorly, from below elbow level with the normal ray almost parallel with the trunk, again using a small extension cone (189)

Bicipital Groove

2

On occasion it is necessary to examine the bicipital groove to exclude soft tissue opacities in the end-on profile projection of the bicipital groove. The patient may stand or sit sideways to the tube with the trunk rotated towards the tube and bent forward, each by approximately 10°, and with the hand facing the trunk.

■ Centre with the vertical beam almost parallel, but with possible angulation not greater than 15° to the shaft of the humerus, and directed towards the depression between the tuberosities in line with the end of the acromion (190, 191)

Note—Figure (191) shows a normal bicipital groove.

				LAT Infero-Superior		
kVp	mAS		Film	Screens	
Inf/Sup	Inf/Sup	FFD	ILFORD	ILFORD	Grid
70	30	100 cm (40″)	RAPID R	SUPER HD	—

			Bicipital Groove		
kVp	mAS	FFD	Film ILFORD	Screens ILFORD	Grid
65	15	100 cm (40″)	RAPID R	SUPER HD	

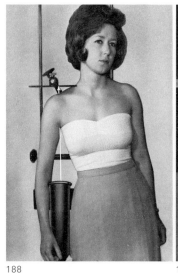
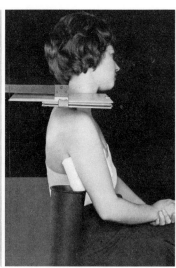

188　　　　　　　189

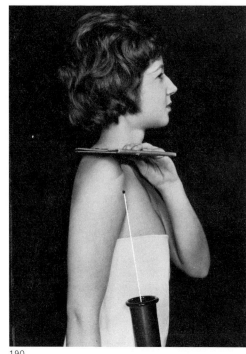

190

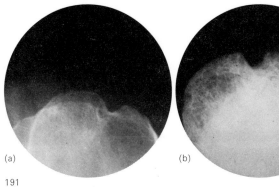
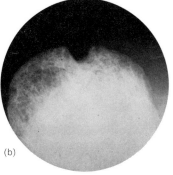

(a)　　　　　　　(b)

191

Supero-inferior

(6) When the arm is not in a splint or plaster a curved cassette may be used.

Seated at the couch and leaning forward with the arm over the cassette, which fits snugly into the axilla, the patient assumes a comfortable position for the axial projection of the shoulder joint and upper humerus.

■ Centre from above to the acromion (192, 193)

Lateral—Supero-inferior

(7) When only limited abduction is possible the patient is seated and leans approximately 10° towards the couch; the cassette is placed between the trunk and elbow and rests on the couch top (194). A modified lateral projection is obtained but with magnification.

■ Centre over the head of the humerus. Some tube angulation may be necessary to coincide with the 10° angle of the median plane of the trunk. Use a small extension cone (194, 195)

Note—With the increased object-film distance producing enlargement a fine-focus tube should be used.

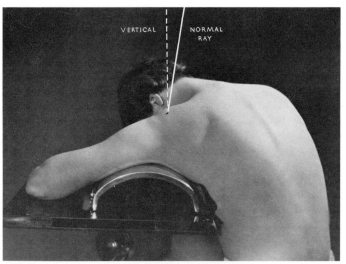

192

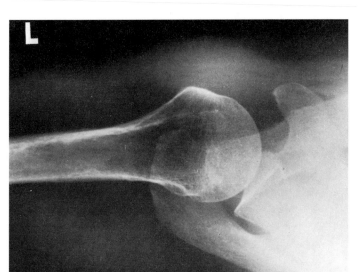

193

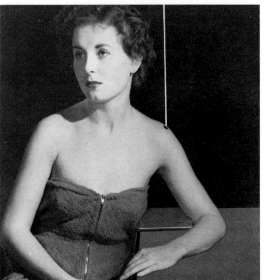

194

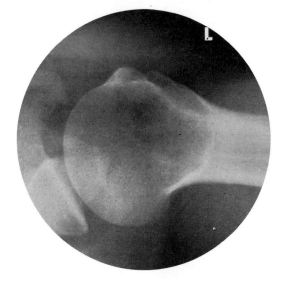

195

Modifications in Technique
Fracture Radiographs

Two right-angled projections of a fracture of the humerus are shown in (196,197) where the method of splinting complicates positioning of the limb for lateral and antero-posterior projections.

Multiple fractures of the humerus are visible in radiographs taken before (198) and after splinting (199).

The radiograph of a baby (200) shows birth injuries to the clavicle and humerus. The limb is supported in a plaster splint. An exposure time of 0·05 second is the maximum which should be used in a young child where there is difficulty in controlling its movements.

With fractures of the humerus modifications of the basic positions (164,167) will frequently be needed. A technique suitable for an individual patient may produce diagnostic radiographs although they may be of poor image quality.

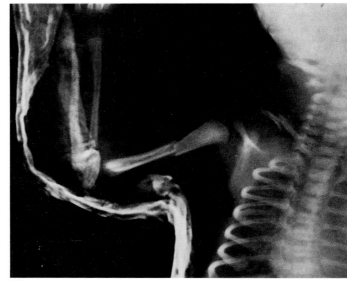

200

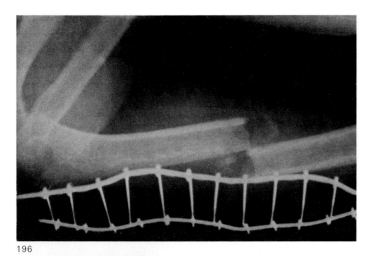

196

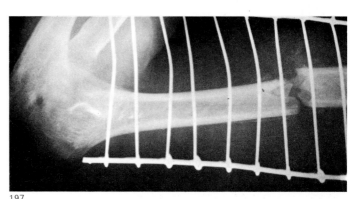

197

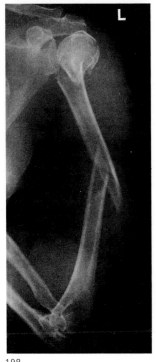

198

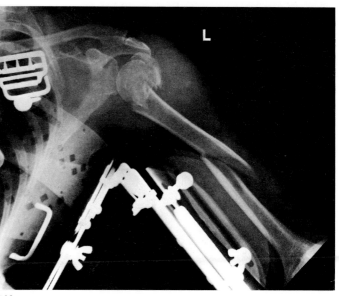

199

Shoulder

Antero-posterior—Supine (basic)

The patient is supine, faces the tube, with the opposite shoulder raised and the head turned toward the affected side to bring the shoulder close to the film. When possible the arm is supinated and slightly abducted.

The patient must be firmly supported behind the shoulders when lowered onto the couch to avoid strain or jarring of the injured limb.

■ Centred over the coracoid process (a bony prominence below the outer third of the clavicle) (201, 202)

Lateral—Supine (basic)

For a modified lateral projection with the patient in the supine position the injured side is raised a little away from the couch with the limb adequately supported on sandbags. The cassette and stationary grid are placed slightly obliquely against the lateral aspect of the shoulder, conforming to the obliquity of the trunk. The X-ray tube is lowered for horizontal projections.

■ Centre with the X-ray beam perpendicular to the obliquely placed film and thus passing through the adjacent chest wall (203, 204)

Alternatively, the patient may be returned to the horizontal position and the sound arm placed over the head for direct centring through the axilla, as for the erect position (176).

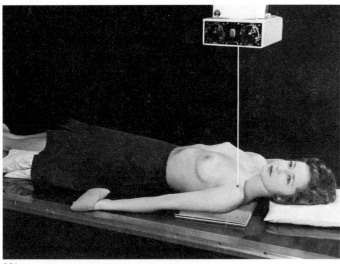

201

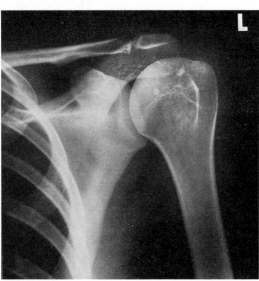

202

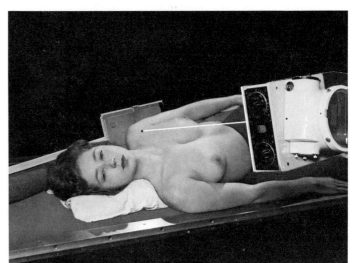

203

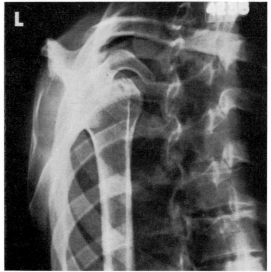

204

Antero-posterior—Erect (basic)

The patient is seated against the cassette and grid and turns slightly toward the injured side for good contact. To aid immobilization, the arm is held on the lap or on an adjacent support (205).

Note—Normal radiographs taken in the horizontal position are shown on page 54 (202, 204). Radiographs taken at right angles to each other (178a, b) show a fracture of the upper end of the humerus.

2

Shoulder							
kVp		mAS			Film	Screens	
AP	Lat	AP	Lat	FFD	ILFORD	ILFORD	Grid
60	65	40	50	100 cm (40″)	RAPID R	SUPER HD	—

Lateral-oblique—Erect (basic)

The seated patient is turned to bring the outer side of the injured shoulder against the cassette and grid. The injured arm is supported. Slight backward rotation of the sound side avoids superimposition of both shoulders on the film (206). The humerus is seen through the rib cage (178).

■ Centre to just below the coracoid process.

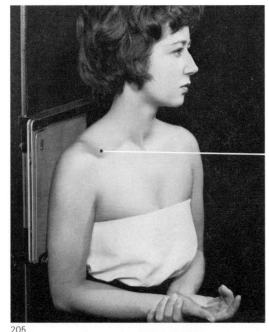

205

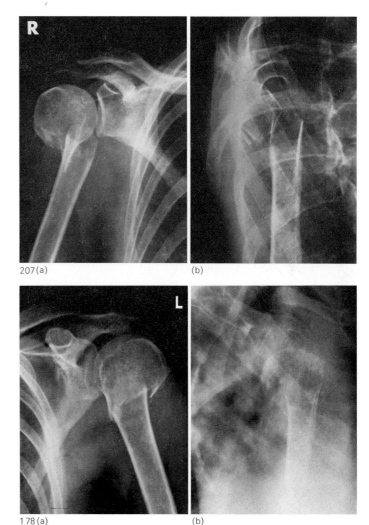

207 (a) (b)

178 (a) (b)

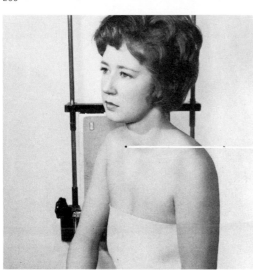

206

Complementary Projections

A combination of the four positions can be used to give a survey
of the various aspects of the head of the humerus (pathology)
and the relationship to the glenoid cavity.
Supine or erect positioning is equally suitable.

(208) The arm is slightly abducted and supinated—palm up.
(211) The arm is slightly abducted and pronated—palm down.
(214) With some abduction the elbow is flexed with external
rotation of the humerus. The hand is palm up on the table top at
the level of the head.
(217) With some abduction and the elbow flexed with internal
rotation of the humerus. The hand is palm down on the table
top lying under the loin.

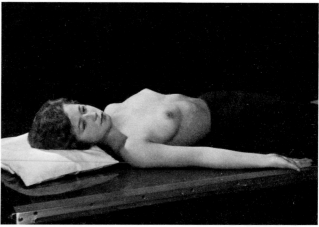

208

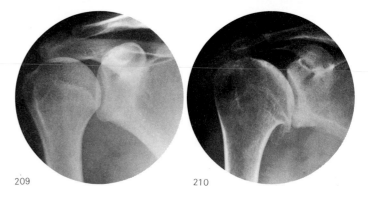

209   210

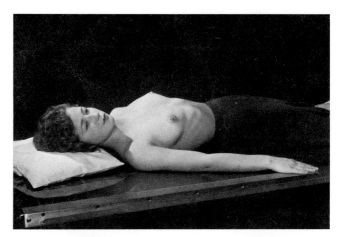

211

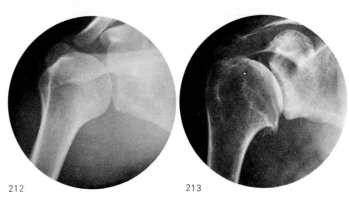

212   213

Two sets of four radiographs; one set of a normal subject (209, 212, 215, 218) and the other with pathology (210, 213, 216, 219) are shown.

These radiographs have been taken with a small localizing cone.

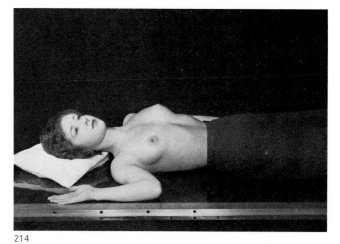

214

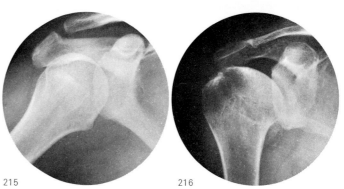

215   216

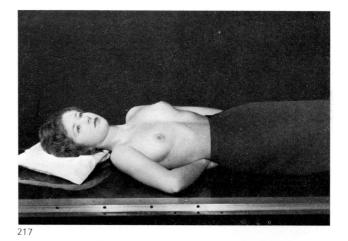

217

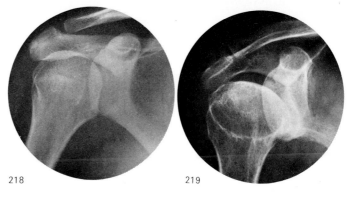

218   219

Dislocation

The deformity of the head of the humerus caused by recurrent dislocation of the shoulder produces a notch at the lateral margin of the head of the humerus and flattening of the upper end of the shaft of the humerus (220a, b, c). This series of radiographs show the antero-posterior (a) and two axial projections taken with the palm facing forward (b) and with the palm facing downward (c).

A further series (221) shows the less common posterior dislocation and once more shows the importance of the axial projection, (6); before (a, b) and after reduction (c).

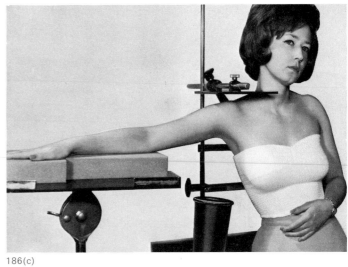

186(c)

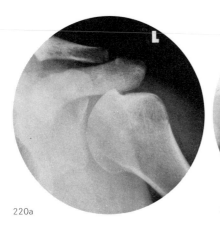

220a

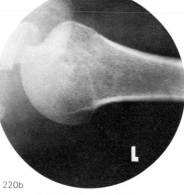

220b
PALM FORWARD

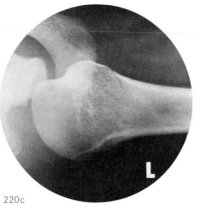

220c
PALM DOWNWARD

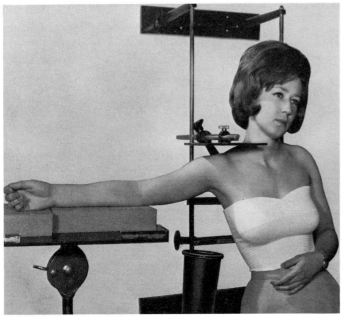

186(b)

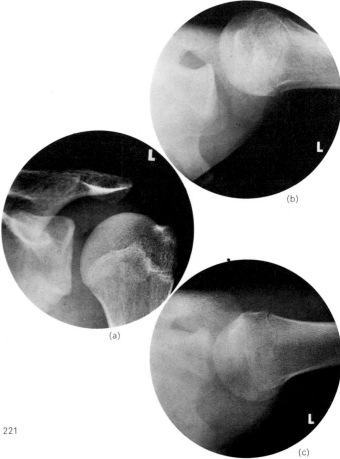

(b)

(a)

(c)

221

Recurrent Dislocation

To determine the possibility of and reason for recurrent dislocation, one or other of the two following views should be taken to complement the basic shoulder joint views.

With the patient supine the arm is raised with the palm of the hand resting on top of the head; the elbow faces forwards.
■ Centre to the coracoid process with the tube angled 10° cephalad (222, 223)

In recurrent dislocation it may be necessary to show the humeral defect in profile (224). Position the patient as for the antero-posterior position of the shoulder joint (201). Direct the tube caudally at an angle of 45° with the central ray going through the coracoid process to show the compression indentation in profile which is produced by the sharp lower glenoid rim, and sometimes referred to as a "hatchet-shaped" defect.

Two radiographs show the difference between the projections with the tube straight (225a) and with the tube angled (225b)

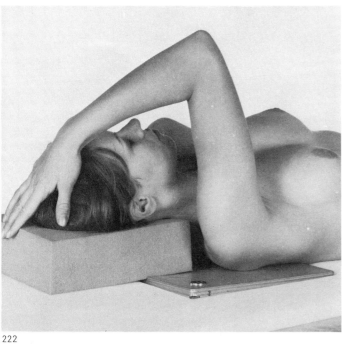

222

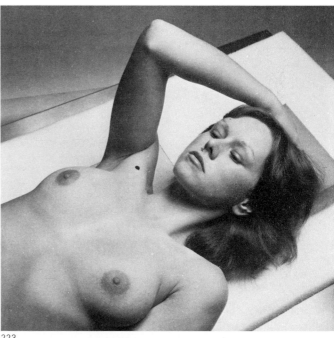

223

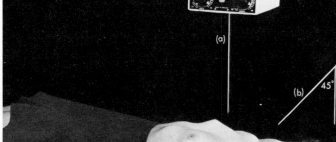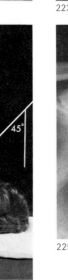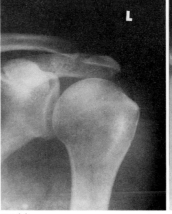

224

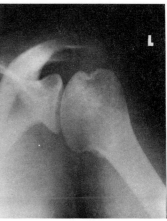

225 (a)   (b)

Calcifications of Tendons

If the shoulder is examined for tendon calcification or for an avulsion fracture of the humerus, each area should be shown in profile. Opacities in the tendons will then not be obscured by overlying bone and will be shown clearly. The exposure factors must be adjusted from those given on page 55 to demonstrate the soft tissues. The diagram (226) is of the shoulder as viewed from the posterior aspect and shows the insertions of the tendons of the supra-spinatus, infraspinatus and teres minor muscles. To appreciate the direction of the X-ray beam in order to take these profile radiographs refer to the axial projection shown in (162).

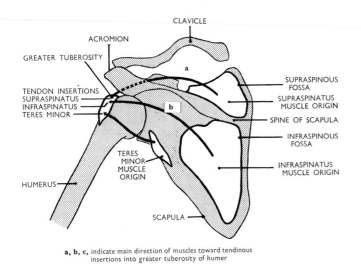

a, b, c, indicate main direction of muscles toward tendinous insertions into greater tuberosity of humer

226

The subscapularis muscle and tendon and the subacromial bursa anterior to the scapula have not been included in the diagram (226).

The first (survey) film taken is a routine antero-posterior view of the shoulder with the arm in supination (227a). To see calfciation which in this view may overlie bone, an increase of 10 kilovolts is required with the milliampere seconds halved. This is needed for two reasons, a) the higher kilovoltage gives sufficient penetration of the humeral head to show underlying calcification, b) there is more uniform contrast between the bone and soft tissue structures.

To show calcification away from bony structure one or more of the following complementary views will be needed.
(227b) as above with 25° caudal angulation of the tube.
(229) antero-posterior with arm in extreme medial rotation.
(231) axial projections with the arm in supination.
(233) the elbow is flexed with some abduction and external rotation of the arm to bring the back of the hand resting on the couch at the level of the head.
The supraspinatus: The tendon crosses the upper part of the shoulder joint to be inserted into the highest part of the three impressions on the greater tuberosity of the humerus, and may

be shown in radiographs taken in the antero-posterior position of the humerus (227a).
Teres Minor. The upper fibres of muscle terminate in a tendon which is inserted on the greater tuberosity of the humerus and the lower fibres of the muscle are inserted immediately below the impression. The termination of the muscle is, therefore, shown along the margin of the bone in antero-posterior radiographs taken in full medial rotation (229).
The subscapularis tendon is inserted into the lesser tuberosity of the humerus and into the front of the capsular ligament of the shoulder joint. It is shown in lateral radiographs of the humeral head when the arm is abducted and supinated; the tube being directed toward the axilla (231).
The Infraspinatus tendon glides over the lateral bone of the spine of the scapula and passes across the posterior part of the capsule of the shoulder joint to be inserted into the middle impression on the greater tuberosity of the humerus. With the patient in the antero-posterior position (227a), it may be better shown if the tube is angled approximately 25° caudally (228b). The tendon is also shown with the humerus in the lateral position (233).

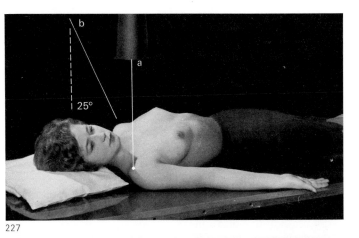

227

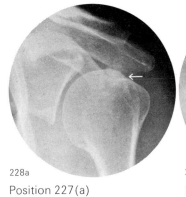

228a
Position 227(a)

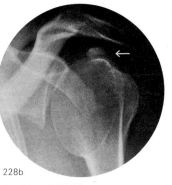

228b
Position 227(b)

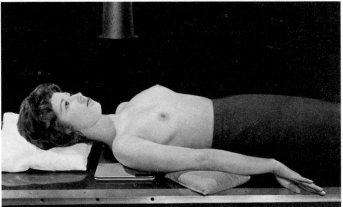

229

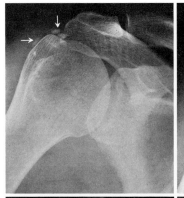

230a
230b

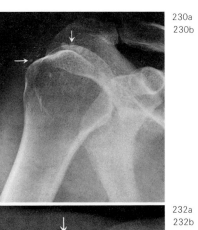

232a
232b

Position 227a (top)
Position 227(a) (above)

Position 229 (top)
Position 231 (above)

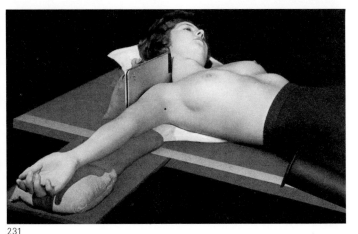

231

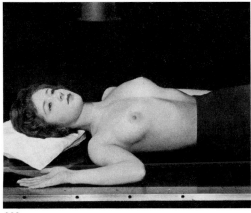

233

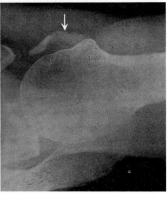

234a
Position 227a

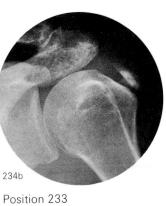

234b
Position 233

Acromio-Clavicular Joint

Subluxation

The same positioning may be used as for the shoulder joint, (page 54) but to show subluxation at the acromio-clavicular joint (236b) the patient is examined in the erect or sitting position (235a) and shows the gravity effect of the unsupported humerus when a sandbag is held in each hand. Comparative radiographs are taken of right and left sides separately (235b).

■ Centre above the head of the humerus radiographing each side in turn (235a, 235b)

A reduction of 5 kilovolts should be made on the figures shown in the exposure table given on page 55.

Two additional radiographs (236) as taken in (235a) but with separate exposures of right and left joints, show the effect of gravity on (a) the normal and (b) the abnormal condition of the joints in a patient with subluxation at the acromio-clavicular joint.

The acromio-clavicular joint may be hidden in the routine antero-posterior radiograph of the shoulder joint (237a). To then show the joint adequately the tube is directed in line with the joint surfaces (237b). Note there will be a slight variation in the direction of the tube angle from subject to subject.

When a patient is round-shouldered the postero-anterior view is more suitable as the joint space is in better alignment with the X-ray beam in this position.

■ Centre in the midline at the level of the humeral head to show both joints (238)

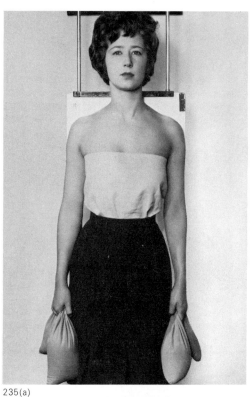

235(a)

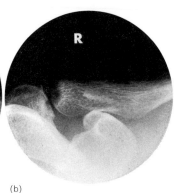

a

b

236

235(b)

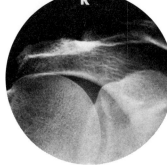

237(a)   (b)

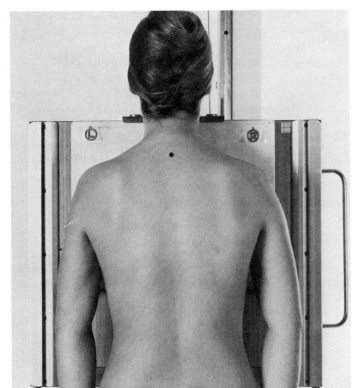

238

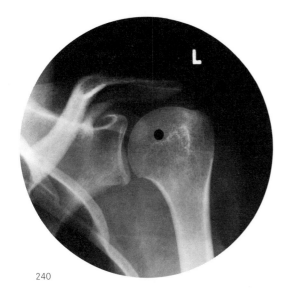

240

Antero-posterior

Normally the broad plane of the scapula lies obliquely to the posterior and lateral aspects of the trunk. Therefore, in order to obtain true antero-posterior projections of the gleno-humeral joint, the median plane of the trunk is ignored and the subject adjusted so that the scapula is parallel to the film.

The patient is supine on the X-ray table and then rotated to bring the trunk to an angle of 25° to the film by raising and supporting the unaffected side on sandbags, the arm is held in partial abduction and the elbow flexed (239). In this position the glenoid cavity is at right angles to the film and a clear projection of the joint space is shown on the radiograph. Erect and horizontal positions are equally satisfactory.

■ Centre over the head of the humerus (239, 240, 241)

Note—(241) shows an abnormal shoulder joint.

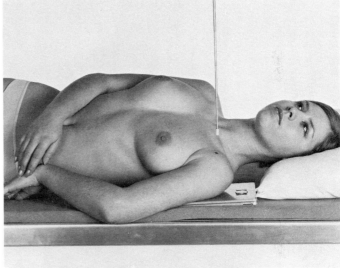

239

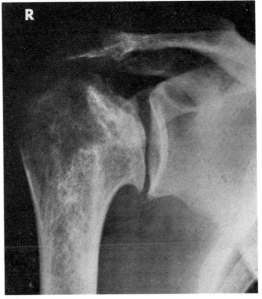

241

Arthrography

As for the elbow joint (page 30) the opaque medium is a 35% water soluble organic iodine compound. (For proprietary names refer to Supplement 1.) Six millilitres of opaque medium are mixed with one millilitre of novocain for injection into the joint space from a point anterior to the acromio-clavicular joint and directed toward the head of the humerus. The arm is abducted and externally rotated. Radiographs, possibly stereographs, are taken from several aspects of the joint—anterior, posterior, oblique and infero-superior.

Scapula

Note—The scapula varies markedly in position with regard to the thorax as the arm moves through rotation, abduction and adduction, flexion and extension. When the shoulders are pressed back with the arms adducted the medial borders are parallel and near to the vertebral column. When the arms are brought forward and upward the scapulae glide over the ribs in the same direction so that the medial borders are oblique to the vertebral column. In radiography of the scapula only a selected range of scapular movements is used, with careful centring of the X-ray tube making use of the oblique rays and carefully positioning the trunk.

Antero-posterior (basic)
The patient is placed in the supine position (242), with the arm supinated and slightly abducted; the opposite shoulder is raised on a small sandbag.

Too great a rotation of the body, as in (239), allows the mediastinum to overshadow the medial margin of the scapula. A 20° angle is therefore recommended.
■ Centre over the head of the humerus (242, 253, 243)

Note—Both the shoulder region and most of the body of the scapula are shown in this projection. The medial border is overshadowed by the ribs, but is visible owing to its close contact with the cassette (244). The cross-sectional diagram shows the method of projecting the scapula almost clear of the rib shadows (243).

Breathing Technique—Antero-posterior
To blur out the superimposing rib shadows a comparatively long exposure is made during quiet respiration. With the patient supine to immobilize the scapula, instructions are given to breath gently and smoothly during an exposure of approximately 5 seconds at the appropriate milliamperage. This shows greater detail in the scapula than with a short exposure technique.

The lateral radiograph (245b) confirms the presence of pathology.

242

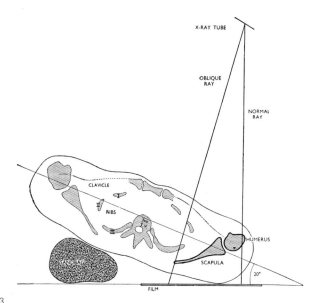

243

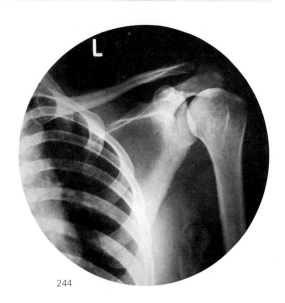

244

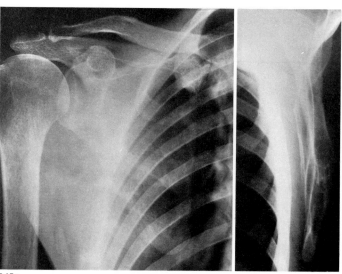

245a   245b

Lateral (basic)

The patient faces the film, with the opposite shoulder raised until the broad plane of the scapula is at an angle of from 75° to 80° to the film. The head naturally rotates away from the affected side for comfort. The affected arm is slightly abducted and the elbow flexed in order to separate the humeral shaft from the blade of the scapula.

■ Centre over the fourth to fifth thoracic vertebra, so that the oblique ray gives a true lateral projection of the scapula (246, 247, 248, 249, 250)

With a localizing cone the tube is angled approximately 15° away from the mid line toward the medial border of the scapula, for the central ray to pass through the scapula from the medial to the lateral border.

The cross-sectional diagram (246) shows the method of projection in the horizontal position used in (247, 248).

The lateral projection (249) shows the head and upper third of the shaft of the humerus, with the scapula edge on, from medial to lateral border, and with the coracoid process medial and the acromion lateral, to the superior angle. In (250) there is a vertical fracture of the body.

Note—The horizontal position appears to be drastic for an injured patient, but there is no difficulty once the patient has been carefully lowered on to the couch. The erect posture is equally satisfactory, and alternative positions are shown in (251) and (252).

2

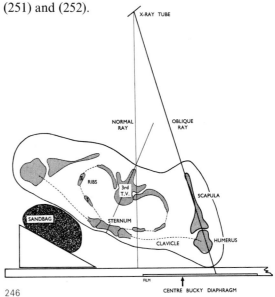

246

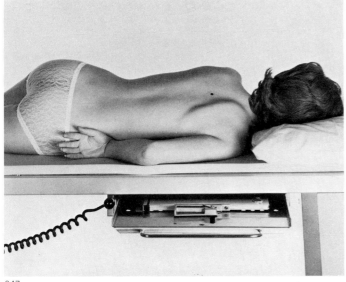

247

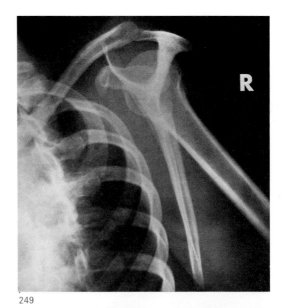

249

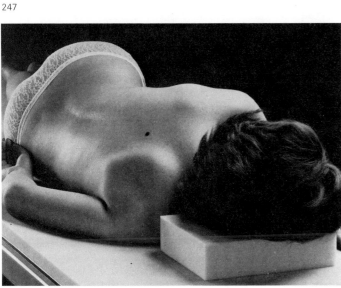

248

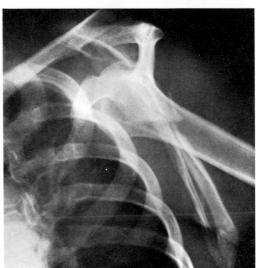

250

65

Scapula—Lateral Erect

With the patient erect or sitting in the lateral position and the injured side toward the film, the trunk is rotated forward by approximately 20° to allow separation of the two sides, and to bring the lateral aspect of the scapula in profile (251). The arm on the injured side can either, (a) be moved forward across the trunk or (b) be moved away from the trunk with slight abduction and flexion of the elbow (252); to separate the humeral shaft from the blade of the scapula, depending on which is more comfortable for the patient.

■ Centre over the fourth thoracic vertebra, so that the oblique rays give a true lateral projection of the scapula (253) which shows a fracture of the lower part of the scapula.

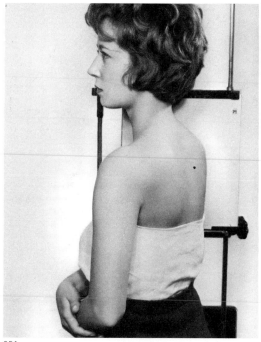

251

Scapula

kVp		mAS			Film	Screens	
AP	Lat	AP	Lat	FFD	ILFORD	ILFORD	Grid
70	80	100	120	100 cm (40″)	RAPID R	SUPER HD	Grid

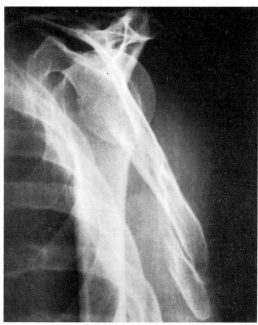

253

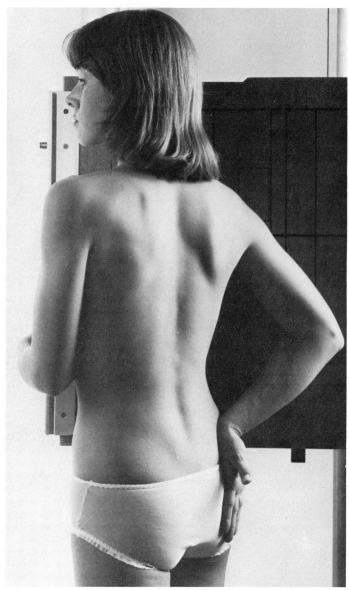

252

Coracoid Process
The coracoid process is visible when the arm is abducted to above the level of the shoulder (254), and also in the lateral projection of the scapula (252).

Antero-posterior
In the antero-posterior position the arm is raised beside the head and the patient is turned slightly forward away from the cassette to separate the lateral border of the scapula from the rib cage.

■ Centre medial to the head of the humerus for the coracoid process, and over the head of the humerus for the scapula (254, 255, 256)

This position (257) also gives a clear view of the acromio-clavicular and shoulder joints, and of the lateral border and inferior angle of the scapula.

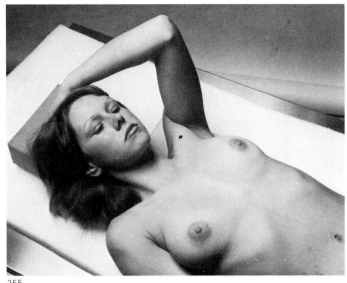

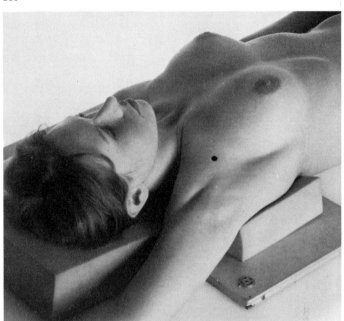

255

256

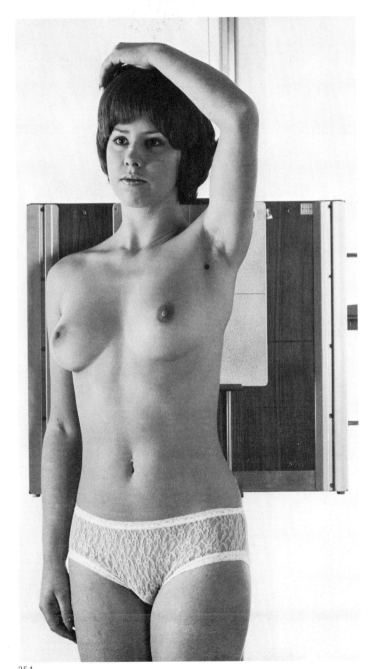

254

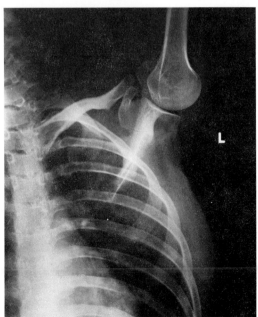

257

Acromion

The acromion is shown in two positions; either a horizontal or vertical technique may be used.

Antero-posterior

In the erect or sitting position the patient faces the tube and is rotated a little toward the affected side to bring the scapula and the acromion nearer to the film (258). The arm is slightly abducted and the forearm supinated to limit overshadowing of the humerus on the acromion.

■ Centre over the coracoid process (258, 261a)

Lateral

With the injured side towards the film and the arm raised and folded over the head, the patient is rotated obliquely forward from the true lateral position by approximately 30° to show the scapula in profile.

■ Centre to the medial border at the level of the spine of the scapula (259, 260)

(261a, 261b) show a fracture at the base of the acromion

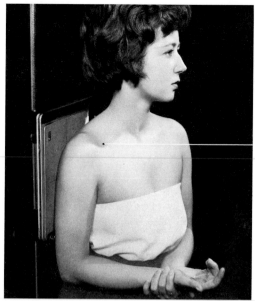

258

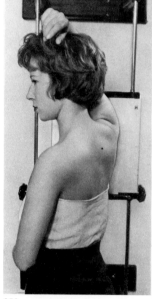

259

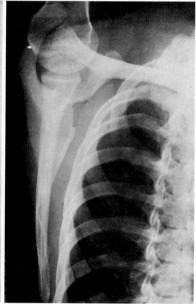

260

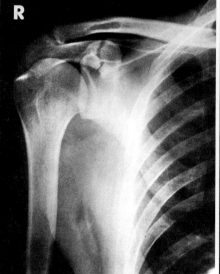

261a

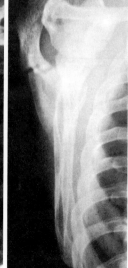

261b

Clavicle

Antero-posterior (basic)

The antero-posterior position is generally used to provide a satisfactory projection of both the clavicle and the shoulder joint. It is easier for the injured subject than the postero-anterior position.

The patient is supine with a small sandbag under the sound shoulder and the head turned toward the injured shoulder, the arm being in a relaxed position beside the trunk (262).

■ Centre to the middle of the clavicle (262, 263).

Postero-anterior (basic)

The patient is placed facing the film, with the head turned away from the affected side to allow the clavicle to make good contact with the cassette. The arm is rotated medially until the palm of the hand faces upward, and the opposite shoulder is raised and supported on a small sandbag (264).

■ Centre to the superior angle of the scapula (264, 265).

Note—In this position the clavicle is oblique to the long axis of the body; the acromio-clavicular joint being more cranial than the sterno-clavicular which lies at the level of the fourth thoracic vertebra. Particular care must be taken to include the medial end of the clavicle on the film.

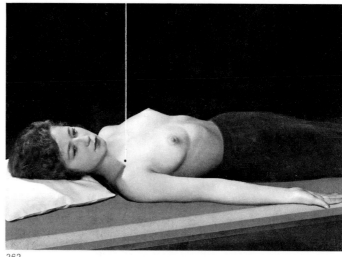

262

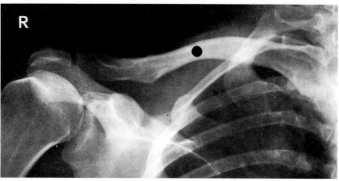

263

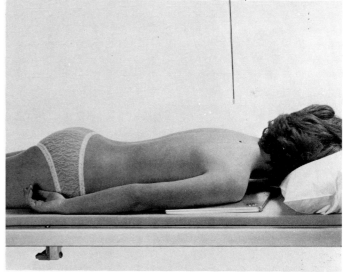

264

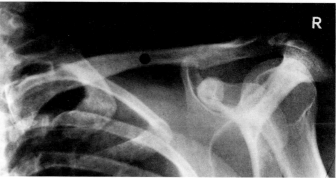

265

Erect

The postero-anterior projection is more easily done with the patient in the seated or standing position. However, on occasion, immobilization is less satisfactory than in the relaxed horizontal position. A short exposure time may be necessary to avoid movement.

The patient faces the tube for the antero-posterior position (266) and has his back to the tube for the postero-anterior position (267).

Clavicle Erect

kVp		mAS			Film	Screens	
AP	Inf. Sup.	AP	Inf. Sup.	FFD	ILFORD	ILFORD	Grid
55	60	40	40	100 cm (40″)	RAPID R	SUPER HD	—

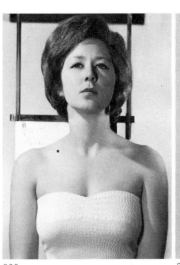
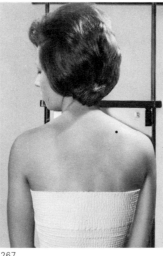

266

267

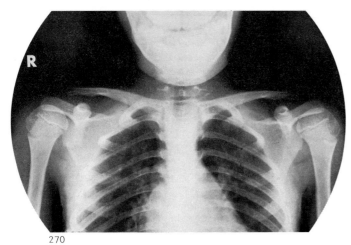

270

Fracture Radiographs

An injury before and after reduction is shown in (268), (269). As will be seen (268) was taken in the postero-anterior position and (269) in the antero-posterior position.

Simultaneous exposure of both clavicles for comparison is shown in radiograph (271). In this instance a fracture of the right clavicle is demonstrated.

Children

For the examination of the shoulder girdle in young children, it may be necessary to include both sides on the one film for comparison, with the patient in the supine position as for the shoulder joints (270) and the clavicles (271).

After making adjustments for a short exposure time, a cassette bearing an identification marker is placed on the couch and the tube centred above. For comfort cover the cold cassette with a thin cushion of plastic sponge. Finally, the child is placed in position so that the mid-line of the thorax at shoulder level is approximately central to the tube and film (270, 271) and the exposure is made immediately. See also birth injuries, page 53.

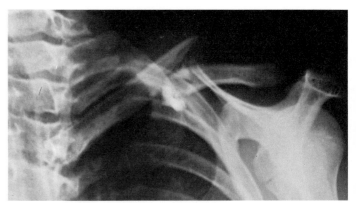

268   POSTERO-ANTERIOR

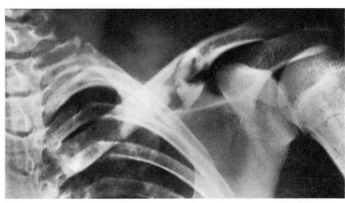

269   ANTERO-POSTERIOR

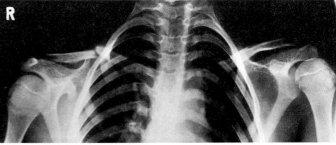

271

Infero-superior—Supine
The patient lies supine on the couch; the shoulder of the affected side is raised on a non-opaque pad and depressed, with the arm adducted and the hand facing the trunk. The head is rotated well over to the opposite side, with the chin in contact with the shoulder.

■ Centre 2·5 cm (one inch) from the sternal end of the clavicle, with the tube angled 35° to the horizontal and 15° outward toward the shoulder (272, 273)

Clavicle Supine							
kVp		mAS			Film	Screens	
AP	Inf. Sup.	AP	Inf. Sup.	FFD	ILFORD	ILFORD	Grid
55	60	40	40	100 cm (40")	RAPID R	SUPER HD	—

Infero-superior—Erect
The infero-superior projection is only used when the patient can stand.

The cassette holder is attached to the vertical support and the tube lowered for upward projection. The patient faces the tube with the shoulders drooping forward and the neck bent away from the affected side.

The cassette-holder is brought forward above the shoulder, keeping well into the neck, and tilted to be parallel to the superior aspect of the clavicle. Using a localizing cone, the tube is angled to approximately right angles to the cassette.

■ Centre to the inner one-third of the inferior surface of the clavicle with the tube direction at an angle of 90° to the film and directed 15° outward toward the shoulder to project the sternal articulation away from the vertebral column (274, 275a,b).

Fracture Radiographs
(275a,b) demonstrates the degree of displacement of the fracture fragments from the two aspects.

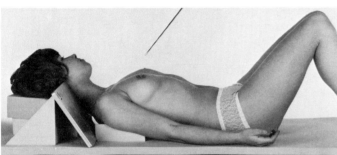

272

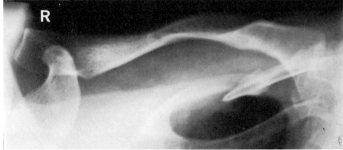

273

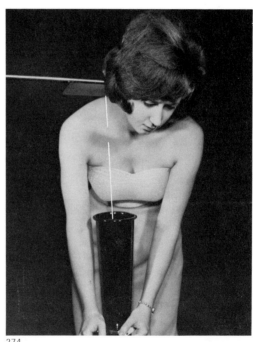

274

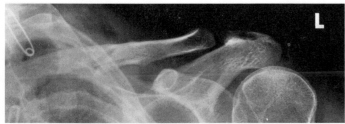

275 (a)

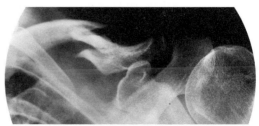

275 (b)

Sterno-clavicular joint

In the true antero-posterior or postero-anterior projection, the sterno-clavicular joints will be hidden by the vertebral column. Oblique projections are therefore required to show the sterno-clavicular joints. A short distance technique to diffuse the shadows of the vertebral column has also been used.

Postero-anterior
Trunk rotated, Tube straight
With the patient facing the bucky, the tunk is rotated to an angle of 45°, so that the vertebral column and the sternum are separated on the film. This allows the clavicle and the sterno-clavicular joint of the one side to be near the film, with the vertebral column over-shadowing part of the shaft of the same clavicle. Erect and horizontal positions are shown.

■ Centre at the level of the fourth thoracic vertebra 10 cm (4 ins) from the mid line and to the side turned away from the film (276, 277, 278, 279, 280, 281, 282)

			S-C Joint		
kVp	mAS	FFD	Film ILFORD	Screens ILFORD	Grid
60	60	100 cm (40")	RAPID R	Standard	Grid

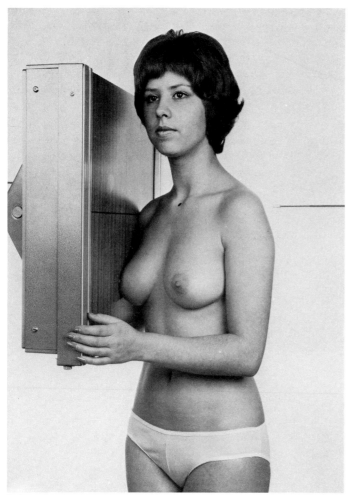

276

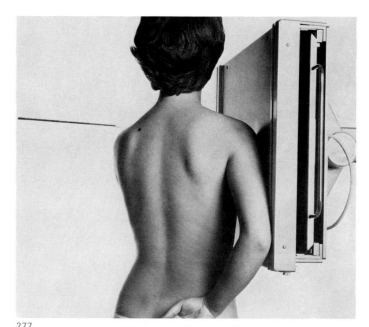

277

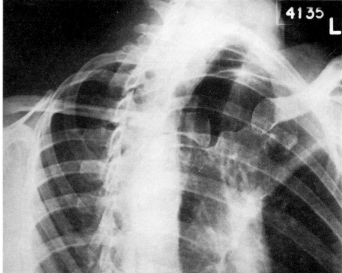

278

The right and left sides are exposed separately. Although both sides are included in each projection the joint nearer the vertebral column and the film is satisfactorily shown whereas the further joint is foreshortened and distorted. An open field has been used in taking radiograph (278) to enable the relationship between the various structures in the oblique aspect to be appreciated, but a small localizing cone improves definition and is used for (281). The right or left marker indicates the joint shown to advantage.

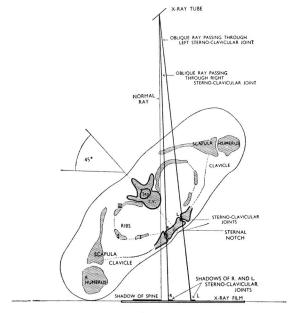

282

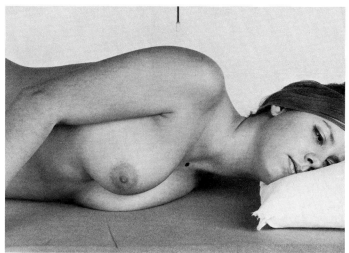

279

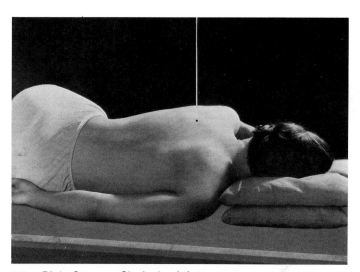

280   Right Sterno—Clavicular Joint

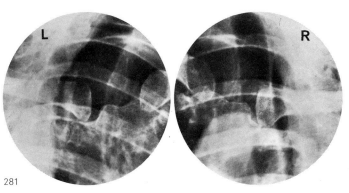

281

Right and left joints for comparison

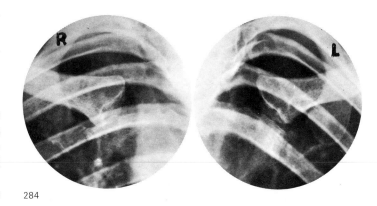

284

Postero-anterior
Trunk straight, Tube angled

The antero-posterior thickness of the patient is measured at the level of the sternal angle. The focus film distance is three times this measurement; this measurement also indicates the necessary tube displacement from each side of the vertebral column in turn before angling the tube toward the vertebrae.

The patient faces the film with the chin over the edge of the cassette, to minimize the subject-film distance.

■ Centre the tube over the right or left shoulder, as required, at the level of the third thoracic vertebra, allowing the necessary measured displacement, and from this off-centre position, angle the tube 18° toward the vertebrae (283, 284, 285)

The cross-sectional diagram (285) shows the method of projection and the significance of the calculated tube displacement and focus-film distance according to the thickness of the patient.

By this method only one sterno-clavicular joint is shown on each exposure, which is clearly defined and free from distortion. This technique may be applied equally well with the patient in the erect position.

On employing a compressor band for skeletal immobilization, prolonged exposure (10 seconds at the appropriate milliamperage) may be made during quiet respiration to diffuse the shadows of lung detail which would otherwise obscure the bones.

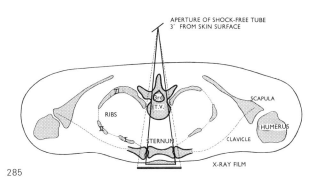

285

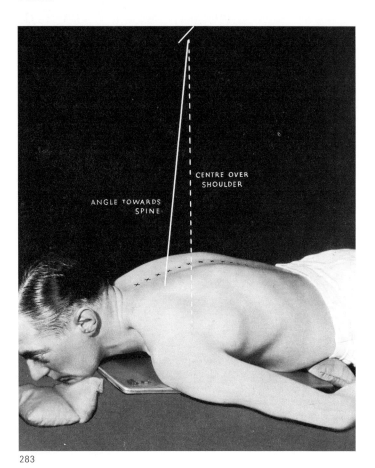

283

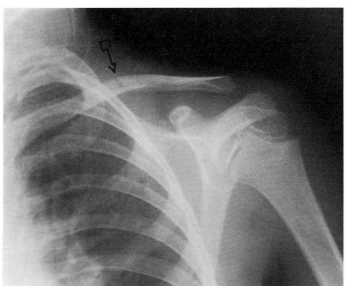

286

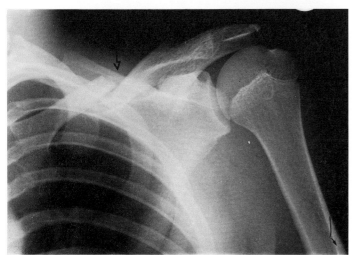

287

288

Lateral

The patient is placed in the true lateral position, with shoulders and arms well back. The exposure is made on inspiration.

■ Centre through the sterno-clavicular joints (288,289)

Radiographs (286, 287, 288) show 3 separate cases of clavicular fractures of varying severity. In (286) there is a minimal greenstick fracture, in (287) a slight crack fracture and in (288) a fracture with downward displacement of the outer half of the clavicle.

S-C JT Lateral

kVp	mAS	FFD	Film ILFORD	Screens ILFORD	Grid
80	80	150 cm (5')	RAPID R	Standard	Grid

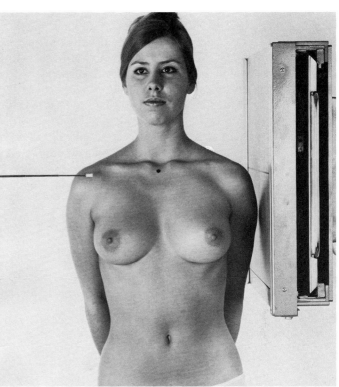

289

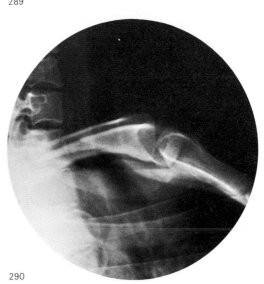

290

Group Investigations

Serial examinations may be required for industrial diseases, e.g. Caissons disease, referred to as the 'bends' (290) or chronic illness, e.g. marble bone disease (293). Radiograph (291) shows localised disuse osteoporosis associated with calcific tendinitis of the tendo Achilles (arrow).

A standard technique will be needed if there is to be accurate comparison of sequential radiographs and can be obtained by carefully instructing radiographers in the required technique. The same radiographer should preferably be used for each examination.

A check on standard contrast and density may be achieved by using a static type of densitometer, such as an aluminium graded step wedge. For thinner regions, a bone density comparator is acceptable. From the comparable recording shown on each radiograph, a standard of contrast and density can be established throughout a long term investigation. To achieve a uniform quality all variables that could materially alter the accepted standard must be avoided. In particular the same personnel and equipment must be available over the period and the same X-ray unit should be used throughout keeping filtration constant with identical exposure factors. The subject area covered should be similar in each examination and the same type of film should be used throughout.

Cassettes and screens should be tested for speed, similarity, and contact discrepancy, and when matched should be used specifically for the serial or group investigation.

Automatic processing has achieved standardization not previously possible,—nevertheless there must be a careful check on the chemicals, especially the rate of replenishment and careful temperature control throughout the project.

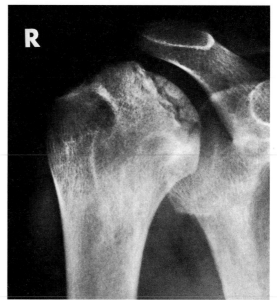

291

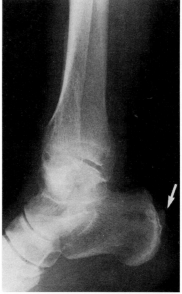

292

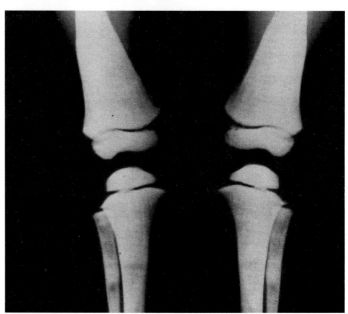

293

3

LOWER LIMB

LOWER LIMB

Anatomical Nomenclature

There has been only one minor change in the names of the bones of the lower limb in the last report (Paris 1955). Namely calcaneous replaces calcaneum.

As there may be some confusion with the tarsal bones, the most commonly used names are given below with the older names in brackets.

Talus (Astragalus)	Calcaneus (Calcaneum) (Os Calcis)	Navicular (Scaphoid)	Cuboid
Cuneiforms—Medial (Internal)		Intermediate (Middle)	Lateral (External)

Radiographic Appearances

Lettered radiographs are provided to assist the student in following the anatomical reference in the text:

Page 79	of the foot dorsi-plantar oblique (295) oblique (296) lateral (297)
Page 99	of the ankle joint antero-posterior (378) lateral (379)
page 107	of the knee joint antero-posterior (411) lateral (412) oblique (413)

General and technical

A unit in which the tube is readily adjusted to any position in relation to the patient is particularly desirable in radiography of the lower limb. With such a unit much unnecessary discomfort may be avoided, both in not having to transfer the patient from the casualty trolley to the X-ray couch, and in not rotating the limb during the examination. With the need for two or more assistants to move a heavy patient, economy in time and labour is also a consideration.

Comfortable relaxation in the various positions is important in order to immobilize the limb adequately. A back-rest should be provided to support the patient in the sitting position for antero-posterior projections and there should also be support for a limb for lateral projections. It is most uncomfortable for a patient to sit without a back support on a hard table-top with legs extended, and it is difficult to keep still in such a position during the X-ray exposure. The recumbent position may be used, but most patients like to see what is happening and if at all nervous they will have more confidence if allowed to remain in a sitting position.

Splints and appliances are never removed without permission from the doctor attending the patient. In these cases, and when plaster has been applied the correct centring point and position for the film may be determined by comparison with the sound limb (294). It is essential to show the relationship between the adjacent joint and the site of fracture, and exclusion of the essential area through faulty centring is inexcusable.

With few exceptions, as indicated, the exposure factors given for each position refer to an adult subject of average physique. For convenience of reference, the exposures for the four general positions of the foot are shown in each table where applicable.

Basic Positions

Again, to avoid confusion from the many alternative techniques included in the text, the basic projections for each region are indicated accordingly as (BASIC).

Varying Tissue Densities

Radiographs for trauma and pathology must show adequate detail of both soft tissue and bone and soft tissue detail is particularly important in bone tumours where the information is essential for diagnosis.

A number of different pathologies change the density of bone and need the exposure factors adjusted accordingly to produce good quality radiographs. A series of radiographs showing some of the conditions is included for guidance on page 80 (298–302).

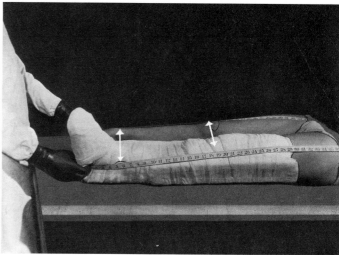

294

Right Foot
Dorsi-plantar
Oblique

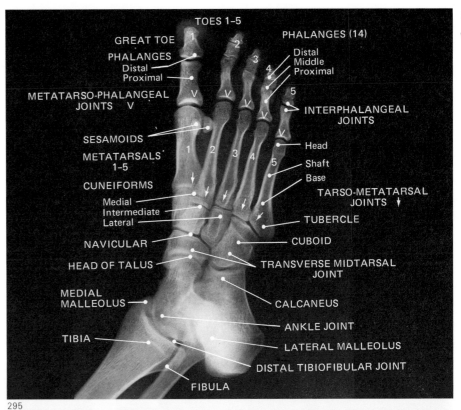

TOES 1-5
GREAT TOE
PHALANGES
Distal
Proximal
1
2
3
4
5
PHALANGES (14)
Distal
Middle
Proximal
METATARSO-PHALANGEAL
JOINTS   V
V
V
INTERPHALANGEAL
JOINTS
SESAMOIDS
METATARSALS
1-5
1 2 3 4
5
V
Head
Shaft
Base
CUNEIFORMS
Medial
Intermediate
Lateral
TARSO-METATARSAL
JOINTS ↓
TUBERCLE
NAVICULAR
CUBOID
HEAD OF TALUS
TRANSVERSE MIDTARSAL
JOINT
MEDIAL
MALLEOLUS
CALCANEUS
ANKLE JOINT
TIBIA
LATERAL MALLEOLUS
DISTAL TIBIOFIBULAR JOINT
FIBULA

295

Right
Foot
Oblique

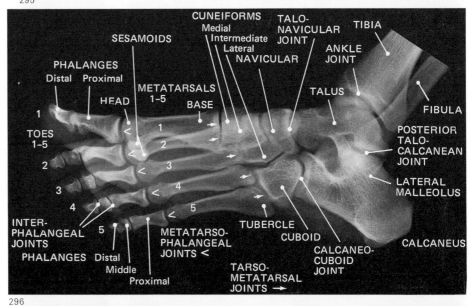

CUNEIFORMS
Medial
Intermediate
Lateral
TALO-
NAVICULAR
JOINT
TIBIA
SESAMOIDS
NAVICULAR
ANKLE
JOINT
PHALANGES
Distal   Proximal
METATARSALS
1-5
BASE
TALUS
FIBULA
HEAD
1
TOES
1-5
2
3
4
1
2
3
4
5
POSTERIOR
TALO-
CALCANEAN
JOINT
LATERAL
MALLEOLUS
INTER-
PHALANGEAL
JOINTS
5
TUBERCLE
CUBOID
CALCANEO-
CUBOID
JOINT
CALCANEUS
PHALANGES   Distal
Middle
Proximal
METATARSO-
PHALANGEAL
JOINTS <
TARSO-
METATARSAL
JOINTS →

296

Right
Foot
Lateral

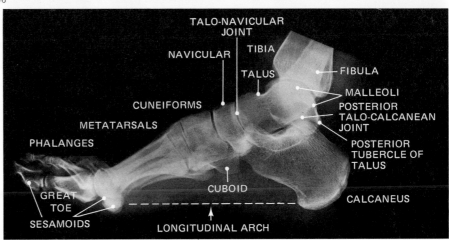

TALO-NAVICULAR
JOINT
NAVICULAR
TIBIA
TALUS
FIBULA
MALLEOLI
POSTERIOR
TALO-CALCANEAN
JOINT
CUNEIFORMS
METATARSALS
POSTERIOR
TUBERCLE OF
TALUS
PHALANGES
CUBOID
CALCANEUS
GREAT
TOE
SESAMOIDS
LONGITUDINAL ARCH

297

Where decalcification of a limb is present as in a radiograph of the ankle joint (298) the exposure must be modified. A deficiency of bone calcium greatly diminishes bone density leaving only thin cortices to be shown radiographically. A normal exposure would provide a useless over-exposed film and in this instance half only of the normal milliampere-seconds was necessary.

On the other hand, in the pathological condition as shown in (300) there is added density often unsuspected in advance. The aim in this subject is not necessarily to penetrate the bone, as the added density is in itself under normal exposure conditions the radiologist's clue to the pathology. However, when there is an indication that an abscess may be present in the bone providing added local density (299), it is necessary to increase the kilovoltage in order to record the transradiant outline of an abscess within the dense area.

In some conditions, such as rickets in an infant, (302), the examination may be restricted to taking films of the long bones.

A single antero-posterior radiograph of each upper limb, and of both lower limbs simultaneously (302) shows the condition caused by a deficiency of Vitamin D in the child's diet.

The need to visualize the soft tissues is shown in the condition of cysticercosis (301), in which there is calcification of a parasite in muscles.

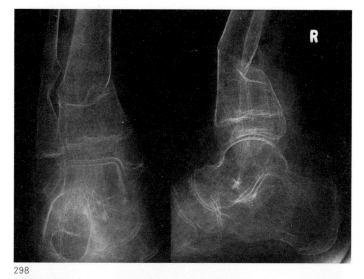

298

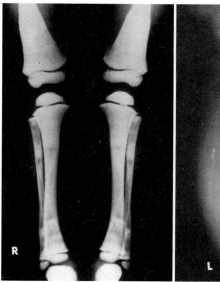

300

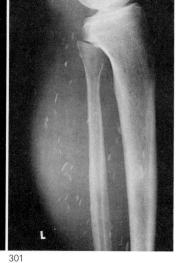

301

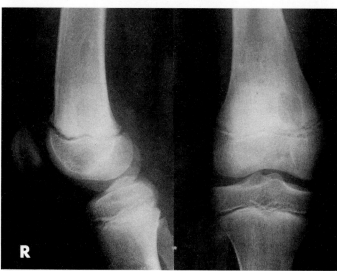

299

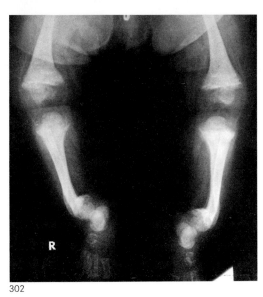

302

Foot

The bones of the foot form a series of curves called the transverse and longitudinal arches. The foot is thicker in the proximal part than the distal and in the medial than the lateral parts so that the dorsal surface slopes from the medial side of the ankle joint at its highest to the fifth toe at its lowest. These differences in thickness will produce variations in radiographic density when radiographing the foot and is one of the reasons for having four basic positions which are used in pairs to meet diagnostic requirements (303, 304, 305, 306).

To avoid excessive variations in density between the thick and thin parts of the foot, either a high kilovoltage can be used or a graduated thickness wedge on the film. However, in practice, separate exposures are usually made for the fore-foot and the hind-foot.

Four of the general positions described on the following pages are shown below.

(**303**) dorsi-plantar—when the foot is bearing the full weight of the body or with the foot in a similar position on the cassette when the patient is supine.

(**304**) lateral—when the sole of the foot is at right angles to the film:

(**305**) dorsi-plantar oblique—when the plantar aspect of the foot is at 40° to the film using a vertical ray from the X-ray tube:

(**306**) oblique—when the sole of the foot is oblique in relation to film and to the vertical X-ray beam.

The term dorsi-plantar replaces the term 'antero-posterior' as applied to the joints generally.

Note—Inversion and eversion of the foot are movements which occur mainly at the midtarsal joint when the sole of the foot is turned in a medial or lateral direction, respectively.

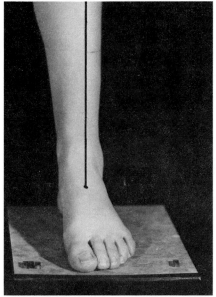

303

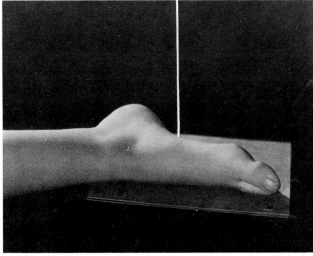

304

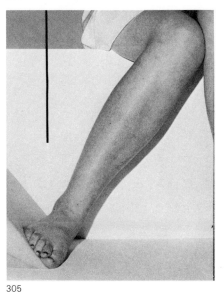

305

306

Dorsi-Plantar—Oblique (basic)

With the patient supine or sitting semi-recumbent, the knee is flexed with the plantar aspect of the foot in contact with the film.

The knee is allowed to lean medially to offset foreshortening of the transverse aspect of the dorsum of the foot. The opposite limb acts as a support to assist immobilization.

■ Centre to the cuboid-navicular region with the central ray vertical.

In a general survey of the foot, the kilovoltage requires to be in the region of 80 kVp to reduce the difference in subject contrast between the thickness of the toes and tarsus to a more uniform radiographic contrast over the range of foot densities.

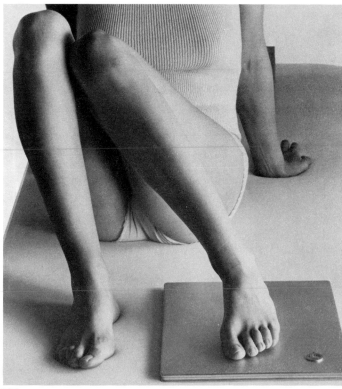

307

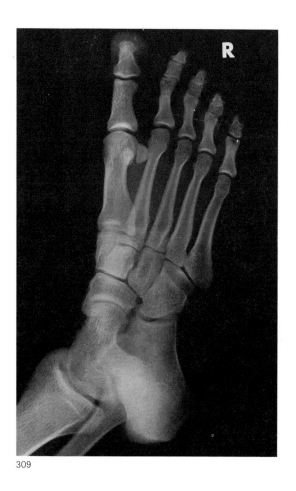

309

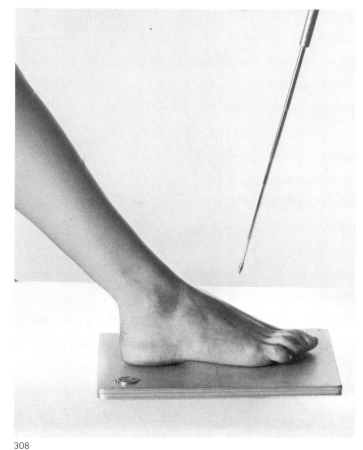

308

Dorsi-Plantar (basic)

With the patient sitting or semi-recumbent, the foot is placed with the plantar aspect in contact with the film. The leg being supported in the vertical position by the other knee (310).

■ Centre over the cuboid-navicular region with the central ray perpendicular to the film (310, 311a)

Note—This position does not show the tarso-metatarsal articulations clearly as the bones overlap in the direction of the X-ray beam. These joints can be shown by either angling the X-ray beam 10–15° toward the ankle joint or by placing a 10–15° wedge under the cassette—its thicker part being toward the toes (311a, 311b).

Dorsi-Plantar (Hallux-valgus)

Both feet are radiographed standing on the film with the weight equally distributed.

■ Centre between the feet at the level of the first metatarso-phalangeal joints with the central ray perpendicular to the film (312).

Foot									
kVp			mAS				Film	Screens	
AP	Obl	Lat	AP	Obl	Lat	FFD	ILFORD	ILFORD	Grid
60	60	70	10	10	10	100 cm (40″)	RAPID R	SUPER HD	—

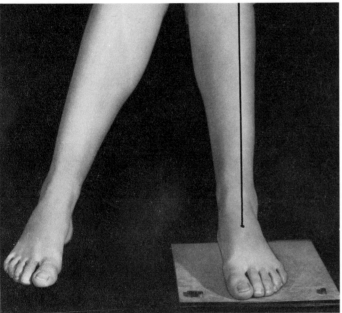

310

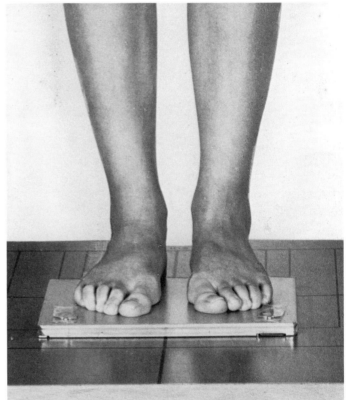

312

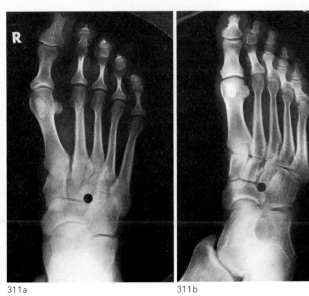

311a   311b

3 Lower limb
Foot

Oblique (basic)

The patient is rotated on to the affected side, with the hip and knee joints flexed. The sound limb is flexed and brought over to make contact with the table in front of the injured limb. This brings the injured limb semi-oblique in position with the lateral aspect of the patella in contact with the table. This position of the limb allows the foot to fall obliquely forward (313).

■ Centre over the base of the fifth metatarsal bone with the central ray perpendicular to the film (313, 314, 315)

The tube may be angled from 5 to 10° to compensate for inadequate obliquity of the foot.

Note—The metatarsal bones are shown in a slightly oblique position, but clearly separated one from the other, permitting minor injuries to be demonstrated satisfactorily.

The two appropriate projections of the foot, dorsi-plantar and oblique, or dorsi-plantar and lateral, may be exposed on a single film 24 × 30 cm (12 × 10ins) or 18 × 24 cm (10 × 8 ins) according to size of the foot.

Injuries

Radiographs (316) show lateral dislocations and fractures at the second to fifth-tarso-metatarsal region. When the site of the injury has been identified it may not be necessary to include the whole of the foot for repeat examinations.

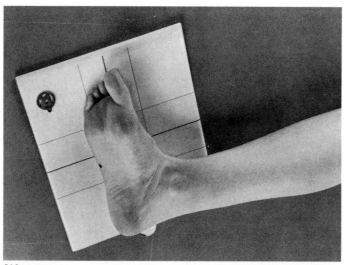

313

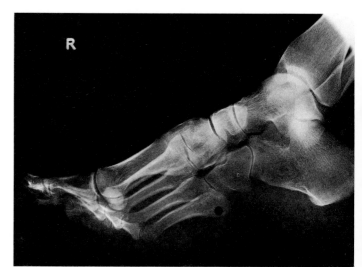

314

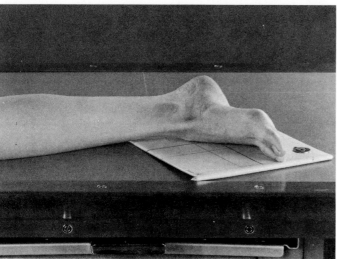

315

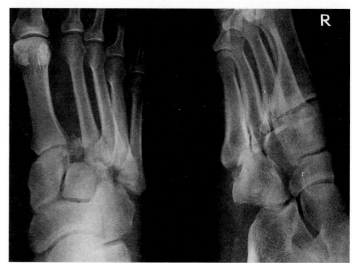

316

Lateral (basic)

The patient is moved into the general lateral position, with the knees flexed and the sound limb raised on sandbags behind the injured limb. A sandbag is placed under the anterior aspect of the affected knee so that the ankle and foot are tilted backward into the true lateral position, with the plantar aspect of the foot at right angles to the film. The position of the limb should be compared in photographs (317) and (313), and in the radiographs (318) and (315).

■ Centre to the navicular-cuneiform region (317, 318)

	Foot							
kVp			mAS				Film	Screens
AP	Obl	Lat	AP	Obl	Lat	FFD	ILFORD	ILFORD —
60	60	70	10	10	10	100 cm (40")	RAPID R	SUPER HD —

Note—This position gives a true lateral projection of the tarsal bones and mid tarsal joints. The five metatarsal bones overshadow each other so that minor injuries in this region will not be visible. The longitudinal plantar arch is shown as well as the underlying soft tissues and in conjunction with the dorsi-plantar position, foreign bodies in this region can be demonstrated clear of bone.

Fracture Radiographs

The lateral radiograph of the foot (319a) suggests a fracture of the calcaneus which is confirmed in the oblique projection when the shadows of the talus and calcaneus are separated and the fracture becomes clearly visible.

These radiographs show the value of the oblique projection.

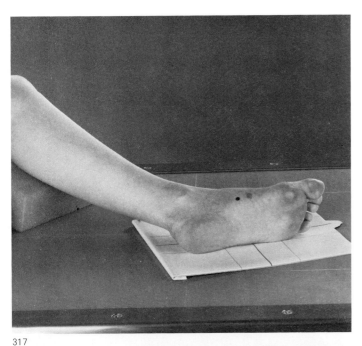

317

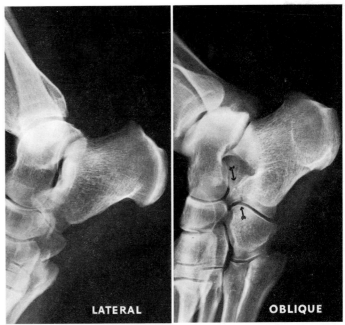

LATERAL   OBLIQUE

319a   319b

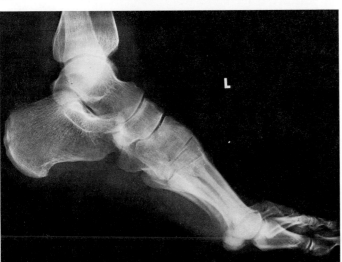

318

Foot—General Note

Comparison dorsi-plantar radiographs are shown in (320a) which demonstrates the condition of osteochondritis (Kohler's disease). Similar comparative oblique projections may also be required. Films should be marked carefully to indicate right and left sides.

Sesamoid Bones—Oblique views

Sesamoid bones occur in the tendons of muscles. Radiographs (321a, 321b, 322) show examples of sesamoid bones in the tendon of peroneus longus.

Note—that they are best shown in oblique views.

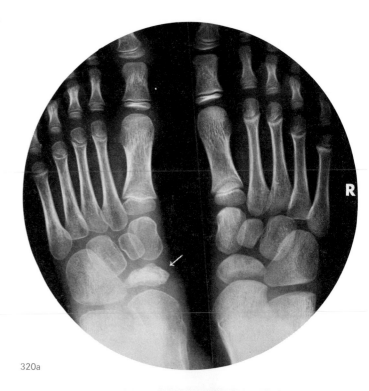

320a

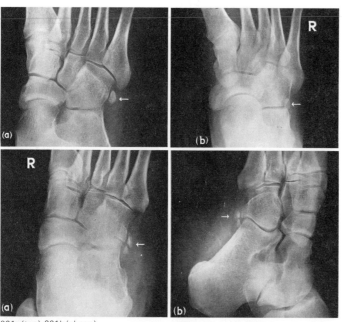

321a (top) 321b (above)

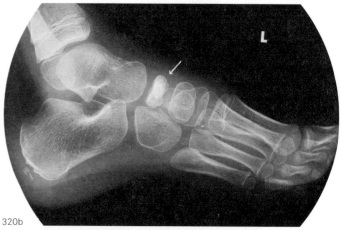

320b

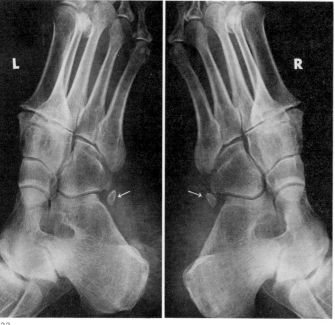

322

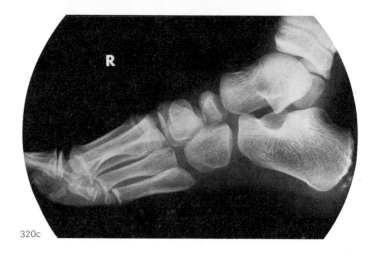

320c

Flat Foot

To show the condition of the longitudinal arches when the feet are bearing the full weight of the body the patient is examined in the erect position (323), a lateral projection is taken of each weight-bearing foot in turn (using a horizontal beam) with the film supported in the vertical position.

Lateral

For convenience in making the projections the patient stands on a low platform; each foot is placed on a separate piece of balsa wood or other transradiant material, leaving a shallow gap between. Two film packs separated by protective lead sheet are placed vertically between the feet and ankles to rest on the platform surface. On bringing the feet together close contact is made with the film packs, the weight of the trunk being supported equally by the feet. To aid general immobilization the patient's hands rest on a convenient vertical support.

■ Centre to the lateral aspect of each foot in turn using horizontal tube projection (323)

The resultant radiographs provide a comparison of the longitudinal arches of the right and left feet (324), as required for an investigation of flat foot.

kVp	mAS	FFD	Film ILFORD	Screens ILFORD	Grid
70	10	100 cm (40″)	RAPID R	SUPER HD	—

Radiograph (325) is taken erect and weight bearing and (326) with the patient lying on a couch as in (317). Compare the different appearance of the arches of the foot in these two radiographs.

Note—It is interesting to see the appearances of the bones of the foot in relation to the high heel (327).

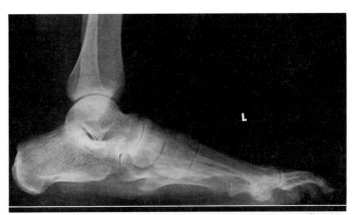

325

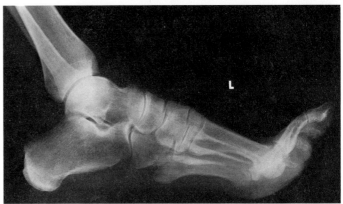

326

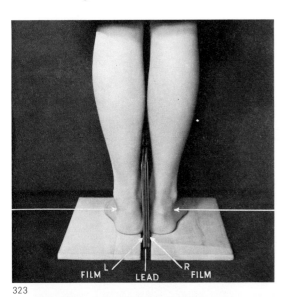

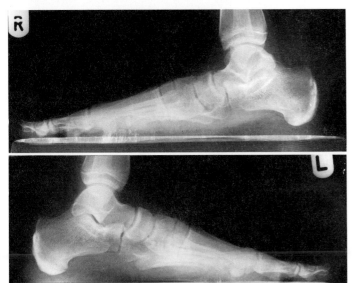

323

324

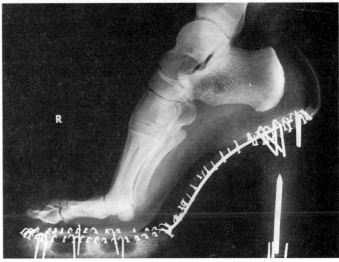

327

Os Trigonum

Occasionally an additional centre of ossification develops in place of the posterior tubercle of the talus, forming a separate bone known as the os trigonum. This fragment of bone may lead to confusion when an injury is suspected. Comparative lateral projections of the two feet may be needed.

Lateral (1)
Both feet may be exposed separately and positioned as for the lateral projection of the foot (317).
■ Centre to the posterior tubercle of the talus (317,318)

Lateral (2)
With a reasonably supple patient both heels may be exposed simultaneously, in many instances, by positioning the sitting patient with flexion at both hip and knee joints and support under the knees, for the soles of the feet to face each other.
■ Centre between the heels (328,329)

			Os Trigonum		
kVp	mAS	FFD	Film ILFORD	Screens ILFORD	Grid
60	20	100 cm (40")	RAPID R	SUPER HD	—

In radiograph (329) the posterior tubercle of the talus is shown in the right foot and the os trigonum in the left foot.

In radiograph (330) the posterior tubercle is detached on both sides giving rise to a bilateral os trigonum.

The same positioning technique (328) may be conveniently employed to show a spur of bone on the inferior aspect of the calcaneus which may cause a painful heel. In (331) both heels are affected. However, in (330,331) the heels were exposed separately.

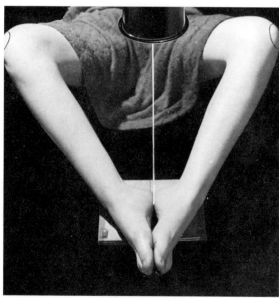

328

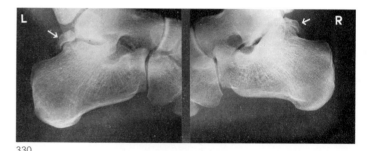

330

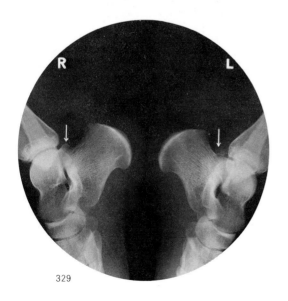

329

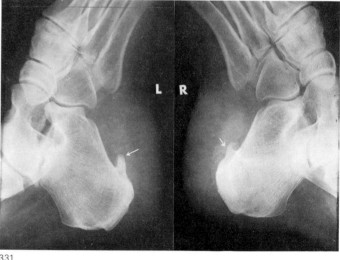

331

Toes

Lateral

The toes are so variable in length and direction that the position for the lateral projection must be adapted to each patient, using modified oblique profile projections as for (334, 335) or, indeed, any of the four general positions of the foot (page 81) may be applicable. For the middle and distal phalanges, place a dental film between individual toes extending to the mid-proximal phalanx; flexion of adjacent toes will often be required and an occlusal film is necessary for the phalanges of the great toe (333).

			Film	Screens	
kVp	mAS	FFD	ILFORD	ILFORD	Grid
50	8	100 cm (40″)	RAPID R	SUPER HD	—

Toes

Fracture Radiographs

When there is doubt as to the presence of a fracture in the dorsi-plantar projection, a lateral view may prove conclusive as shown in (334, 335).

Pathology

Two projections are necessary to show the pathology affecting the third and fourth proximal phalanges which is also present in the third metatarsal (336).

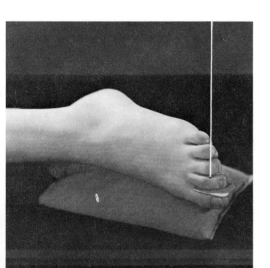

332

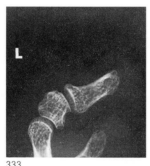

333

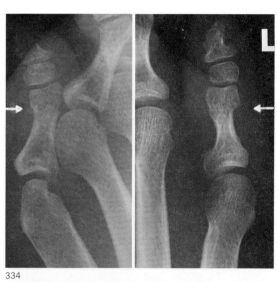

334

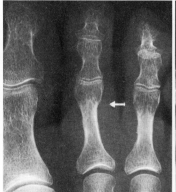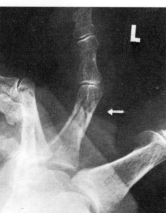

335

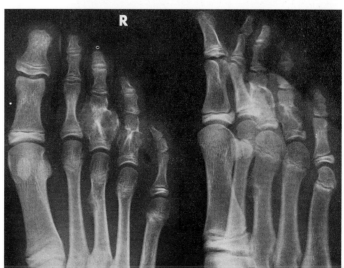

336

Great Toe

Dorsi-Plantar (basic)

The foot is placed with the plantar aspect on the film, the leg being maintained in the vertical position.

■ Centre over the first metatarso-phalangeal joint (337, 338)

Great Toe

kVp		mAS			Film	Screens	
D-P	Lat	D-P	Lat	FFD	ILFORD	ILFORD	Grid
50	50	12	12	100 cm (40″)	RAPID R	SUPER HD	—

The two projections, dorsi-plantar and lateral are usually taken side by side on one film as in (336).

Lateral (1) (basic)

The limb should be placed with the great toe and medial aspect of the leg, including the patella, in contact with the couch. The heel is raised on a sandbag and the film supported in contact with the foot. The sole of the foot is obliquely forward in relation to the film.

■ Centre over the thenar eminence of the great toe (339, 340)

This position gives the most satisfactory lateral projection of the great toe from the base of the metatarsal bone.

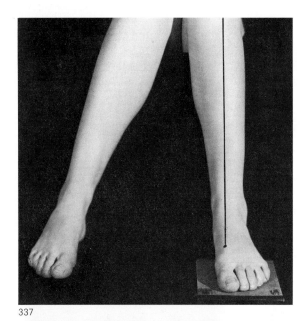

337

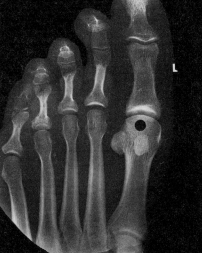

338

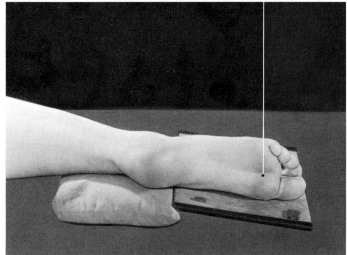

339

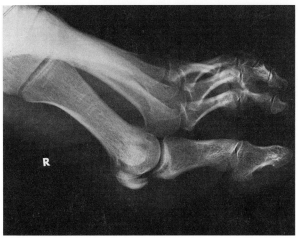

340

Lateral (2)

Alternatively, the knee is raised on a sandbag and the foot tilted backward so that the sole of the foot is oblique to the film.

■ Centre over the first metatarso-phalangeal joint (341, 342)

Great Toe (Lateral)

kVp	MAS	FFD	Film ILFORD	Screens ILFORD	Grid
50	20	100 cm (40″)	RAPID R	SUPER HD	—

Fracture Radiographs

Fractures of the proximal and distal phalanges of the great toe are demonstrated in (343).

Radiographs (344), dorsi-plantar and lateral, show a fracture of the tip of the distal phalanx of the great toe.

A fracture at the base of the first metatarsal is shown in the dorsi-plantar and lateral projections (345a). After reduction, the improved alignment of the fracture fragments is clearly shown through the plaster splint (345b) for which the exposure, was increased by 50%.

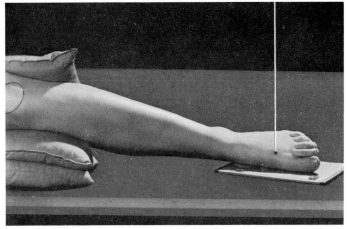

341

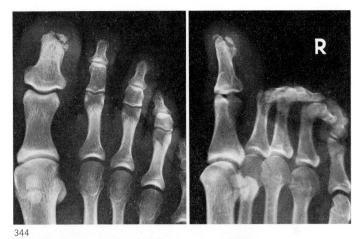

344

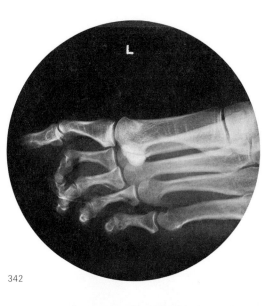

342

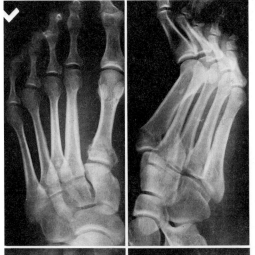

345a

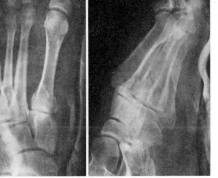

345b

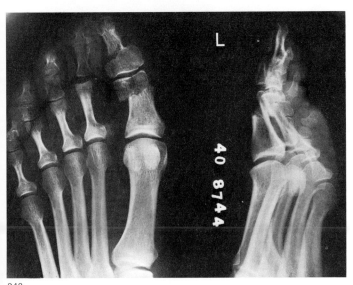

343

First Metatarso-Phalangeal Sesamoid Bones

The sesamoid bones at the first metatarso-phalangeal joint are visible in both lateral and axial projections.

Lateral

With the foot in the lateral position shown in (317), page 85, the sesamoid bones are shown in profile (349b).

■ Centre over the sesamoid bones (317,349b)

Axial

There is the choice of three projections:

(1) With the patient sitting on the couch and with the film held firmly against the instep, flexion at the joint is produced by a tightened bandage passed round the great toe (346,348a).

(2) With the limb lateral and the great toe pulled forward, the film is placed vertically and well into the instep for horizontal tube projection (347,348a).

(3) With the patient in the prone position, pressure of the plantar aspect of the phalanges on to the couch and film promotes flexion at the joint (348b).

■ Centre through the sesamoid bones (346,347,348a,b)

			Sesamoids		
kVp Axial	mAS Axial	FFD	Film ILFORD	Screens ILFORD	Grid
65	10	100 cm (40")	RAPID R	SUPER HD	—

Abnormality

(349a,b) shows a large overgrowth of bone on the medial sesamoid of the big toe.

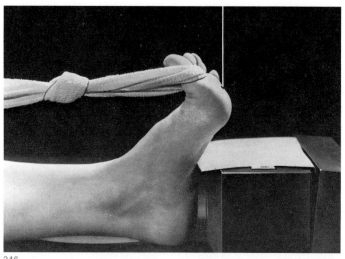

346

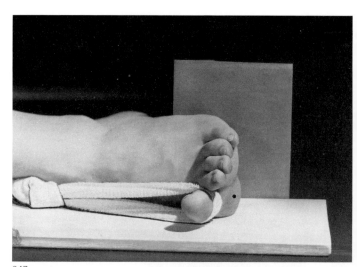

347

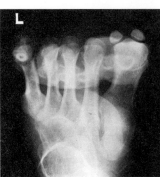

348a

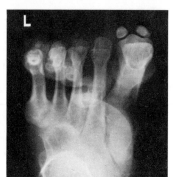

348b

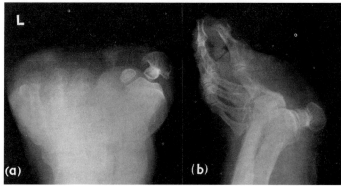

(a) 349a   (b) 349b

Calcaneus (os calcis)

kVp	mAS	FFD	Film ILFORD	Screens ILFORD	Grid
60	12	100 cm (40″)	RAPID R	SUPER HD	—

The calcaneus, which is the largest of the tarsal bones, forms the heel of the foot. It articulates anteriorly with the cuboid, and superiorly, through three articular surfaces, anterior, middle and posterior, with the talus (368, 369). Of these, the sustentaculum tali provides the middle articulation. The complete radiographic examination includes lateral, axial and oblique projections.

Following a fracture, accurate alignment must be re-established; it is essential, therefore, to place the film correctly in relation to the bone at each examination in spite of the presence of awkward appliances (362).

Axial (1) (basic)
The patient is seated or lying with extended limbs in the antero-posterior position; the heels are separated by a small non-opaque pad and the great toes are touching one another. The ankles are flexed and held in dorsi-flexion by a bandage round the forefeet. The film is placed under the back of the heels to include the calcaneo-cuboid joints (353).

Lateral (basic)
The lateral position of the ankle with a sandbag under the knee also shows the calcaneus in a true lateral position.
■ Centre over the talo-calcaneal articulation (350, 351)

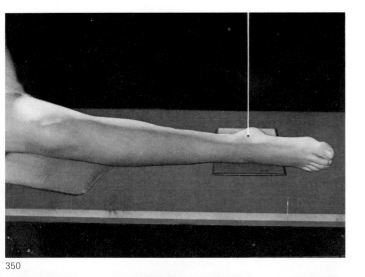

350

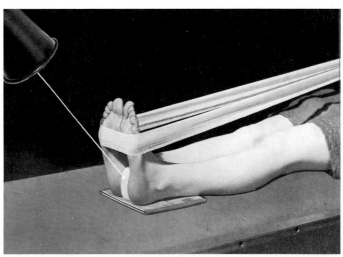

352

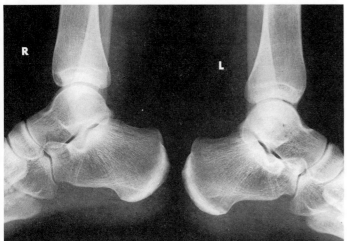

351

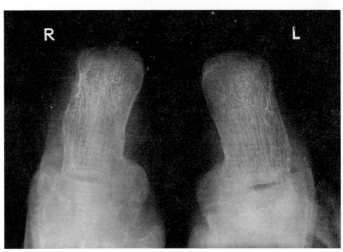

353

Axial (2)

With the patient prone the legs are raised on sandbags and the feet allowed to extend over the end of the couch; the soles pressing against the film, which is supported in the vertical position.

■ Centre between the posterior aspect of the heels, with the tube angled 55°–60° from the vertical (354, 355)

Axial (3)

When it is easier to examine the patient in the lateral position, the limbs are raised for horizontal alignment and separated by non-opaque pads between the heels and the knee joints. This allows symmetrical positioning of the legs without discomfort to the patient while the position is maintained. The film is supported against the heels for horizontal tube projection.

■ Centre at an angle of 60° to the film (355, 356)

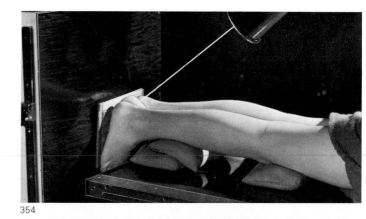

354

Calcaneum Axial

kVp Axial	mAS Axial	FFD	Film ILFORD	Screens ILFORD	Grid
70	12	100 cm (40″)	RAPID R	SUPER HD	—

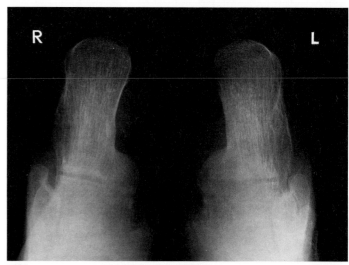

355

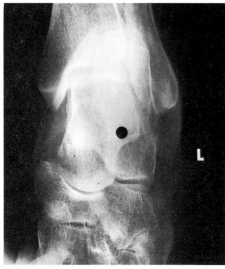

358

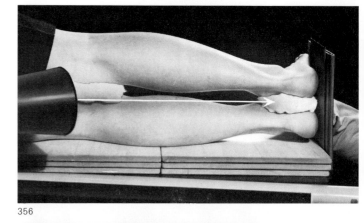

356

Fracture Radiographs

In radiograph (357) the fracture is not well shown on the lateral view but is clearly defined on the axial projection. The thicker, front part of the calcaneus is under-exposed compared with the region of the fracture which is correctly exposed.

Note—To show the calcaneo-talus relationship through the superimposed tibia and fibula, the dorsi-plantar oblique position (307 page 82) can be used but the tube must be centred to the talus and the exposure increased by 50% (358).

94

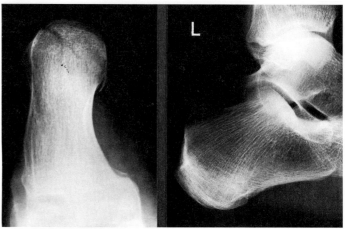

357

Axial (4)

To exclude a fracture of the calcaneus in ambulant patients it may be convenient for the examination to be done in the erect position. This position cannot, of course, be used for non-ambulant patients whether in a wheelchair or on a stretcher-trolley.

The patient stands with both heels on the film, the body leaning forward with the knees slightly flexed and with the hands resting on a table or chair for support. If weight-bearing on the heels is too uncomfortable, a small 15° angle block is placed under the film.

■ Centre between the heels, with the tube angled at from 10 to 15° from the vertical (359, 361).

If the patient cannot flex at the ankles then the tube may be angled 30° to the heels (360). The result is the same as obtained in axial (2) radiograph (355).

■ For **Exposure Factors** see page 93.

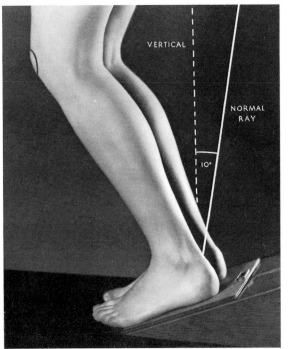
359

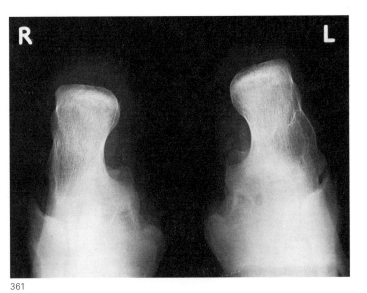
361

Note—Radiograph (361) is a badly positioned film with foreshortening of the calcaneus, the talo-calcaneal joint is also obscured; and can occur in any of the axial projections.

Radiographs (362) show an intramedullary pin in the calcaneus with the foot in plaster and demonstrate that satisfactory routine projections can be obtained under difficult circumstances. With the foot in plaster the exposure must be increased by 60 to 70% compared with the normal.

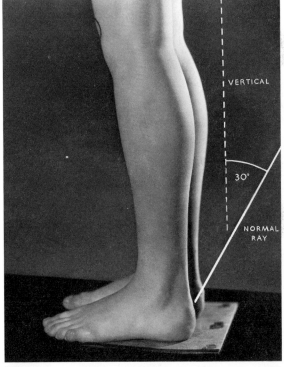
360

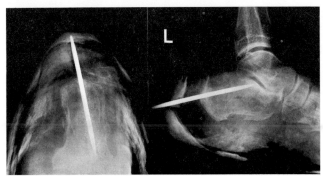
362

95

Talo-Calcaneal Joints
Radiographs of dry bones (368, 369) show the position of the three superior articular surfaces of the calcaneus—anterior, middle and posterior—and must be studied in conjunction with the oblique projections.

Oblique
Oblique projections are essential to show the posterior talo-calcaneal joint and the middle sub-taloid joint with the sustentaculum tali (368, 369). Two positions of the foot are used oblique-medial and oblique-lateral, with varying tube angulation toward the head.

Oblique-medial
With dorsi-flexion at the ankle joint the limb is rotated medially to an angle of 45° to the couch surface (363, 364). The Potter-Bucky compression band helps to immobilize the foot in this position.

■ Centre 3 cm (1¼ ins) below the lateral malleolus with the tube angled for each exposure in turn:
40°—to show the anterior part of the posterior talo-calcaneal articulation (363, 365);
30° to 20°—to show the articulation between the talus and sustentaculum tali (363, 366);
10°—to show the posterior part of the posterior talo-calcaneal articulation (363, 367).

Note—In the appropriate dry bone radiograph, page 97, the wire is at the position of the posterior edge of the posterior talo-calcaneal joint surface.

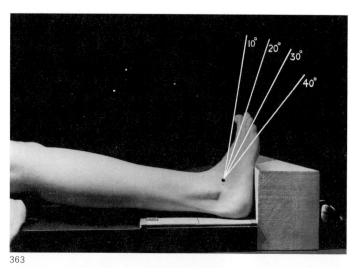

363

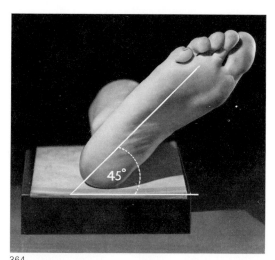

364

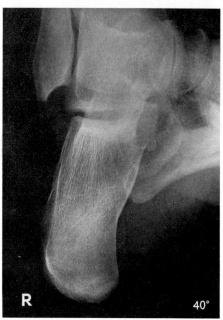

365

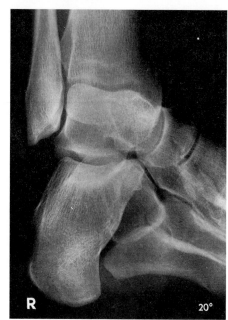

366

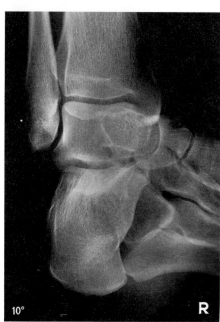

367

96

Oblique-lateral

Maintaining flexion at the ankle joint, the limb is rotated laterally until the foot is again at an angle of 45° to the couch (370, 371), and is then immobilized.

■ Centre 2·5 cm (1 in) below and just in front of the medial malleolus with the tube angled 12° to 18° towards the head (370, 371, 372).

This projection is used to confirm a fracture, to disclose dorsi-plantar compression, and to show the calcaneal sulcus.

kVp	mAS	FFD	Film ILFORD	Screens ILFORD	Grid
60	16	100 cm (40″)	RAPID R	SUPER HD	—

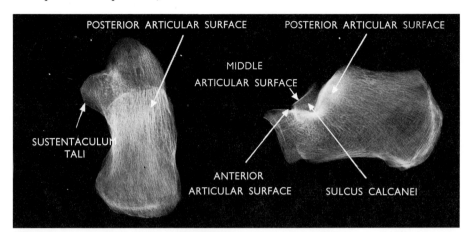

368

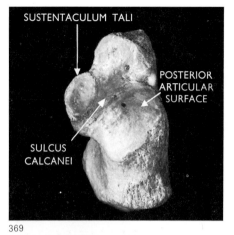

369

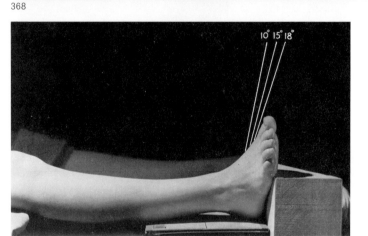

370

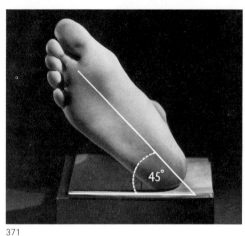

371

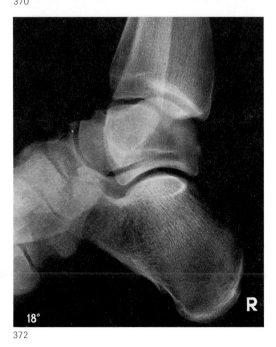

372

Oblique-Lateral

From the lateral position the limb is rotated toward the film to be at an angle of approximately 40°, the patella being in contact with the couch.

■ Centre to the ankle joint with the tube angled 20° downward (373)

Arthrodesis

Arthrodesis is the surgical fixation of a joint resulting in bony ankylosis. The joint is immobilized in plaster until the radiograph shows bony fusion is complete.

A triple arthrodesis involving the talo-calcaneal, talo-navicular and calcaneo-cuboid joints may need radiographic demonstration.

For a complete survey of this area the following positions can be used
(a) Oblique foot, concentrating over the ankle (375)
(b) Oblique foot 20° caudal tilt (374).
(c) 45° oblique medial, 10° cephalic tilt (376).
(d) 45° oblique lateral, 15°–18° cephalic tilt (377).

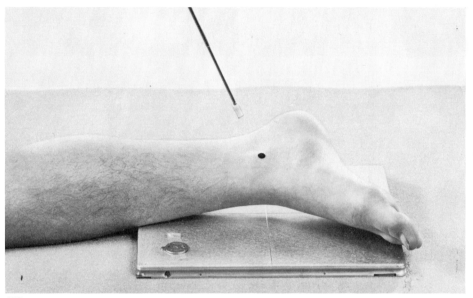

373

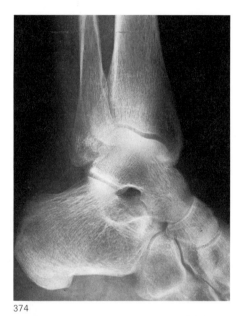

374

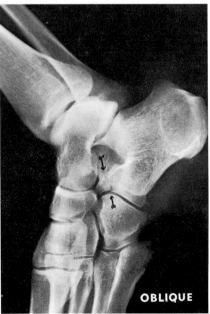

375

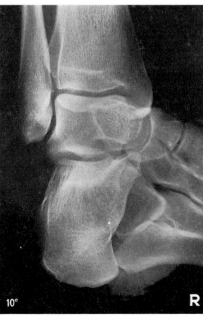

376

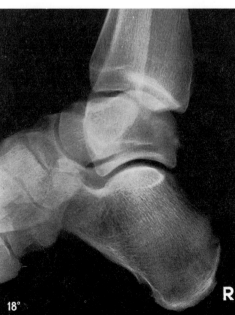

377

3

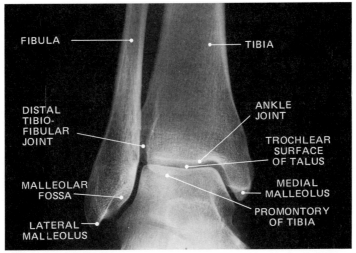

RIGHT ANKLE
378
ANTERO-POSTERIOR

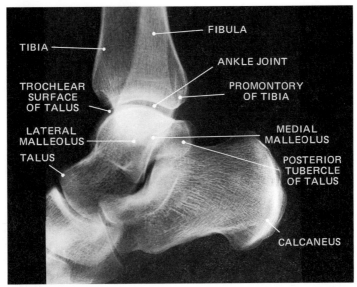

RIGHT ANKLE
379
LATERAL

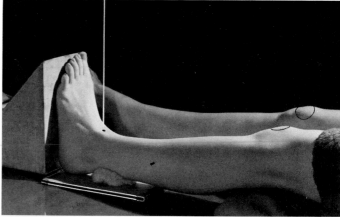

380

Ankle Joint

Radiographic Appearances

Lettered radiographs, antero-posterior (378) and lateral (379), are included to help the student with anatomical references in the text.

Antero-posterior (basic)

This examination may be done with the patient seated with a back-rest support or the patient supine with a small sandbag under the knees to allow slight flexion for comfort and a small non-opaque pad under the tendo-achilles to prevent undue pressure of the heel on the couch. The ankle is supported in flexion, and the limb rotated medially until the medial and lateral malleoli are equidistant from the film, this ensures a clear joint space in the radiograph between tibia, fibula and talus (381).

A 90° angle block, supported by sandbags, is used to steady the foot in position (380).

The foot is placed so that the joint space is one-third of the film length above the lower border of the film, as it is more important to include the lower third of the leg than the region below the level of the malleoli.

■ Centre midway between the malleoli (380, 381, 382)

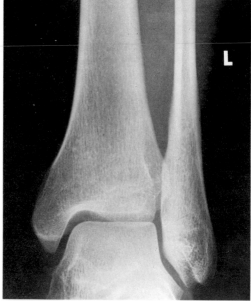

381

Ankle

kVp		mAS			Film	Screens	
AP	Lat	AP	Lat	FFD	ILFORD	ILFORD	Grid
60	60	12	10	100 cm (40″)	RAPID R	SUPER	—

The photograph of the soles of the feet (382) shows the method of centring according to the position of the foot. For the left foot (382) the limb is rotated medially, so that the intermalleolar line is parallel to the film, and the tube is straight (380). The right foot is straight, with the tube angled to bisect the line between the malleoli at right angles to provide a similar result to (381).

The fibula in profile may have no surrounding soft tissues, therefore, the lateral malleolus may be over-exposed appearing too black on the radiograph. Increased kilovoltage will reduce the contrast producing a more even exposure across the ankle joint; the miliampere seconds must be correspondingly reduced.

Note—Whenever possible the two projections—antero-posterior and lateral—should be exposed side by side on a single film (387).

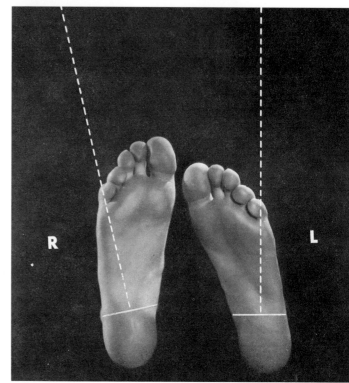

382

Lateral (basic)—Medio-Lateral

The patient is in the lateral position, on the injured side, with a pad under the anterior aspect of the knee to tilt the ankle into the true lateral position.

To include the maximum length of bone above the ankle joint to show the general alignment of the bones, the cassette is positioned so that its lower edge is half an inch higher than the sole of the foot. When the patient cannot be moved into the lateral position, a horizontal projection is used, the film placed vertically against the ankle.

■ Centre over the medial malleolus (383, 384)

Note—The film should include the lower third of the tibia and the fibula, the talus and the calcaneus. The joint space of the ankle is overshadowed by the malleoli.

Latero-Medial—Ankle

The patient lies on the unaffected side, and the injured limb is brought over in front of the sound limb, with the lateral aspect of the patella in contact with a pad to tilt the ankle into the true lateral position.

■ Centre over the lateral malleolus with the central ray perpendicular to the film (385)

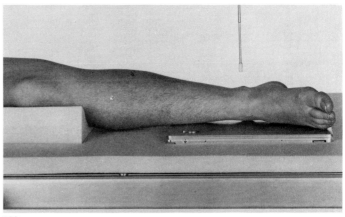
383

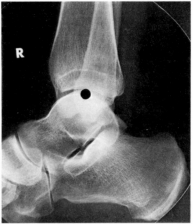
384

Ankle

| kVp | | mAS | | | Film | Screens | |
AP	Lat	AP	Lat	FFD	ILFORD	ILFORD	Grid
60	60	12	10	100 cm (40″)	RAPID R	SUPER	—

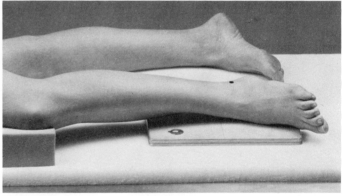
385

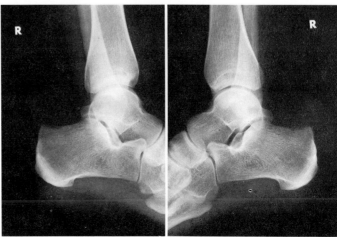
LATERO-MEDIAL
386a
MEDIO-LATERAL
386b

101

Fracture Radiographs

A Pott's fracture is shown in (387). The two radiographs (388) show a spiral fracture of the tibia, note that its upper end must be included in the film. At the initial examination when the extent of the fracture is not known, care must be taken to include a sufficient length of the tibia and fibula so as not to miss a fracture or to include its full extent. However, in follow up examinations, only the affected area need be included on the radiographs. Again, whenever possible, the two projections should be made side by side on a single film.

Oblique—Antero-posterior

From the antero-posterior position the limb is rotated medially through 45° (389) and supported in position by a non-opaque triangular pad.

■ Centre to the ankle joint (389, 390)

Oblique—Lateral

From the lateral position the limb is rotated toward the film to be at an angle of approximately 40°, the patella being in contact with the couch.

■ Centre to the ankle joint with the tube angled 20° downward (391, 392)

Arthrography

See also pages 30, 62, 118. For the ankle joint 3 ml of a 35% solution of water soluble organic iodine compound is injected anteriorly, with the needle directed toward the articular surface of the talus. Radiographs are taken from the antero-posterior (380) and lateral (383) aspects.

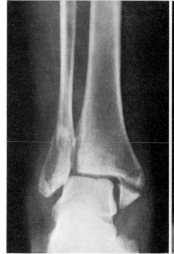
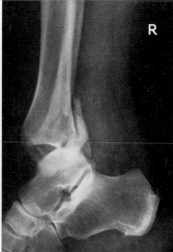

387

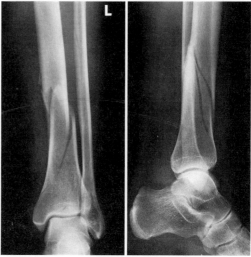

388

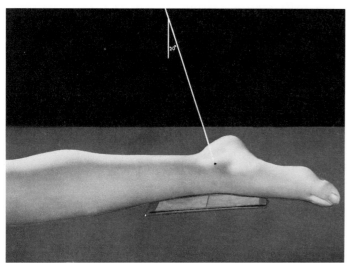

391

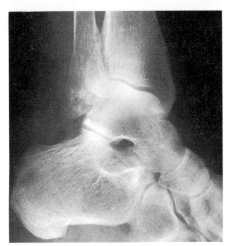

392

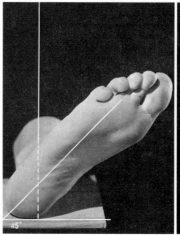
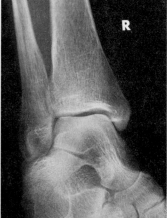

389   390

Subluxation

Subluxation at the ankle joint may be due to rupture or stretching of the lateral ligaments. A modified technique is required to show this condition.

With the limb in the antero-posterior position, the foot is inverted—turned medially—at the midtarsal joint. To maintain the foot in this position, a sling round the foot is weighted with a sandbag at its free end, which hangs over the side of the couch, or the foot is held in this position by a doctor wearing lead apron and lead gloves.

Special Note—The adjustment of the foot to forced inversion should not be undertaken by the radiographer.
■ Centre midway between the malleoli (393, 394, 395)

When the ligaments are stretched or torn, this positioning has the effect of widening the joint space on the outer side (395b); compare this radiograph with (395a) taken of the same foot without inversion of the foot, when the joint space appears to be normal.

A radiograph of the normal ankle with the foot inverted shows the joint surfaces parallel when the ligaments are undamaged (395a).

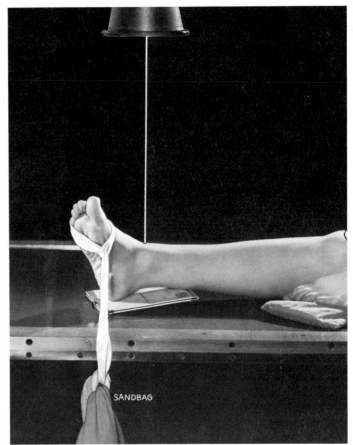

393

Ankle Subluxation

kVp		mAS			Film	Screens	
AP	Lat	AP	Lat	FFD	ILFORD	ILFORD	Grid
60	60	12	10	100 cm (40″)	RAPID R	SUPER HD	—

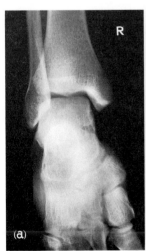

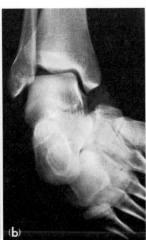

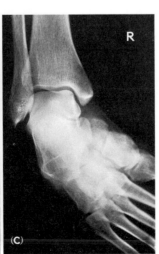

395

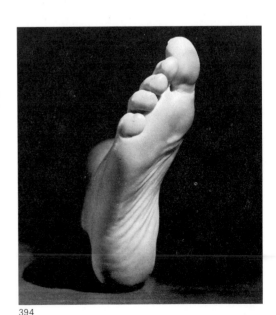

394

Leg

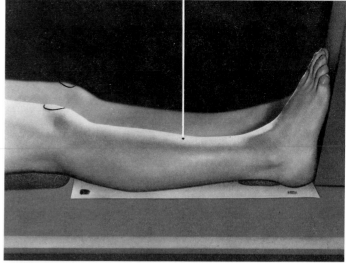

396

For gross injuries to the leg the knee and ankle joints must be included to show the general alignment of both tibia and fibula. Only in children will it be possible to do this on one film (397a, b); for adults, two radiographs are usually required, one from the ankle upward (399), the other from the knee downward (400). The middle third of the leg will be included on each film.

The film should be placed well above the knee and well below the ankle because the great divergence of the peripheral radiation will tend to project the joints beyond the edge of the film.

In case of an obvious fracture to the lower leg, the proximal tibio-fibular joint should always be included as there may be another fracture in this area (402).

Guide to Appropriate Positions

For the general examination of the leg use positions (396) and (398), or to avoid movement of the limb (400) should replace (398). To show the proximal tibio-fibular joint use positions (405) or (407).

Antero-posterior (basic)

The patient should be supine, with the limb slightly rotated medially and supported in position. When the patient is to be re-examined following a fracture then only the joint nearest to the fracture site need be included, the film should be placed well below or above the joint to allow for projection displacement.
■ Centre to the middle of the film (396, 397a)

Lateral (basic)

The patient is turned on to the affected side, with the limb in the true lateral position. The film is positioned so that the joint adjacent to the site of injury is included on the film. If it is necessary to include the whole limb and adjacent joints, two films will be needed as shown in (399, 400).
■ Centre to the middle of the film (397, 398)

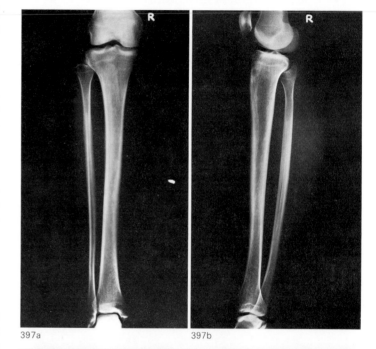

397a   397b

Leg							
kVp		mAS			Film	Screens	
AP	Lat	AP	Lat	FFD	ILFORD	ILFORD	Grid
60	60	20	20	100 cm (40″)	R	HD	—

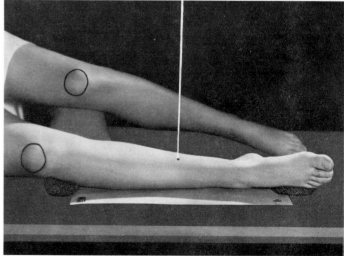

398

Stretcher Patients

If the patient's leg is on a splint or has an obvious fracture, the limb must not be moved into the lateral position. After exposing for the antero-posterior position (399), the tube arm is adjusted to the horizontal ray position and a lateral radiograph is taken keeping the patient supine (400).

Leg							
kVp		mAS			Film	Screens	
AP	Lat	AP	Lat	FFD	ILFORD	ILFORD	Grid
65	65	16	16	100 cm (40″)	RAPID R	SUPER HD	—

Fracture Radiographs

The four radiographs (401) show a fracture of the tibia and fibula in the middle third as well as of the lateral condyle of the tibia and were taken as described in (399,400). In the illustration (401) the overlap for each pair of films has been removed and the extent of the overlap is indicated with arrows. Radiograph (402) shows an additional fracture to the proximal end of the fibula.

Radiographs (403) were taken initially in the Accident and Emergency department and (404) following reduction of the fracture and immobilization in plaster of Paris. By increasing the exposure and using correct positioning the bones can be adequately demonstrated.

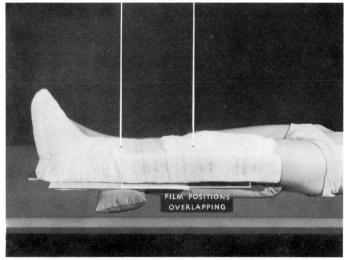

399

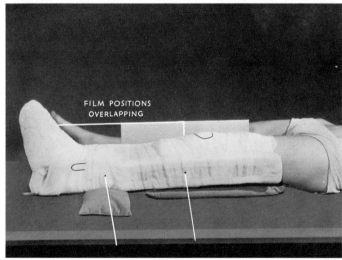

400

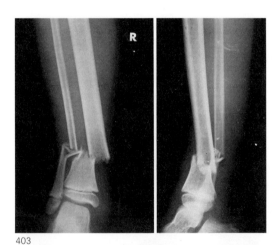

403

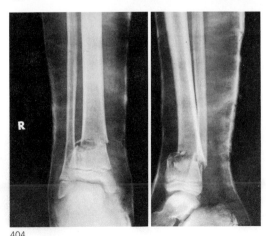

404

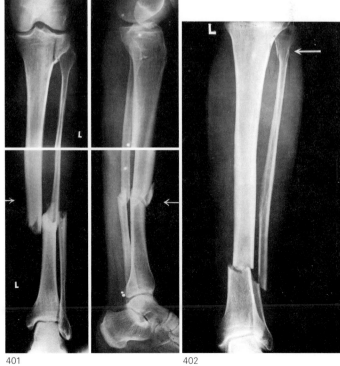

401　　　402

Proximal Tibio-Fibular Joint

A small degree of obliquity is needed to show the tibio-fibular joint as it is obscured in both the antero-posterior and the lateral projections of the legs when using the routine positions (396, 397a, b, 398).

Antero-posterior oblique

From the antero-posterior position the limb is rotated medially 20° to show the tibio-fibular joint clear of the tibial condyle.
- Centre over the head of the fibula (405, 406)

Lateral oblique

From the lateral position the leg is rotated laterally 20° so that the head of the fibula is in profile.
- Centre over the head of the fibula (407, 408)

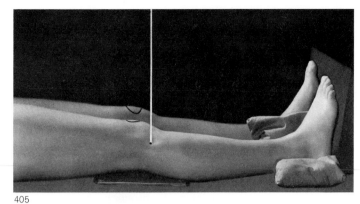

405

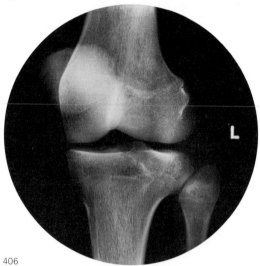

406

Tibio-Fibular Joint

kVp	mAS	FFD	Film ILFORD	Screens ILFORD	Grid
60	24	100 cms (40″)	RAPID R	SUPER HD	—

Note—The exposure is reduced (e.g. 65 kV to 60 kV) from that used for the basic positions of the knee joint to show the less dense area around the tibio-fibular joint.

Positive and Negative

Two examples are given to show the meaning of positive and negative images. On the left the positive image (409)—as would be seen on a fluorescent screen without a television monitor, the bones appearing black. On the right the familiar negative image, the bones appearing white.

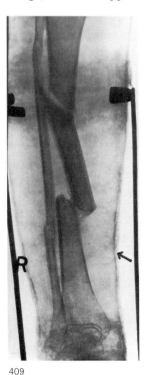

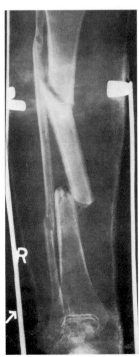

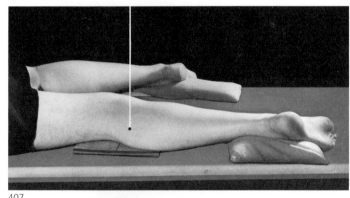

407

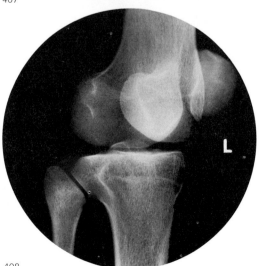

408

409

410

Knee Joint

Radiographic Appearances

Three lettered radiographs, antero-posterior (411), lateral (412) and lateral oblique (413), show the anatomical references in the text.

The anatomy of the joint should be fully understood before radiographic examinations are attempted.

The choice of screen or non-screen film and the use of a grid are matters for the individual worker to decide.

With larger subjects there may be considerable scattered radiation when non-screen film is used, and although this effect can be minimized by using a grid, the exposure must then be increased. The tendency therefore, is to use intensifying screens, when the increased contrast will off-set the effect of scatter which would otherwise occur if non-screen film without a grid was used.

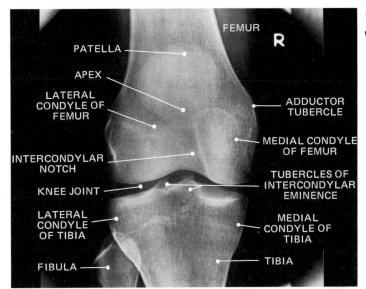

RIGHT KNEE
411

ANTERIOR-POSTERIOR

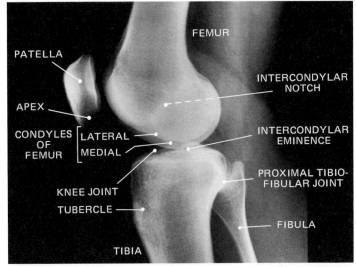

RIGHT KNEE
412

LATERAL

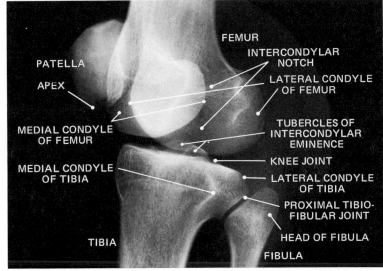

RIGHT KNEE
413

LATERAL OBLIQUE

Antero-posterior (basic)

With the patient supine or sitting on the couch with a back rest, the knee is relaxed. It may be necessary to rotate the leg slightly outward to centralize the patella over the femur, the limb being held in position by sandbags.

■ Centre 2 cm (1 ins) below the apex (lower level) of the patella (414, 415)

With slight flexion at the joint or by angling the tube 5° upward the central ray is parallel to the joint surfaces showing the true width of the joint.

Knee							
kVp		mAS			Film	Screens	
AP	Lat	AP	Lat	FFD	ILFORD	ILFORD	Grid
60	60	24	24	100 cm (40")	R	HD	

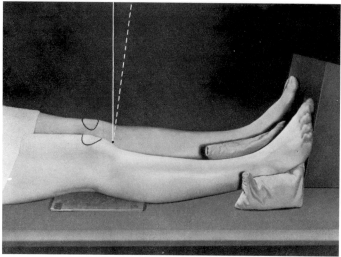

414

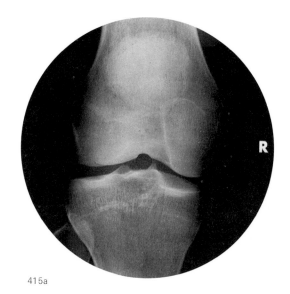

415a

Lateral (basic)—Medio-Lateral

To obtain a true lateral projection the operator must appreciate the general relationship of bone and articular surfaces entering into the joint. When the subject is erect the femur is oblique in direction from hip to knee joint, lateral to medial, (415b). Since the articular surfaces of the knee joint are horizontal they are not at right angles to the shaft of the femur. These facts will help the operator to place the knee in the true lateral position so that the condyles are superimposed and the patella seen in profile.

The patient is turned on to the affected side, with the limb flexed at hip and knee; the sound leg is brought well forward and raised on a sandbag in front of the injured limb (416). The ankle on the injured side is raised on small sandbags to bring the long axis of the tibia parallel to the film. Finally, the transverse axis of the patella should be at right angles to the film.

■ Centre over the anterior border of the medial condyle of the tibia which can be felt as a prominent ridge approximately 2 cm (1 in) below and medial to the lower border of the patella when the knee is flexed (416, 417)

Note—On occasion both medio-lateral (416) and latero-medial (418) projections are recommended.

Lateral—Latero-Medial

The patient is turned on the unaffected side with the limb flexed at the hip and knee and with the sound leg brought well forward, the film is raised in contact with the knee. Support is provided at the ankle.

■ Centre to the lateral condyle of the tibia

Note—In cases of fracture of a femur or tibia a lateral view of the knee must be taken using a horizontal ray.

3

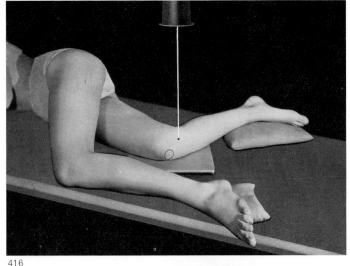

416

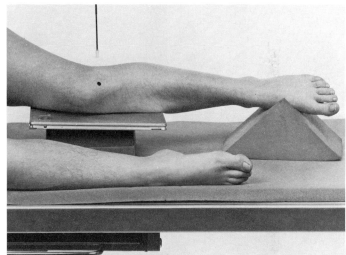

418

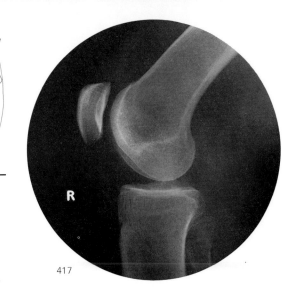

415b

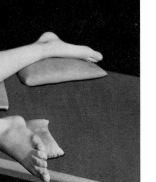

417

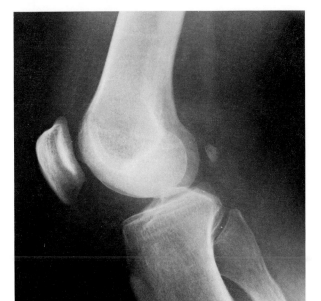

419

109

Tibial Tubercle

For the routine antero-posterior and lateral projections the tube is centred over the knee joint, but when the radiograph is taken specifically for the tibial tubercle exposures are made of each side in turn.

■ Centre over the tibial tubercle (420)

Note—The adjusted lateral centring for the tubercle tends to give a slightly oblique projection of the joint (420).

Sesamoid Bones: Patella, Fabella

The patella is the largest of the sesamoid bones and is developed in the quadriceps femoris muscle. Occasionally another sesamoid appears near to the knee joint—the fabella, which develops in the outer head of the gastrocnemius muscle. In the lateral projection it appears on the posterior aspect and adjacent to the femoral condyle (421). Although not always visible in the antero-posterior projection (422), the fabella may be seen overshadowing and adjacent to the border of the lateral condyle (422,423).

Lateral—Patient Supine
Latero-Medial

In cases of patella fracture, particularly when the fragments are separated by opposing muscle pull, (425), tension is kept to a minimum by examining the patient supine with the knee extended (424). For the lateral projection the cassette is placed vertically against the medial aspect of the joint and the tube lowered for horizontal projection.

For all fractures unnecessary manipulation of a limb must be avoided, the tube and film are placed in appropriate position usually with the patient supine.

(425) shows a fracture of the patella before and after treatment with a wire suture to maintain the fragments in apposition.

Note—(424) shows a bandage twisted round the foot, with the ends weighted by small sandbags to immobilize the leg. Small pads under the knee and heel are used to help relaxation.

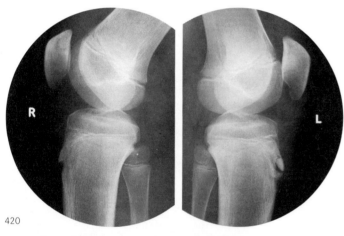

420

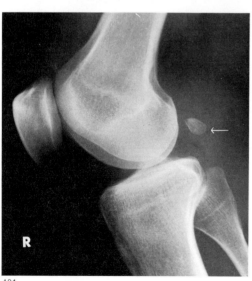

421

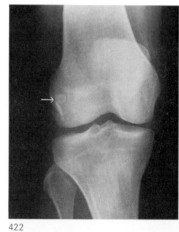

422

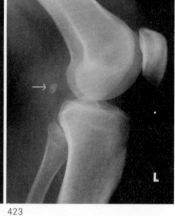

423

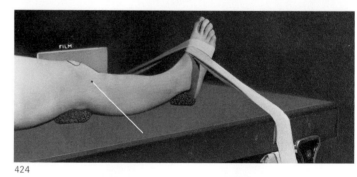

424

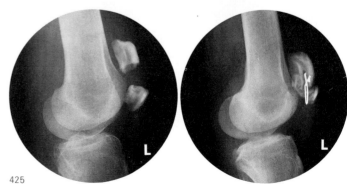

425

Postero-Anterior Patella

This position may be used for a doubtful fracture of the patella. Close contact with the film gives a sharply defined image (427). An increase of 75% on the antero-posterior knee exposure time is essential to show bone detail in the patella. Postero-anterior radiograph (427) should be compared with antero-posterior radiographs (429).

With the patient in the prone position, the knee is slightly flexed by placing a small sandbag beneath the thigh, preventing uncomfortable pressure of the patella on the couch; in addition, a sandbag under the ankle joint raises the toes and adds considerably to the patient's comfort.

■ Centre to the crease of the knee (426, 427)

Antero-posterior

When the knee is too painful for the postero-anterior position a satisfactory result will be obtained with the antero-posterior projection provided:

(a) the focal spot is no greater than 1 mm,

or alternatively,

(b) the focus film distance is increased to 127 cm (48 ins).

The exposure must be increased by 15 kVp compared with the antero-posterior knee (basic) for adequate penetration of the patella through the femur. The leg should be rotated slightly outwards to centre the patella over the femur.

■ Centre 2·5 cm (1 in) below the apex of the patella with the tube vertical (428, 429).

Patella Postero-Anterior

kVp	mAS	FFD	Film ILFORD	Screens ILFORD	Grid
65	24	100 cm (40″)	RAPID R	SUPER HD	—

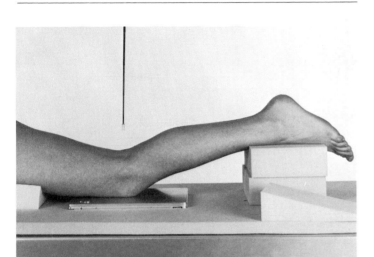

426

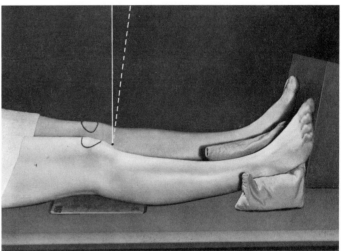

428

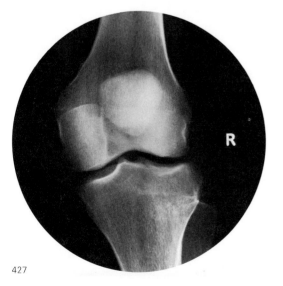

427

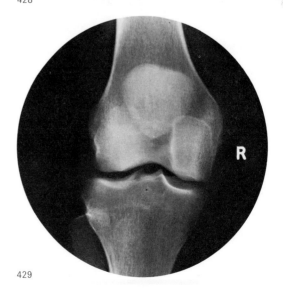

429

Infero-superior

(1) The patient is prone, with right-angled flexion at the knee joint. The limb is steadied by a band round the ankle, which is attached by its free ends to a vertical support. Both knees may be positioned similarly for simultaneous exposure.

■ Centre behind the patella, with the tube angled approximately 15° toward the knee to avoid the toes (430, 432)

(2) With the patient sitting on a couch with the knees flexed, the film is placed on the anterior aspect of the lower thigh and held by the patient over a 45° pad, (or held in position by a long arm cassette holder) (431). The tube is lowered to the appropriate distance and, just avoiding the feet, is angled upwards toward the knee.

■ Centre with the central ray passing immediately behind the patella parallel to its long axis; the cassette must be perpendicular to the central ray with the appropriate right and left letters on the film. The infero-superior projection (434) shows a minor fracture of the patella without displacement of the fragment and could not be shown in the usual antero-posterior and lateral projections.

Patella Infero-superior

kVp	mAS	FFD	Film ILFORD	Screens ILFORD	Grid
65	24	100 cm (40″)	RAPID R	SUPER HD	—

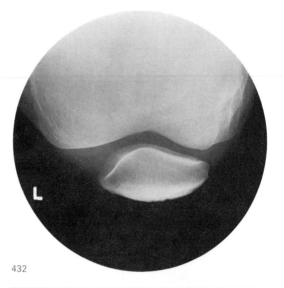

432

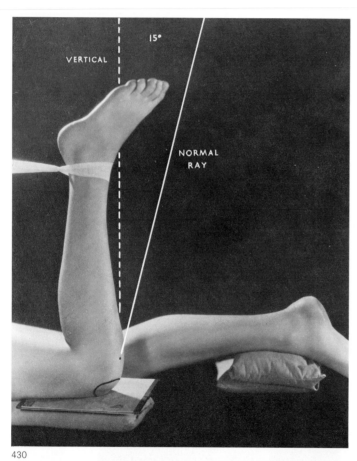

430

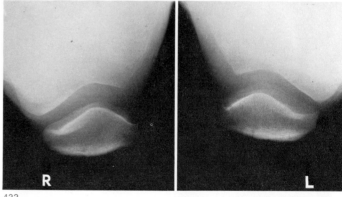

433

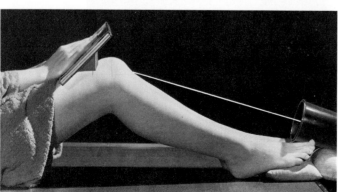

431

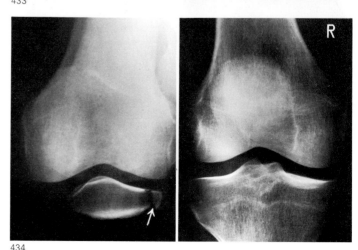

434

Oblique

The lateral and medial oblique positions of the knee joint whether done postero-anteriorly or antero-posteriorly are not used routinely but may be required for special purposes, e.g. to show the shadow of the patella separate from the femur for small fissure fractures or for pneumoarthrography and arthrography to demonstrate the semilunar cartilages. (Pages 116–118).

Oblique—Postero-anterior

With the patient prone an exposure is first made with the limb rotated laterally, and then medially to approximately 45°. For slight flexion at the knee joint place a sandbag under the ankle.

■ Centre over the patella at the level of the crease of the knee on its posterior aspect; each half of the patella is shown in turn separated from the base of the femur. (435, 436a,b).

Oblique—Antero-posterior

When the antero-posterior oblique positions are used for pneumoarthrography three similar projections are made for each semilunar cartilage. Refer to page 116.

3

Patella Oblique

kVp	mAS	FFD	Film ILFORD	Screens ILFORD	Grid
65	10	100 cm (40″)	RAPID R	SUPER HD	—

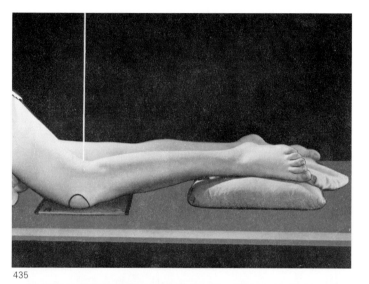

435

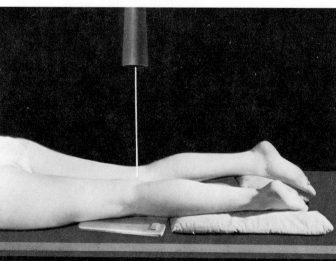

437

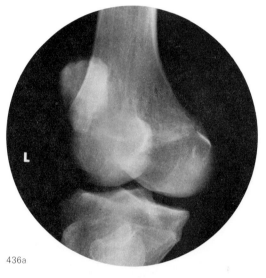

436a

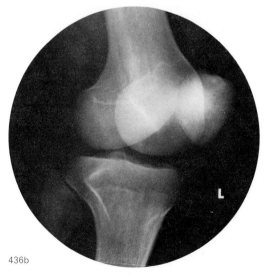

436b

Intercondylar Notch

Views of the intercondylar notch are taken for loose bodies (440) and for a fracture (441) in this region. To show the full axial extent of the notch, two projections are necessary to include the anterior and the posterior aspects.

The knee is flexed over an angle block and a small non-screen film is placed well up under the femur to allow for displacement due to angulation of the X-ray tube (438, 439a,b).

■ Centre immediately below the lower level of the patella with the tube angled towards the knee and the axial ray directed
(a) at 110° to the lower leg to show the anterior portion of the intercondylar notch,
and
(b) at 90° to the lower leg to show the posterior margin of the notch (438, 439a,b, 440).

Abnormality

An abnormality of the intercondylar notch is shown in the two projections (440) and a fracture in (441).

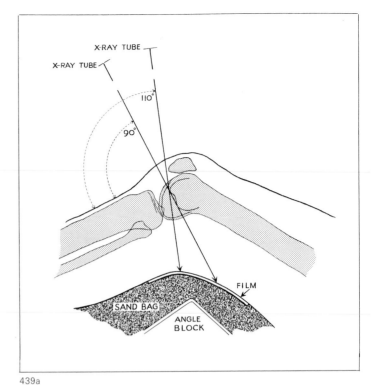

439a

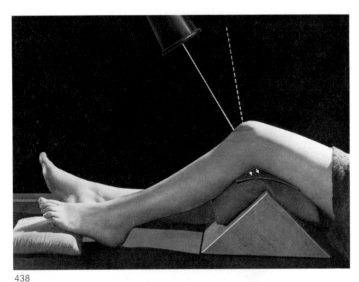

438

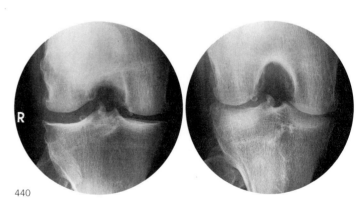

439b

110° ANGLE   90° ANGLE

440

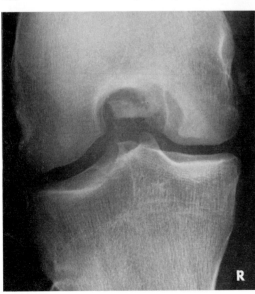

441

Intercondylar Notch

kVp	mAS	FFD	Film ILFORD	Screens ILFORD	Grid
65	30	100 cm (40″)	RAPID R	SUPER HD	—

Subluxation at Knee Joint
Lateral

To demonstrate subluxation at the knee joint use either the gravity effect on a stretched tendon (443) or the weight pressure effect (444).

(1) With the patient supine the leg is raised and supported at the ankle joint in a relaxed state, the film is placed vertically in contact with the medial aspect of the knee.

■ Centre with a horizontal ray to the middle of the lateral aspect of the knee joint (442, 443).

Note—Radiographs (443) show the unusual backward curve of a subluxation as compared with the normal appearance in (417).

(2) With the patient standing, the sound limb is placed in a forward relaxed position and the affected limb a little behind takes the full weight of the body. The cassette is supported vertically against the lateral aspect of the knee joint.

■ Centre with a horizontal ray to the middle of the medial aspect of the knee joint (444).

Subluxation							
kVp		mAS			Film	Screens	
AP	Lat	AP	Lat	FFD	ILFORD	ILFORD	Grid
65	65	24	24	100 cm (40″)	RAPID R	SUPER HD	—

Antero-posterior

Radiograph (445) shows a medial subluxation. The exposure was made with forced abduction to produce widening of the joint space resulting from the injury to medial collateral and anterior-cruciate ligaments. The technique is described in connection with pneumoarthrography on page 117.

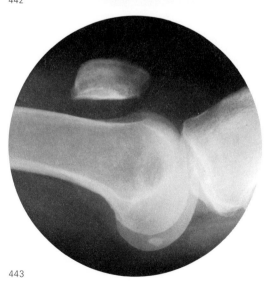

442

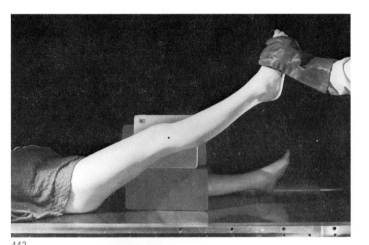

443

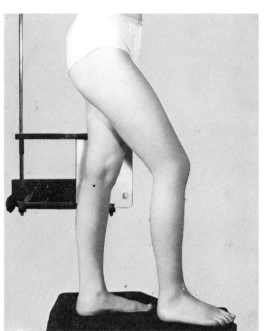

444

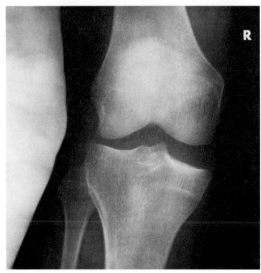

445

Semilunar Cartilages (menisci)

Although the supine position may be used the prone position is preferred by some workers and not infrequently radiographs are taken in both the supine and prone positions, particularly for double contrast arthrography.

After initial viewing on the image intensifier with the patient in the prone position and the knee slightly flexed the level of the joint is marked on the skin for guidance in centring.

Using lead letters, R or L to indicate medial or lateral cartilage, and using appropriate figures for identification, three radiographs are taken of each cartilage in the following order:
(1) postero-anterior with medial rotation (446),
(2) postero-anterior (447),
(3) postero-anterior with lateral rotation (448);
three exposures of each meniscus are made on one 24 × 30 cm (12 × 10 ins) film.

The tube is centred over the cartilage concerned, medial or lateral, for the six postero-anterior projections. Part of the joint under examination being opened by forced abduction or adduction of the tibia on the femur. This manipulation imposes considerable strain on both the operator and the patient necessitating a short exposure time and good team work. Two or three additional exposures are also used—lateral with the knee flexed, either medio-lateral (449), which allows the air to rise and surround the medial cartilage, or latero-medial when the air rises to surround the lateral cartilage; also antero-posterior with the knee flexed as for the posterior intercondylar notch (450), which shows the cruciate ligaments (anterior and posterior) (454).

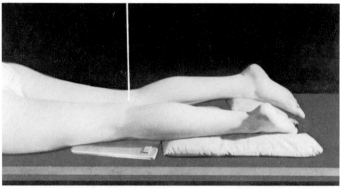

446

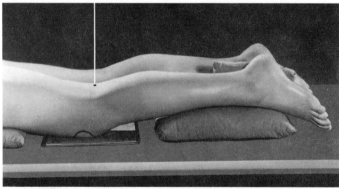

447

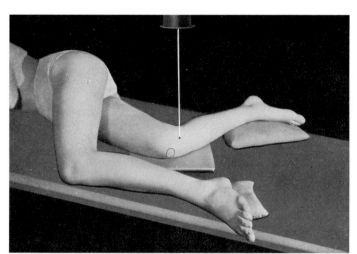

449

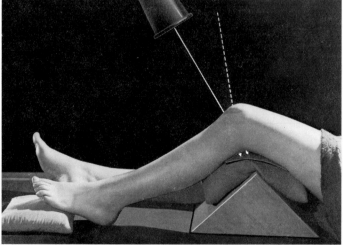

450

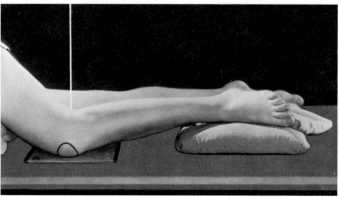

448

The two semilunar cartilages of the knee joint lie between the femoro-tibial condyles. The medial cartilage is C-shaped, and the lateral is more nearly circular: both are thicker at the outer border than at the inner. The medial cartilage is more firmly attached to adjacent structures than the lateral and therefore is more readily injured. Anterior and posterior cruciate ligaments may also need to be shown in this examination. These liagments are named cruciate because they cross each other as the arms of the letter X, extending between the condyles of the femur and the tibia.

For a slipped semilunar cartilage or other abnormality the radiographs are taken to show both bone and soft tissue and serve as a check for possible bony injury; but they will also demonstrate cartilage calcification when present (451).

The normal menisci are not seen except after injection of contrast medium into the joint. They will then appear lighter against an air injection (452) and darker against an injection of positive contrast medium (456). This examination is called arthrography. When air or oxygen is used the procedure is known as pneumoarthrography; when a water soluble contrast medium is injected the general term arthrography is used. However, the modern technique uses both gas and a positive contrast medium to produce the double contrast arthrogram. For pneumoarthrography about 80 to 140 millilitres of air or oxygen is injected into the joint space after adequate aseptic skin preparation. Immediately before the X-ray examination the supra-patellar pouch is compressed by placing an elastic bandage above the knee joint, thus forcing the oxygen in the supra-patellar pouch between the articular surfaces. This shows the light density cartilages against the very dark shadow of the oxygen (452). Considerable oxygen remains in the joint space six hours after injection.

The initial positioning must include three projections for each cartilage with a long localizing cone of 3 inch aperture close to the skin surface. Fine grain intensifying screens and a short exposure time are used with carefully selected exposure factors to give satisfactory definition and suitable contrast.

3

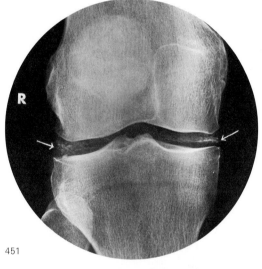

451

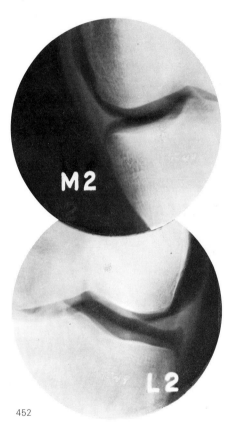

452

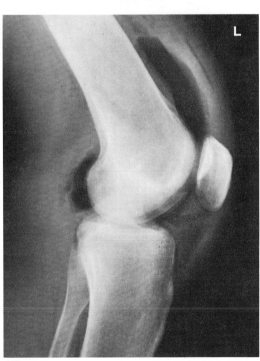

453

117

Semilunar Cartilages (menisci) (*continued*)

The two radiographs (452) show normal semilunar cartilages, M2, medial, and L2, lateral. Series (455) of the medial cartilage taken in the postero-anterior position—M1 with rotation inward, M2 without rotation, and M3 with rotation outward—show a tear through the body of the cartilage. These radiographs (452,455) selected from two original series were taken during the application of forced abduction and adduction to show the medial and lateral cartilages respectively.

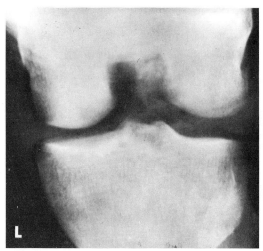

454

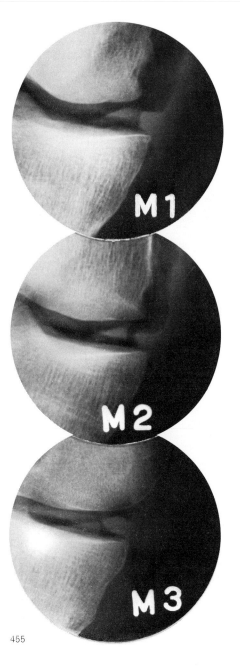

455

Arthrography

Adequate preparation of the skin is required.

If an excess of fluid is present in the joint it is aspirated. Using a water-soluble organic iodine contrast medium 4 to 10 millilitres of a 45% solution is injected from the lateral aspect of the joint.

After the injection the knee is put through a full range of movements several times so that the contrast medium can be distributed throughout the joint. A firm bandage for compression is placed above the patella and maintained there during the radiographic exposure. The routine six views for the menisci are then taken, three for each cartilage namely—antero-posterior with the leg straight; antero-posterior oblique with the leg rotated medially; antero-posterior with the leg rotated laterally. After these views the bandage is removed and then a postero-anterior with the knee slightly flexed, a lateral straight and a lateral with some flexion are taken.

Radiographs (456) show three of a series of exposures of the right knee made with the patient in the supine position, (a) antero-posterior with the limb straight; (b) oblique with the limb rotated medially; (c) oblique with the limb rotated laterally; and (457) lateral, (a) with the knee extended and (b) with slight flexion.

3

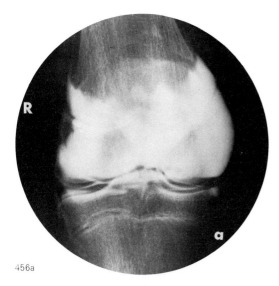

456a

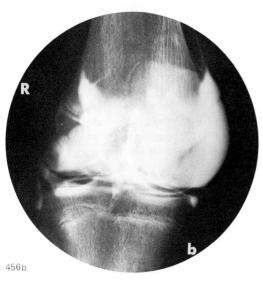

456b

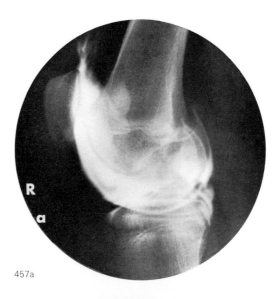

457a

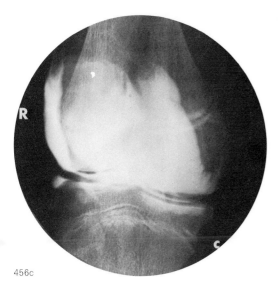

456c

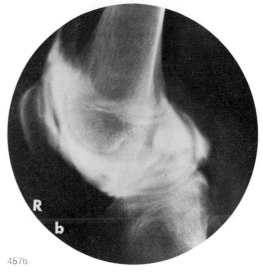

457b

Femur

Lower Two-Thirds
Radiation Protection
When the lower pelvis is included on a radiograph adequate radiation protection by the use of suitably shaped protective shields for the testes and ovaries is essential. Lead impregnated rubber sheeting with a lead equivalent of 2·0 mm is used. See pages 127, 128, for radiation protection when examining the hip joints.

Antero-posterior (basic)
With the patient supine the leg is rotated slightly outwards and the film placed well below the knee to include the joint.
■ Centre to the middle of the film (458,459)

Lateral (basic)
The patient is turned on to the affected side, with the knee flexed and the foot raised on a small sandbag. Support the sound limb either in front of or behind the injured limb. The film should be placed well below the knee again making sure that the knee joint will be included on the radiograph.
■ Centre to the middle of the film (460,461)

				Femur			
kVp		mAS			Film	Screens	
AP	Lat	AP	Lat	FFD	ILFORD	ILFORD	Grid
70–75	70–75	30	30	100 cm (40″)	RAPID R	SUPER HD	—

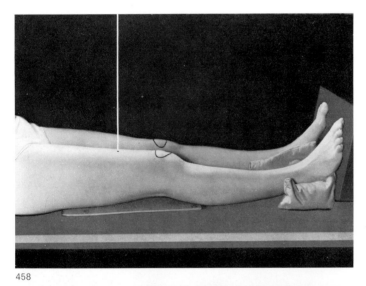

458

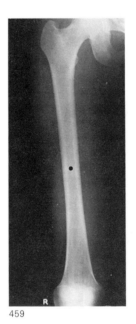

459

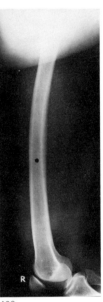

460

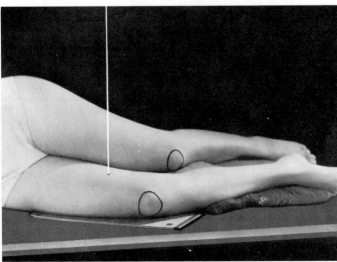

461

Stretcher patients

When the patient cannot be turned on to the side for a lateral projection, the sound limb is raised on a support, the film is placed vertically against the outer side of the injured thigh and a horizontal X-ray beam is projected to the inner side (462). This technique was used for the lateral projection showing a fracture of the lower third of the femur (463).

A diagram of a suitable support is shown in (466). A pad between the support and the limb is essential for the patient's comfort. The support is prevented from slipping forward by placing a sandbag on the cross-bar and also against its base. In many departments a foot-stool is used.

Amputations

The examination of a limb stump may present a special problem, as it is difficult to immobilize the limb in position. The bone may be rarefied; the degree of rarefication depends on the lapse of time since the amputation and the surrounding soft tissue may be less than is usual for the region. The exposure must be adjusted accordingly so that both the bone and the soft tissue are adequately shown.

Pads and sandbags are used to immobilize the stump and the adjacent joint as well as a Potter-Bucky compression band to prevent uncontrolled movements. Standard antero-posterior and lateral projections are taken (465). Special projections to show the cut ends of the bone using a tube tilt of approximately 30° may be required.

The exposure should be adjusted for good bone and soft tissue detail using a short exposure time.

3

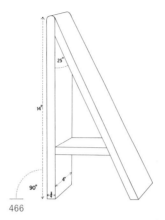

466

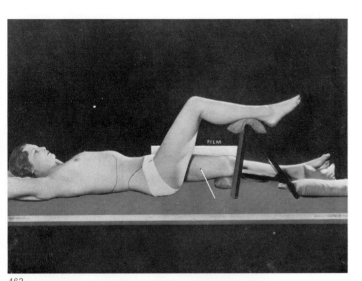

462

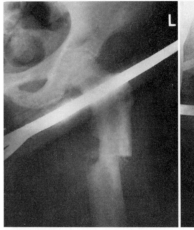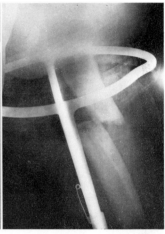

464

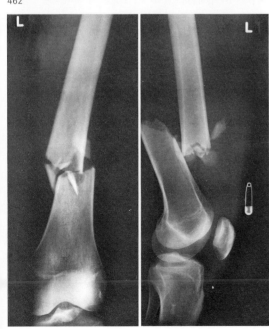

463

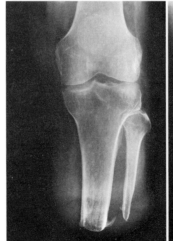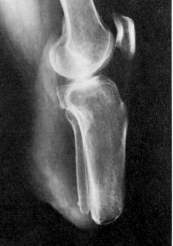

465

121

Measurement of length

In childhood, abnormality at the hip joint may lead to a severe handicap due to the shortening of a limb. To prevent disability due to the limbs being of unequal length, growth of the sound limb is arrested at the knee joint by the surgical insertion of four or more staples about the epiphyseal line, usually of the femur (471), but sometimes of the tibia (470). This retards the growth of the sound limb, giving it a similar length to that of the affected limb. Periodic X-ray examinations are required to record the comparative growth of the limbs.

Both limbs are radiographed simultaneously and geometric enlargement of the bone shadows is prevented by using a perpendicular X-ray beam centred over each joint in turn. The patient is supine, the limbs, as far as possible, in similar relationship to the pelvis; the feet are separated by approximately 6 inches. Two methods of carrying out this examination in the antero-posterior projection can be used, either by localized separate exposure or by a scanning technique.

Localized exposures

A 35 × 85 cm (14 × 36 ins) film is placed to include both limbs from the hip to the ankle joints, using a small tube aperture and centring directly over each of the joints in turn. Radiograph (467) shows that the relative level of right and left sides, for hips, knees and ankles, and the total length of the bones is indicated. If a long cassette is not available two 35 × 43 cm (14 × 17 ins) cassettes may be used. These are butted together to give the full length coverage as shown for the vertebral column, page 225. A clearly labelled radio-opaque ruler lies across the junction of the two cassettes to show the degree of overlap or separation for accurate measurement of the differences between the two radiographs. However, the two radiographs are usually joined together with sellotape for convenience of viewing and subsequent filing.

A scanning radiograph is preferable and is taken simultaneously of both limbs from hips to ankle joints; called a scanogram.

Note—In (467) the rings show the position of the localized exposure for each joint superimposed on a scanogram and a scanogram is shown in (470).

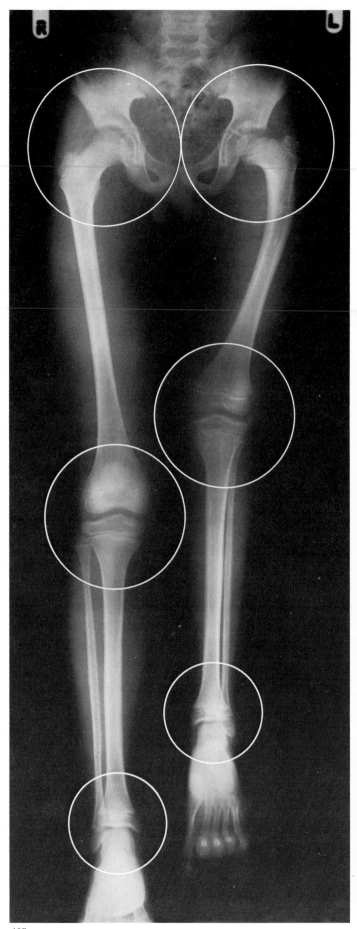

467

Scanography

A scanogram is a radiograph taken with a narrow aperture while the tube is moved the length of the cassette. Each small area is scanned briefly by the X-rays from the moving tube and differs from cineradiography since the exposure source moves along a stationary continuous film instead of the moving film being exposed frame by frame by a stationary X-ray tube.

The narrow tube-diaphragm aperture, 1/16th-inch in width at a focus-film of 100 cm (40 ins) or 1/8th-inch width at 85 cm (36 ins) to cover both limbs from side to side, is at right angles to the direction of the tube movement (468).

It is essential for the depth of the narrow diaphragm aperture to be at least double its width to avoid a penumbra effect (469). The two exposures (469) taken at 100 cm (40 ins) distance with a 1·5 mm (1/16th-in) aperture, show in (a) the result of an aperture depth of 1·5 mm (1/16th-in) with the accompanying penumbra and (b) the effect of an aperture depth of 3 mm (1/8th-in) being double the width of 1·5 mm (1/16th-in). The latter provides a well defined all-over density coverage so essential to the provision of a satisfactory scanogram.

continued overleaf

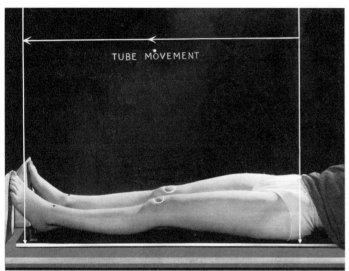

TUBE MOVEMENT

468

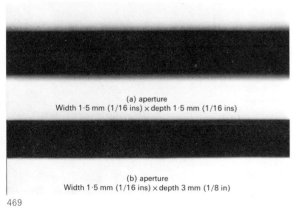

(a) aperture
Width 1·5 mm (1/16 ins) × depth 1·5 mm (1/16 ins)

(b) aperture
Width 1·5 mm (1/16 ins) × depth 3 mm (1/8 in)

469

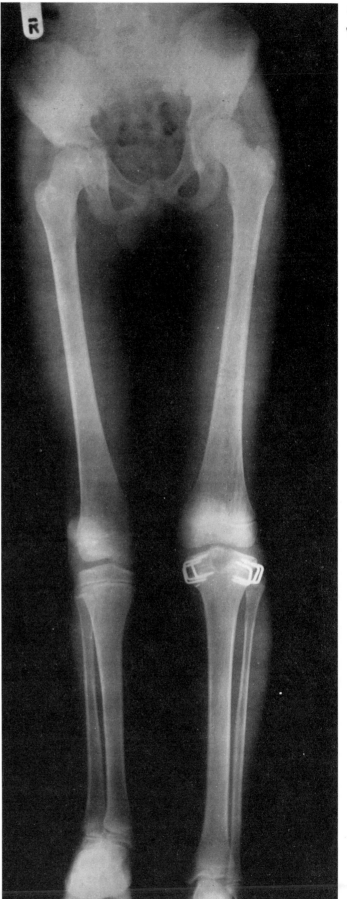

470

Scanography (*continued*)

A small ½ hp motor may be used to move the parallel tube stand along a floor rail. Alternatively, if movement of the X-ray couch, either as a whole or just the couch top, can cover the 85 cm (36 ins) distance required, combined movement of patient and film in relation to the stationary tube is simpler than installing a special small motor for moving the tube.

A uniform density from hip to ankle joints during an 8-second or 10-second run, is necessary and may be achieved by increasing the speed of the tube movement, or alternatively, the appropriate couch-patient-film movement, thus gradually reducing the exposure time—approximately 5 seconds from hip to knee joints and 3 seconds from knee to ankle joints. Manual control of timing and varying speed of movement is a matter of experience but quite readily achieved.

When a small motor is employed, the rate of tube movement can be automatically adjusted by means of a differential speed ratio control, providing both a slower movement for the thicker parts from hip to knee joints, and the faster movement which is required for the smaller lower limbs from knee to ankle joints.

Alternatively, the milliamperage may be modified at pre-arranged intervals, so that either way the milliampere seconds are reduced appropriately to give a uniform density over the lower limbs. For a child of ten years, at 65 kVp and 100 cm (40 ins) focus-film distance, the total exposure is for 10 seconds, using Rapid R film and Standard Tungstate screens. When current is the variable factor the milliamperes are gradually adjusted from 100 to 20; thus 100 mA at the hip joint, 75 mA at mid thigh, 50 mA at the knee joint and 20 mA at the ankle joint.

On the other hand, a piece of washed-off film base placed in the half of the cassette relating to the lower leg, achieves the necessary reduction in density by limiting the effective fluorescence, thus providing the over-all density required without the necessity of using manual, motorized or electric control of the rate of movement.

The procedure can be simplified by using graduated intensifying screens with the fastest point of the screen placed under the hip joint and the slowest point under the ankle joints. The exposure is then kept constant at approximately 65 kV, 100 mA and 100 cm focus-film distance. Radiograph (471) shows surgical staples across the epiphysis of the femur for prevention of growth on the left side in an attempt to equalize the length of the limbs.

Note—Unless there is a smooth movement of tube or couch a stroboscopic effect is produced (471).

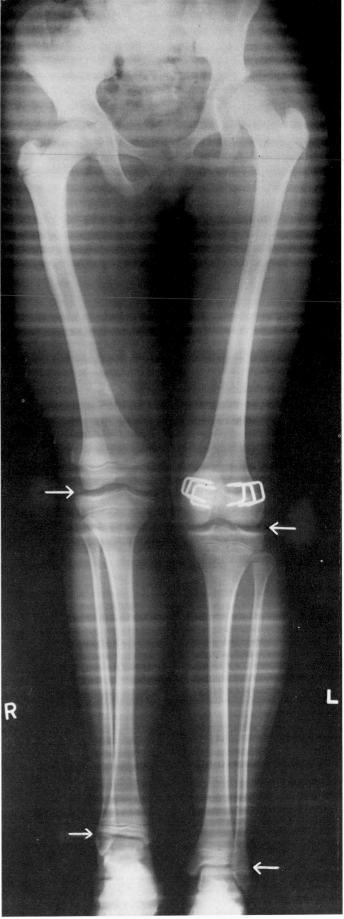

471

4

HIP JOINT AND UPPER THIRD OF FEMUR

SECTION 4

HIP JOINT AND UPPER THIRD OF FEMUR

The hip joint is a ball and socket joint in which the smooth, almost spherical head of the femur articulates with the acetabulum which is formed by the three parts of the innominate or hip bone on the lateral aspect of the pelvis. The proximal end of the femur consists of head, elongated neck and greater and lesser trochanters.

Radiographic appearances
Three, lettered radiographs showing two projections of the hip joint, antero-posterior (473), lateral (474), and lateral of the neck of the femur (475) will help the student to follow the anatomical references in the text.

Radiation protection
Close coning of the hip joint is acceptable for some examinations otherwise suitable protective shields for males and females, which vary in size according to the patient's age should be used. Protection of the gonads is generally provided by lead rubber of thickness equivalent to about 2 mm of lead. Examples are shown for male and female subjects (476, 478, 479). For purposes of hygiene the shields are covered with a plastic washable material. For male subjects a rectangular shield (477a) usually with a slightly larger base, is placed with the smaller upper end just above the symphysis pubis. The larger end is attached to a bar of stiff plastic material which is placed

across the thighs (478a). The dimensions shown are for an adult subject to give ample protection. Examples of shields for use on infants and children are shown in (476a, 478a, 479a). The shield (477b) may also be used in males in the reverse direction at the appropriate level.

For females the applicator is roughly triangular with a convex upper surface (477b) which is placed with its widest diameter at the level of the anterior superior iliac spines and with the blunt apex below the symphysis pubis. Dimensions are given for a female of 16 years (477b) and for an infant (477c). The shield is shown in position in radiographs (476b, 478b, 479b), and provide essential protection of the female gonads.

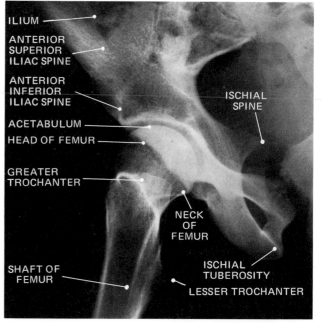

RIGHT HIP
474

LATERAL

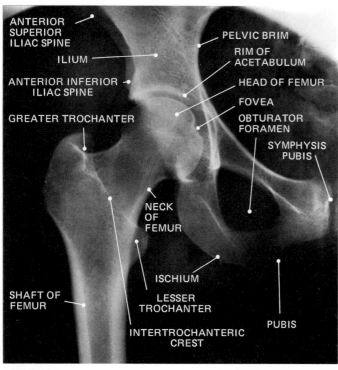

RIGHT HIP
473

ANTERO-POSTERIOR

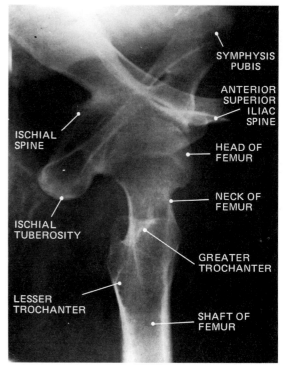

NECK OF LEFT FEMUR
475

LATERAL

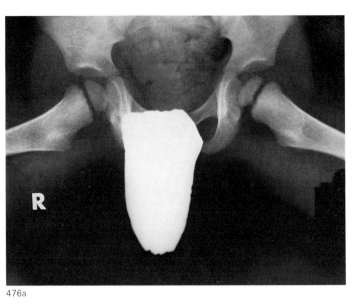

476a

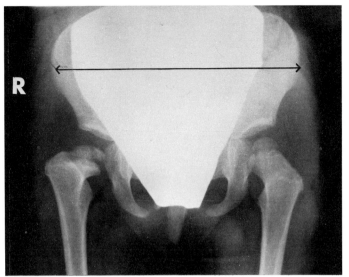

476b

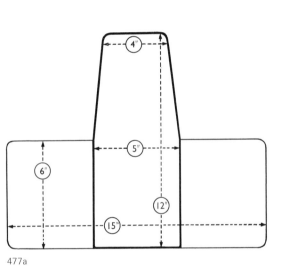

477a

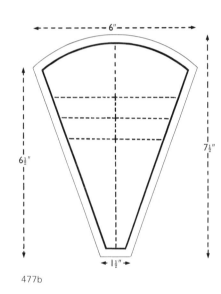

477b

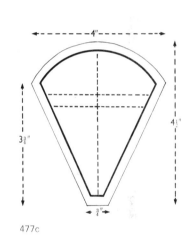

477c

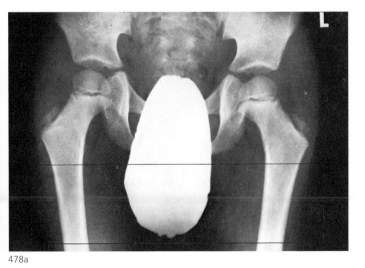

478a

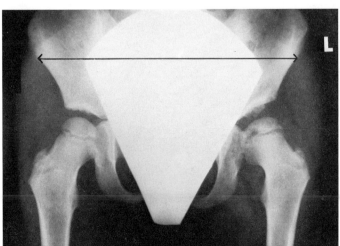

478b

General and technical

Radiographs of the hip joint should include the upper third of the femur, and the pelvis from the level of the anterior-superior iliac spine downwards to show the ischium and pubic bone. Antero-posterior projections are usually made of both hips simultaneously for comparison. Lateral projections are taken as required; in addition, tomography may be used.

Ideally, the pelvis must be placed symmetrically on the couch but where there is wasting of the buttock or swelling on one side, then the pelvis will need to be tilted to compensate and maintained in that position to obtain acceptable radiographs. The alignment of the pelvis may be checked either manually or by using a spirit level between the anterior-superior iliac spine (480).

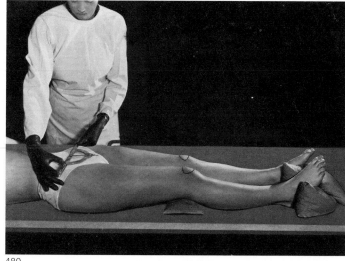

480

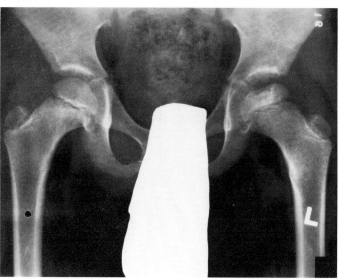

479a

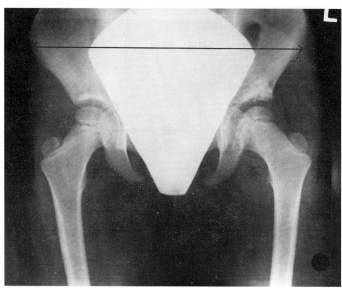

479b

Technical

In examining the hip joint, the use of intensifying screens and a moving or stationary grid is essential. The exposure factors refer to an adult subject of average physique.

Basic positions

The initial routine projections are indicated as (Basic) and several variations are included to show the more difficult projections for lateral positioning particularly in complex abnormalities. A special technique for the neck of the femur from the lateral aspect for use in the operating theatre during a pinning and/or plating operation is given under a separate heading.

Effect of rotation of limb

Rotation of the whole limb on its long axis occurs at the hip joint, the position of the foot usually indicating the relationship between head and neck of femur and the acetabulum. In cases of trauma to the hip joint the position of the foot is a significant clue to the type of injury. The varying radiographic appearances of the hip joint as the limb is rotated medially or laterally can be anticipated by the position of the foot.

With medial rotation the femoral neck is elongated and less oblique in direction, as compared with the foot in a forward position. The greater trochanter is rotated forward, and the lesser trochanter backward being obscured by the shaft of the femur (481,482).

With lateral rotation the femoral neck appears foreshortened and more oblique in direction. The greater trochanter is obliquely over-shadowed by the neck, and the lesser trochanter becomes conspicuous (483,484).

The commonly used position is with the feet straight forward (485,486).

The appearance of the femur also varies with the centring point, whether centred over the femoral head for one hip (500,502), or in the mid line for both hips (488,489).

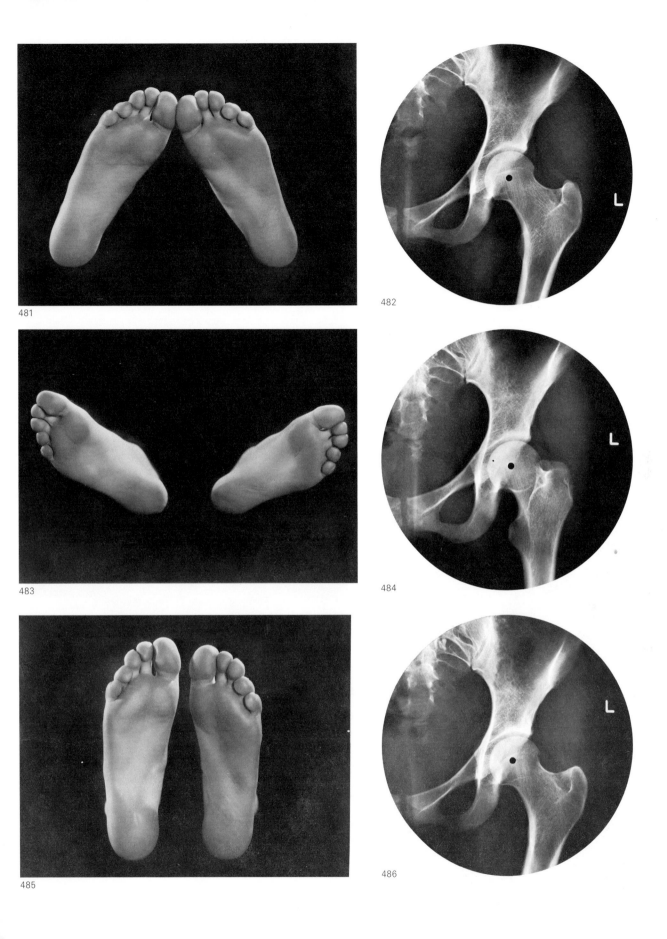

481

482

483

484

485

486

4 Hip joint and upper third of femur

Antero-posterior—Both Hips (basic)

For purposes of comparison it is preferable to include both hips on the same film; especially for Shenton's line (489) and in children to assess small differences in contrast and density which may indicate early disease.

The patient is supine and the pelvis is adjusted so that the transverse plane is parallel to the film. This position may be checked by placing a spirit level across the anterior superior iliac spines; or, with a thumb on each iliac spine and the fingers in contact with the couch, the pelvis is rotated into the correct position and kept there with non-opaque pads. It is important for the pelvis to be central to the couch and film, the film being large enough to include both trochanters. Take care that the radiation protective devices are correctly adjusted. Both feet are sandbagged in similar positions, preferably with the longitudinal axis of the soles of the feet at right angles to the couch and the heels slightly apart (485, 487).

The depression over the greater trochanter on the lateral aspect of the thigh indicates the approximate level of the joint and is at the upper border of the symphysis pubis.

■ Centre for both hips in the mid line, approximately 5 cm (2 ins) below the level of the anterior, superior iliac spines, corresponding to the trochanteric depression, or 2·5 cm (1 in) above the upper border of the symphysis pubis (488, 489)

Note—A line following the curve of the lower border of the superior pubic ramus and the inferior border of the femoral neck (Shenton's line) (489) is used to compare the two sides of the pelvis in the event of an injury (490) or congenital dislocation of the hip.

The patient with a fracture of the neck of the left femur (radiograph 490) would maintain his left leg in lateral rotation as in (483) and it must not be moved for the radiograph.

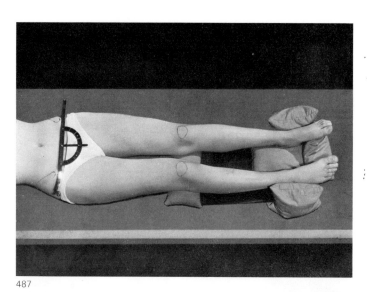

487

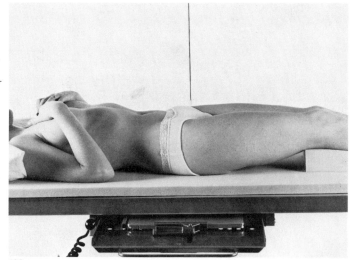

488

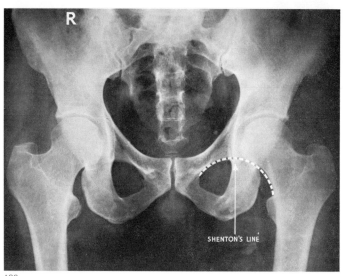

SHENTON'S LINE

489

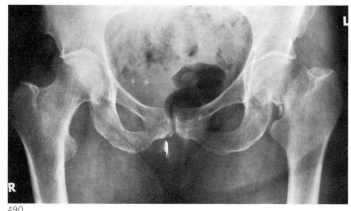

490

Hip AP

kVp	mAS	FFD	Film ILFORD	Screens ILFORD	Grid
70	60	100 cm (40″)	RAPID R	FT	GRID

130

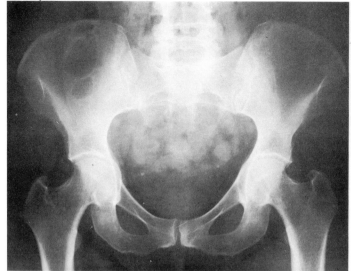

491

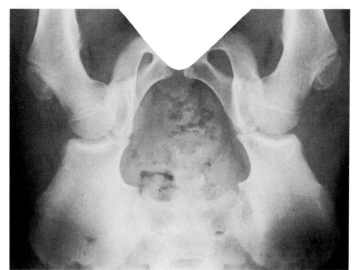

492

(491) Normal pelvis of adult female.
(492) Normal pelvis of adult male.
(493a) Normal pelvis of adolescent male.
(493b) "Frog" view to show lateral aspects
of neck and head of femurs.

493(a)

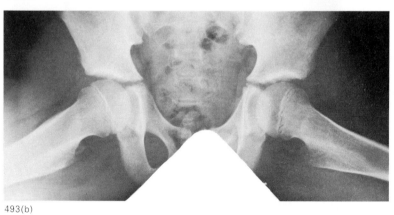

493(b)

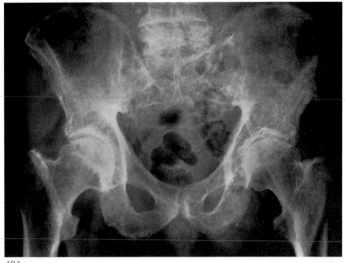

494

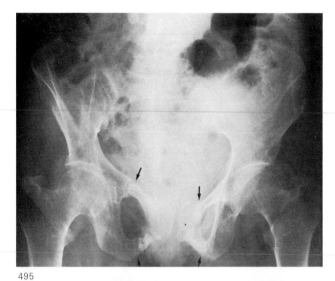

495

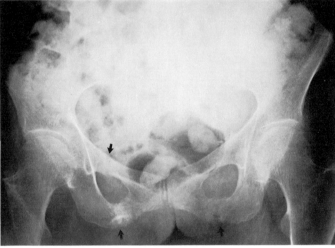

496(a)

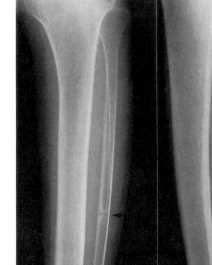

496(b)

(494) Pagets' Disease of left hemi pelvis.
(495) Osteomalacia with Loosers Zones (arrows).
(496a) Osteomalacia with Loosers Zones (arrows).
(496b) AP and Lat. views of leg with Loosers Zone (arrows).

Antero-posterior—Single Hip (basic)

As with the antero-posterior (basic) view for both hips and the pelvis, the limbs are symmetrical, and the transverse plane parallel to the film, but the hip to be examined is central to the couch. Both feet are immobilized as in (487). A small aperture cone to include only the one side is used. The position of the joint may be localized by two methods, (a) the position of the depression over the greater trochanter indicates the level of the lower acetabulum. At this level centre to a point midway between the inner and outer margins of the thigh. (b) Draw a line between the anterior, superior iliac spine and the upper border of the symphysis pubis; then draw a second line perpendicular to the first at its mid point. Centre along this second line 2 cm (¾-in) below the point of the intersection (497, 498) and the second point lies over the middle of the head of the femur.

■ Centre as for method (a) or (b) (497, 498, 499)

Injuries

(503) shows a separated bone fragment of the acetabulum after reduction of an upward dislocation at the hip joint.

A fracture of the neck of the femur causes lateral rotation of the limb (483) which must not be placed in the normally correct

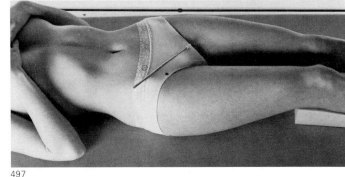

497

position with the toes pointing forward (485). The sound limb should therefore be placed in similar lateral rotation (483) so that the two sides are comparable.

For thin subjects with little overlying soft tissue the greater trochanter may well be over-exposed on the radiograph, showing as a completely blackened area, in sharp contrast to the main bone structures (501a) and may be corrected by using a high kilovoltage (501b) or by reducing the subject's contrast by exposing through a lead filter sheet of thickness 0·0015 inch placed over the film-cassette.

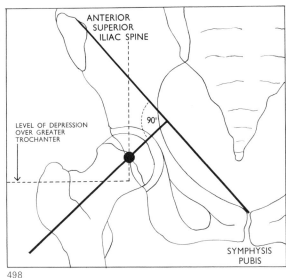

498

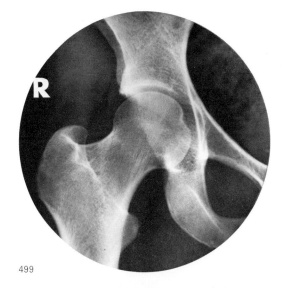

499

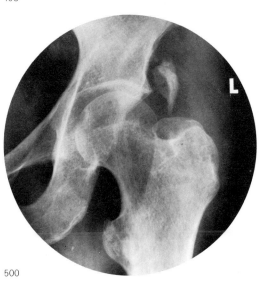

500

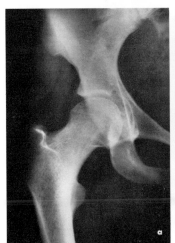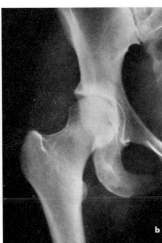

501

Lateral—Single Hip (basic)

When able to be moved without discomfort, the patient is turned on to the affected side with the hip joint in the middle of the table and flexion at hip and knee joints. The pelvis is rotated 45° backwards with the good limb raised and supported in a comfortable position.

■ Centre to the hip joint (501, 502, 503)

In this projection the lateral margin of the pelvis, the acetabulum, the head and neck of the femur, the greater trochanter and the upper third of the shaft of the femur are visible.

Hip Ob/Lat

kVp	mAS	FFD	Film ILFORD	Screens ILFORD	Grid
70	60	100 cm (40″)	RAPID R	FT	Grid

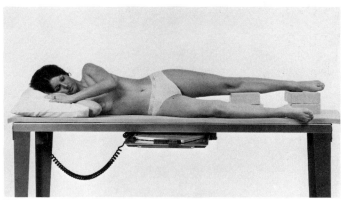

502

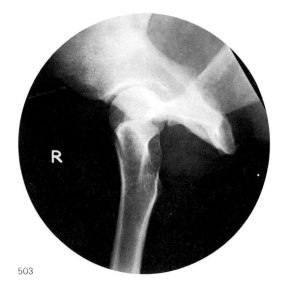

503

Lateral—Both Hips (basic)

When both hips are freely mobile they may be exposed simultaneously (1) for the general lateral projection (507) and (2) for lateral projection of the femur (513). In both instances similar results are obtained to those shown for the single hip.

General lateral (1)

The patient is supine, the shoulders raised on pillows and the hips and knees are flexed. With lateral rotation at the hip joints through approximately 60°, the knees are separated to bring the soles of the feet together (504); the limbs are steadied with non-opaque pads and sandbags under the thighs producing what is aptly described as the "frog position."

■ Centre between the hip joints (504, 505, 507)

Diagram (505) shows the position of the limbs for the general projection with the modified position for the neck of the femur (508) indicated by broken lines.

Note—(507) shows a simultaneous exposure of a normal hip on the right side and an abnormal condition on the left, providing a satisfactory comparison with the antero-posterior radiograph (506).

Neck of Femur (2)

The same technique of simultaneous lateral projection of right and left hips may be used for the neck of the femur.

With the patient in the supine position, the hips and knees are flexed and the limbs are rotated laterally through 15°. The feet are placed side by side, plantar surface to couch. A sandbag against the toes prevents the feet from slipping.

■ Centre between the hip joints (508, 509, 510)

Diagram (509) shows the position of the limbs for this projection with the previous projection (507) indicated by a broken line.

Hip Lat Frog

kVp	mAS	FFD	Film ILFORD	Screens ILFORD	Grid
70	70	100 cm (40″)	RAPID R	FT	Grid

Note—Radiographs (510, 511) compare the two position respectively (508, 509).

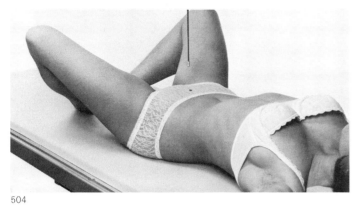

504

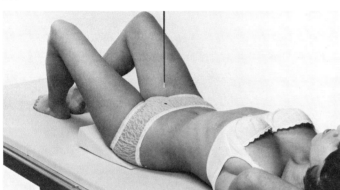

505

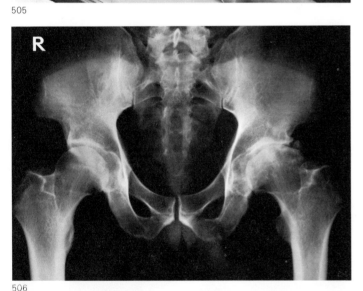

506

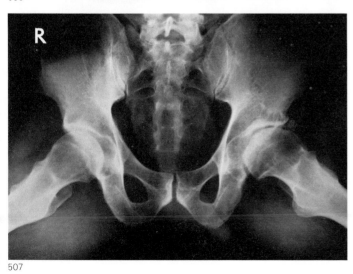

507

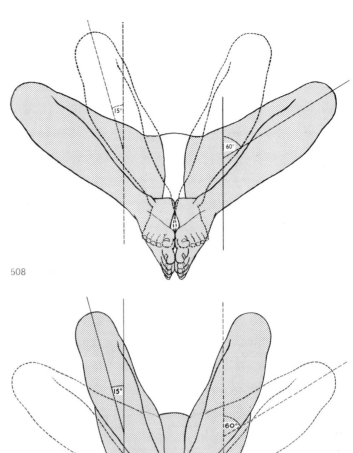

508

509

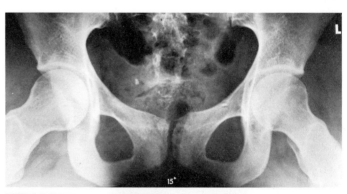

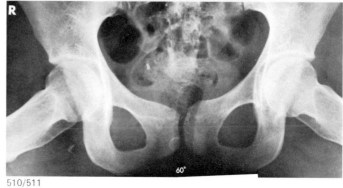

510/511

Abnormalities

Radiographs (512, 513) are the views which are usually done to exclude a minimal subcapital fracture of the neck of the femur which may only be seen in the lateral projection. Radiographs (514, 515) show an exostosis which is projected over the neck of the femur in the antero-posterior view but its true nature is only indicated on the lateral view.

Severe osteo-arthritis of the hip may require the introduction of a prosthesis which is shown in (516, 517). An opaque metal cup has been fitted over the head of the femur. Radiographs (518, 519) show a transradiant plastic cup allowing adjacent bone to be seen on the radiograph but strengthened by metal cross-wires to indicate its position. In all these conditions, two projections, antero-posterior and lateral are essential for the examination.

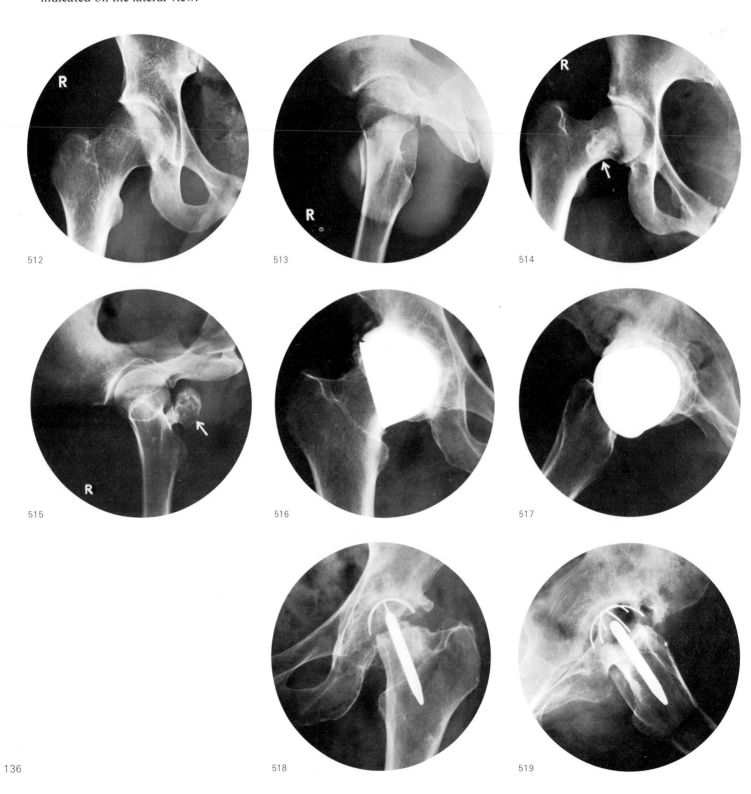

512

513

514

515

516

517

518

519

Stretcher and ward patients

In many instances it is not advisable to move the patient from the stretcher trolley, while in others the examination is made in the ward. In either case the patient remains supine during the complete examination. Both projections may be taken with the mobile unit and a stationary grid is an asset in these circumstances.

Patients referred from the Accident and Emergency department are frequently fully clad and opacities in the clothing may obscure important parts on the film. In raising the pelvis to remove the clothing and to place the film in position great care should be taken to support the injured limb.

Antero-posterior

The antero-posterior view in emergency cases is done using the projection on page 130 (488, 520).

Lateral—Upper third of femur

The film-cassette is placed against the lateral aspect of the thigh well above the hip joint, the sound limb being raised and supported. With a horizontal ray the tube is centred to the medial aspect of the upper third of the shaft of the femur, and is directed obliquely towards the joint.

Satisfactory projections are obtained of the neck and upper third of the shaft of the femur (521, 522). Radiographs (523) show an intertrochanteric fracture of the neck of the femur and were taken antero-posterior (a) as in (520) and lateral (b) as in (521).

Lat Neck Femur

kVp	mAS	FFD	Film ILFORD	Screens ILFORD	Grid
75	80	100 cm (40″)	RAPID R	FT	Stat

Note—The lateral projection of the hip joint is part of a routine examination as for other joints.

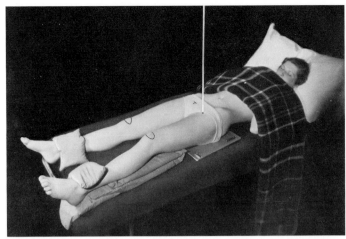

520

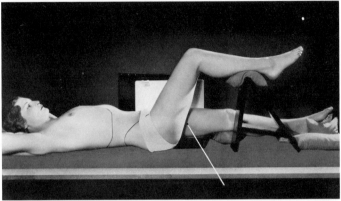

521

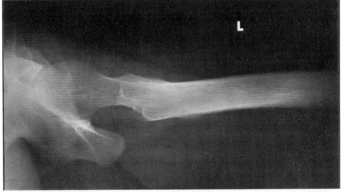

522

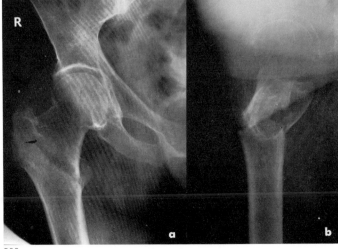

523

Conditions requiring modification in technique

In radiographing a diseased hip, with the affected side fixed in position, it is usual to take both hips for comparison, with both limbs equally abducted (524).

In other circumstances the sound limb is placed in the normal position with the pelvis symmetrical (525). Where the differences in bone density are important both hips must be exposed simultaneously and this also applies in the follow up examinations of slipped epiphysis (526).

Follow up examinations over a long period should be of the same quality, and with comparable positioning of limbs and pelvis. There is no excuse for distorted projection of the pelvis even under the conditions suggested in (525), but where a malformation is present whether congenital or acquired, tomograms may be required (527). To include the whole of the upper third of the femur where there is a dislocation at the hip joint, the film must be at a higher level (528), although centring for follow up examinations should be at the normal hip level.

The exposure factors must be tailored to the individual

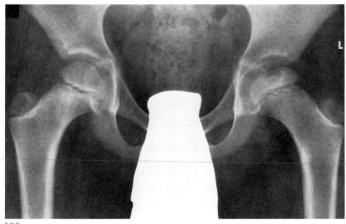
526

patient and examination, for example, where there is loss of bone calcium following a long period of bed rest, a lower exposure is required as compared with the original exposure otherwise the film will be over-exposed.

Hips treated on extension frames or in plaster of Paris present special radiographic problems, particularly for the lateral view. When both hips are in abduction in plaster, it is not possible to obtain a satisfactory lateral projection using the lateral (basic) position.

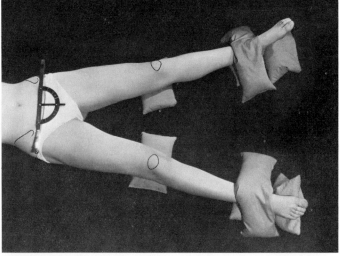
524

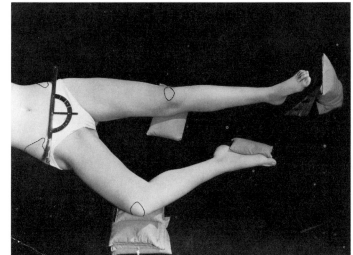
525

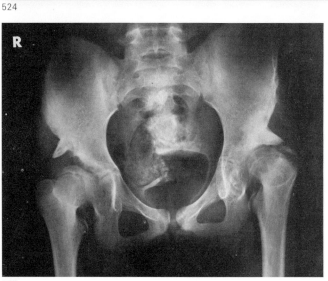
527

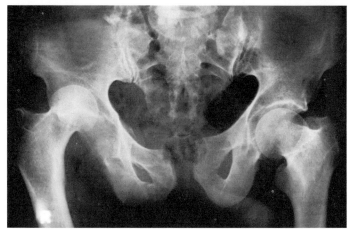
528

Lateral (1)

When the patient cannot be moved from the supine position the film-cassette is placed against the outer side of the thigh, but tilted a little under the thigh and supported at an angle of approximately 25°. The tube is lowered for horizontal projection but with a downward tilt of 25° to coincide with the tilt of the cassette.

■ Centre to the hip joint from the medial aspect of the thigh, the central ray being at a right angle to the oblique plane of the cassette (529, 530, 531).

The cross-sectional diagram (530) shows the relationship between tube, cassette and the affected hip, enabling the two sides to be separated.

Lateral (2)

An alternative lateral view can be obtained by rotating the patient 15° with the affected hip supported on a sandbag.

Using a horizontal beam, centre to the hip which should be at the level of the middle of the cassette (532, 531).

The cross-sectional diagram (532) shows the position of the two hips when the pelvis is tilted, the film in position, and the direction of the X-ray beam.

			Film	Screens	
kVp	mAS	FFD	ILFORD	ILFORD	Grid
80	80	100 cm (40″)	RAPID R	FT	Stat

Lat (2)

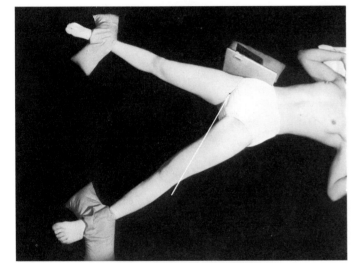

529

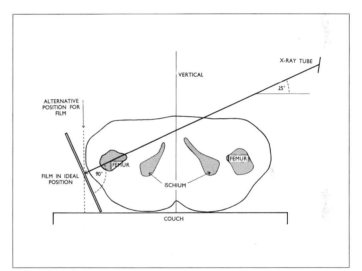

530

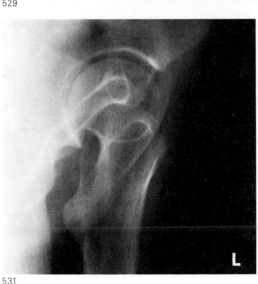

531

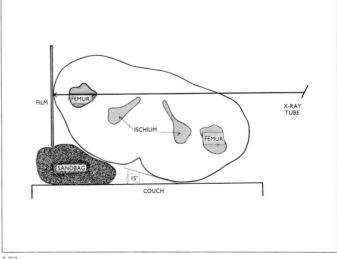

532

Congenital Dislocation of Hip

The series of radiographs are part of a record of a child treated at an orthopaedic hospital showing different stages in the treatment over considerable periods, as indicated, for congenital dislocation of hip, usually referred to as CDH.

A selection has been made of some of the many aspects in radiographic technique required for guidance and for the maintenance of satisfactory records from stage to stage of treatment. The date on which the examination was made is shown on each radiograph.

Series (533) includes in (a) an early radiograph taken before treatment, (b) eight months later with abduction and rotation, in plaster, (c) after twelve months a similar position controlled by a special appliance, and (d) the result of treatment twenty-seven months later.

Radiographs (534,535) are included to show the use of tomography. The heavy plaster in (534) is uneven and it is difficult to differentiate the bone outline, but the tomogram (535) has shown the outline of the heads of the femurs.

Patients continue to be under observation by the orthopaedic surgeon throughout childhood, and so each child becomes well known to the X-ray department where there is a lively interest in following the child's progress over the years.

20.11.52

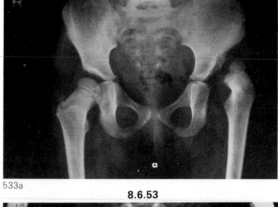

533a

8.6.53

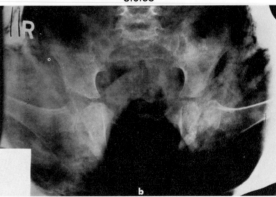

533b

17.6.54

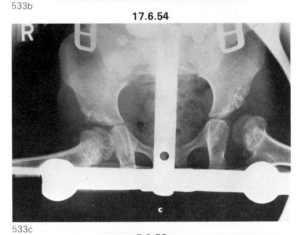

533c

5.9.56

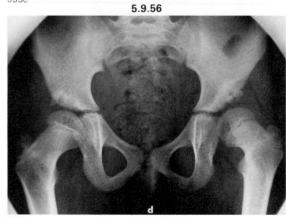

533d

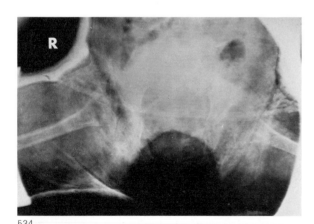

534

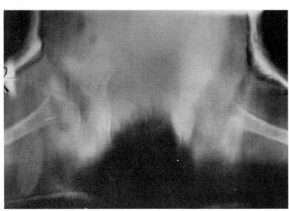

535

Neck of Femur

Two radiographs (536,537) show a Smith-Petersen pin in position following an operation for fracture of the neck of the femur. Such operations follow reduction of a fracture of the femoral neck. The surgeon requires radiographic control for insertion of a stainless steel nail through the greater trochanter and long axis of the neck into the head of the femur.

Careful radiographic preparation is required before a pinning operation if no hitch is to occur during the procedure with the radiographs being produced in the minimum of time. In modern practice a C-arm image intensifier is used for both antero—posterior and lateral viewing of the operative field. A minimum of radiographs are then required, usually only a final check film in the antero-posterior and lateral projections.

When a C-arm image intensifier is not available in the theatre suite two mobile X-ray units will be needed with appropriate accessories and automatic processing including an ample supply of films and cassettes. The X-ray units must be thoroughly cleaned and in working order. It is the duty of the radiographer to test the equipment before the operation and to see that the darkroom is in readiness for speedy and efficient processing. A modern theatre suite should be equipped with an automatic rapid film processor and adequate viewing facilities for the films.

One X-ray unit is placed in position for the antero-posterior view and the other for the lateral view. The first exposures are made immediately after reduction of the fracture, and these radiographs are then used as the control for positioning and exposure for the subsequent series of radiographs.

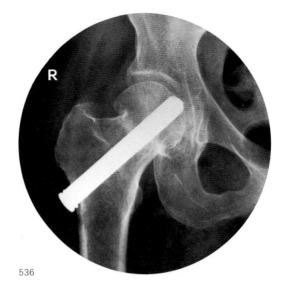

536

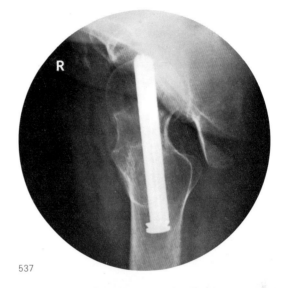

537

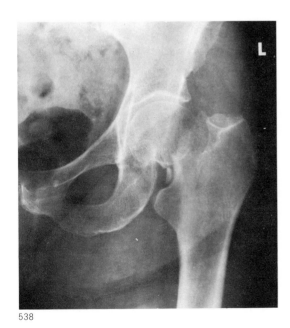

538

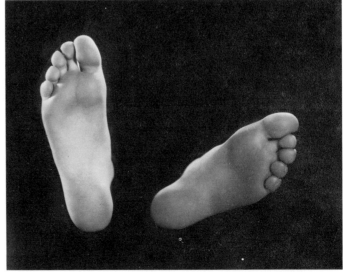

539

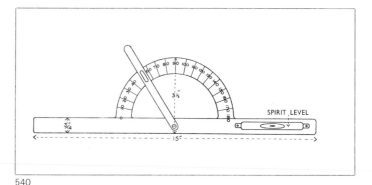

540

Strict asepsis is always required in the operating theatre. Following reduction of the fracture the patient is adjusted on the orthopaedic table with both limbs fixed in abduction and with medial rotation of the injured limb. A slot in the table allows the antero-posterior film-cassette to be placed in position without moving the patient. The pelvic rest and perineal bar are made of a transradient material not of metal, so that the femur is unobscured in either direction.

For the lateral projection, the film is pressed well into the soft tissues of the iliac crest and parallel to the femoral neck. An adjustable cassette support clipped onto the operating table is essential for this projection which is made from the medial side of the thigh. A stationary grid cassette is used.

In the lateral projection, the film-subject distance is considerable in relation to the focus-film distance therefore a relatively fine focus tube is required in mobile units to provide acceptable radiographs.

Antero-posterior

After reduction of the fracture the limb is maintained in the operative position assuring a satisfactory projection in the antero-posterior position.

The film-cassette is inserted in the cassette tunnel beneath the operating table, strict conditions of asepsis being observed.

Antero-posterior radiograph (538) shows the position before a reduction of a fracture. In (539) the sole of the foot is in the typical position of lateral rotation when the patient has a fracture of the neck of the femur.

Diagram (540) shows the size of a suitable protractor. The original model was made of cardboard, with a drawing pin to attach the movable arm to the base. The protractor can be very helpful to a beginner in locating the position of the neck of the femur on the skin surface (540, 542).

Lateral

Positioning for the lateral projection is complicated by the possible varying degrees of abduction of the limb (541), by the degree of medial rotation of the limb (545a,b), and by the injury sustained (538). The principle of the lateral projection is to place the film-cassette parallel to the neck of the femur and to centre the X-ray beam at right angles to both neck of femur and film (544, 545a,b).

Three tracings showing varying degrees of abduction of the limb, with the appropriate position for the film-cassette, have been superimposed to produce illustration (541). From this composite drawing the necessary adjustments in the film position relative to the position of the abducted neck of femur will be appreciated. The contraction of the abductor muscle group on minimum and maximum abduction should be noted (541).

For the beginner to appreciate the surface position of the femoral neck, it is helpful to place the protractor shown in (540) with the base extending from the anterior superior iliac spine to the upper border of the symphysis pubis, first on an antero-posterior radiograph adjusting the moving arm over the neck of the femur, and then transferring the set protractor to the actual position on the subject (542). The following procedure may also be helpful.

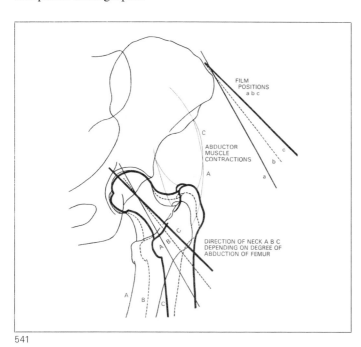

541

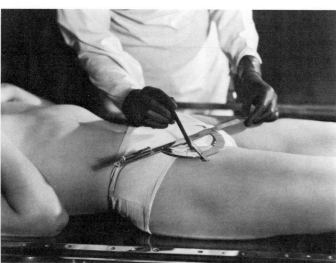

542

The head of the femur is just above the level of the depression in the thigh over the greater trochanter. A small set square is placed with one side of the right angle along the thigh and the other side transversely at hip level, the hypotenuse of the triangle indicates the appropriate direction of the neck of the femur (544). Obviously, the position of the set square and thus the direction of the neck will alter as the limb is abducted (545a,b). On placing a triangular plastic sponge block, to resemble a second large set square, with the apex symmetrical to the smaller set square, the hypotenuse of the triangle is on a level with the iliac crest and indicates the direction and position for the film-cassette (544, 545a,b). With a little practice and an understanding of the theatre set-up for the patient, the relative positions of tube and film are readily appreciated.

In the radiographic tracing (544) the direction of the X-ray beam is indicated. The structures of the thigh show the marked depression in the tissues over the greater trochanter, with the relative anatomical levels of the hip joint and the upper border of the symphysis pubis.

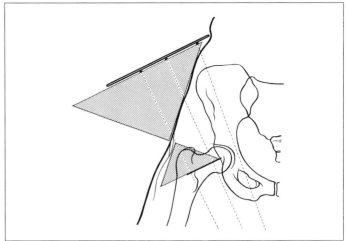

544

For the lateral projection the placing of the film-cassette is the important factor, and to determine the related direction of the neck, a metal bar is clipped on to the cassette and adjusted to the horizontal position as confirmed by means of attached spirit levels (546). The horizontal metal bar shows clearly in the radiograph, and the surgeon is able to estimate the degree of angulation required for the neck of the femur, medial or lateral (547). See also tracing diagrams (548) to (552).

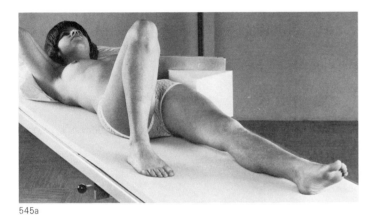

545a

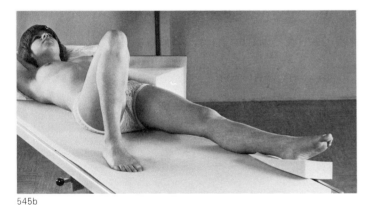

545b

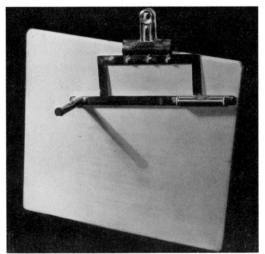

546

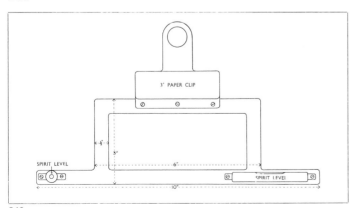

543

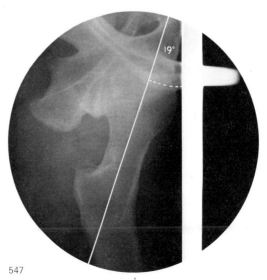

547

Operation procedure

This page will be helpful in giving the usual sequence of radiographs which are taken during a pinning operation. Each surgeon has variations in technique with specific requirements from the radiographer which may be different from those given in this book.

Tracings from a series of radiographs before, and during reduction and fixation of a fractured neck of femur are shown in (548, 549, 550, 551, 552); while the operative technique may vary, the principle of determining the direction of the nail is the same and the radiographic control provides the surgeon with the information required.

(548) Tracings of the initial antero-posterior and lateral radiographs taken in the X-ray department before reduction of the fracture.

(549) Tracings from radiographs taken in the theatre after reduction and insertion of the guide nail.

Calculations for the direction of the nail can be made from the radiographs. The holes in the guide nail are one centimetre apart and, as there is the same degree of enlargement of the Smith-Petersen nail, the length of nail required can be measured from the guide nail allowing one centimetre for impaction of the fragments when the nail is finally driven into position.

(550) The best position for the Smith-Petersen nail is selected from the radiographs of (549) in both antero-posterior and lateral aspects as indicated by a line in the tracings. The angle between line and guide nail is measured which, in this instance, is 30° from the antero-posterior aspect and 9° from the lateral aspect.

(551) Shows the Smith-Petersen nail being introduced at the correct angle using the previous calculations.

(552) Shows the Smith-Petersen nail in its final position.

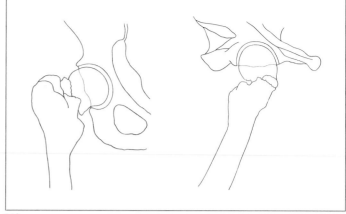

548

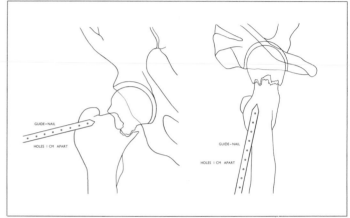

549

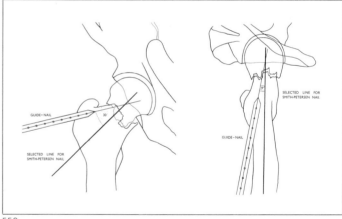

550

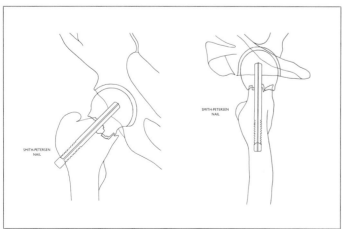

552

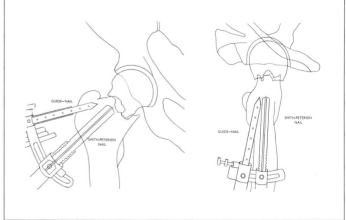

551

Some of the variations and alternatives in the pinning operation are shown on this page.

Kirschner Wires

One or more Kirschner guide wires are driven into the neck of the femur in the required direction for the Smith-Petersen nail. Two radiographs (553) are taken in (a) the antero-posterior and (b) lateral positions and the necessary direction for the nail in relation to the wires is estimated. After withdrawing the wires the nail is driven into the neck of the femur in the same direction (544a,b).

Notched angulator

The angulator is placed over the hip joint with one arm parallel to the femur and an antero-posterior radiograph is taken (555a). An elongated metal pin is placed on the radiograph in the ideal direction for the Smith-Petersen nail (555b). Using the appropriate notches as shown on the radiograph the nail is superimposed on the angulator to provide the correct direction. The nail is then driven into the neck of the femur along the line of the guide as shown on the angulator.

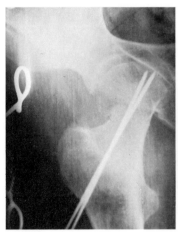
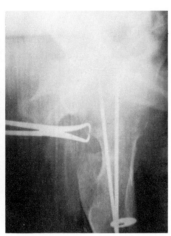

553a/b

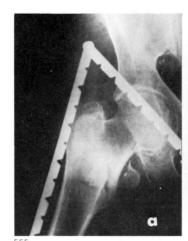
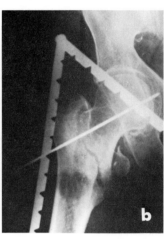

555

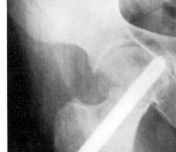
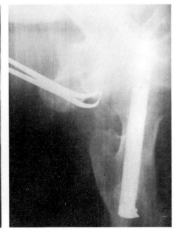

554a/b

Lateral (1) (basic)

(556) The sound limb is abducted and the leg hangs over the side of the couch with the foot on a stool while the upright cassette is supported parallel to the neck of the femur. Using a small aperture the central ray is directed at right angles to the neck of the femur and the film, at the level of the greater trochanter.

Lateral (2)

(558) Using a curved cassette the position of the tube and film are reversed. The cassette is placed well up into the groin between the legs, with the curved surface parallel to the femoral neck. The tube is centred from the lateral aspect of the thigh at right angles to the femoral neck and cassette.

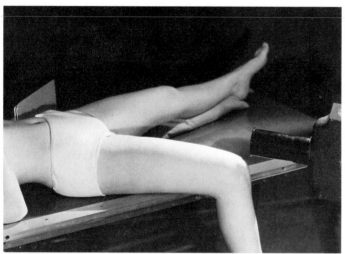

556

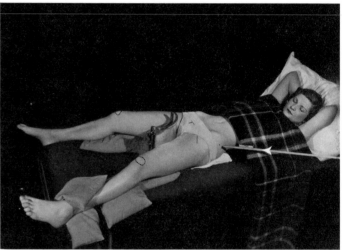

558

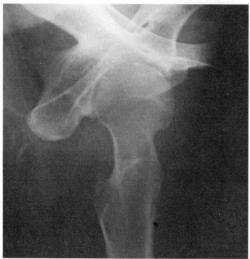

557

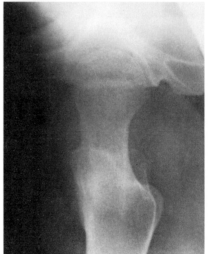

559

Lateral (3)

Another method of applying the technique of the curved film, particularly in the operating theatre, is by using a specially designed combined horizontal cassette holder and vertical film pack holder for taking the antero-posterior and lateral projections, respectively. This piece of apparatus replaces the normal buttock rest and perineal bar.

As shown in diagram (563), this cassette holder, the upper surface of which also forms the buttock rest, is constructed of two five-ply wood surfaces which are separated by three 2 cm ($\frac{3}{4}$ in) high wooden discs, so placed as to establish the position of the cassette for the antero-posterior projection (564). The vertical film support, roughly semi-cylindrical in shape, consists of a block of wood fixed at one side of the surface of the buttock rest, having a hole passing through its centre and continuing through both surfaces of the cassette holder, thus enabling the apparatus to be fitted over the normal perineal bar and locked in position on the theatre table. The curved surface is lead-covered to absorb X-ray scatter, and is surrounded at a distance of 1 cm ($\frac{3}{8}$-in) by a similarly curved piece of three-ply wood, a slot thus being formed to accommodate a special film pack.

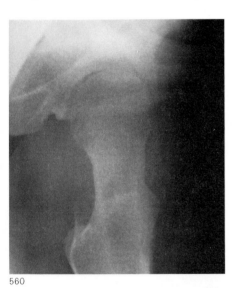

560

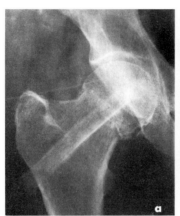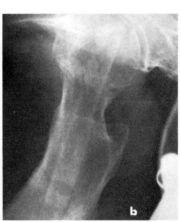

561

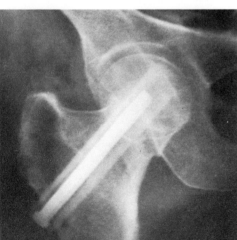

562

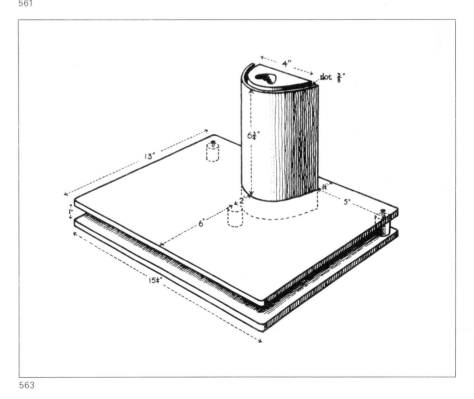

563

As will be seen in diagram (565), this vertical film support forms an adequate 'curved cassette' which, by virtue of its position and of the compression given by the extension of the limbs, is ideally placed for the lateral projection, being the position maintained throughout the operation. The film and the thin flexible screens, in an envelope, are placed in the narrow slot, which is designed to give the necessary screen-film contact. The tube is centred obliquely between the anterior superior iliac spine and the greater trochanter toward the film (565, 560).

Diagram (564) shows the relationship of subject and films for exposure in sequence, with the two X-ray tubes in position where they remain throughout the operation. As will be seen, the cassette and film pack are manipulated from the side of the couch remote from the surgeon.

Diagram (565), prepared from tracings taken from radiographs exposed with the film in position, shows the relative positions of tube, neck or femur and film for the lateral projections.

Radiographs taken by this method show (561) the introduction of a bone graft from the fibula, and (562) the graft reinforced by a central single-fin nail.

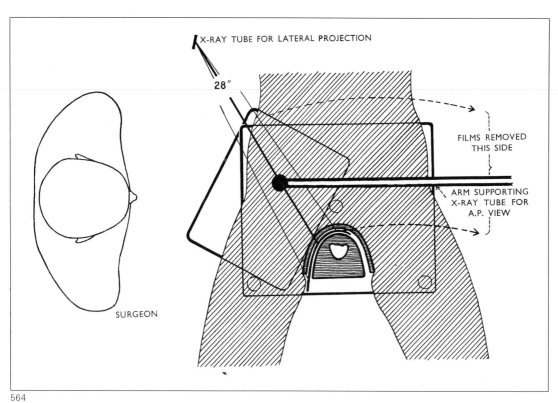

564

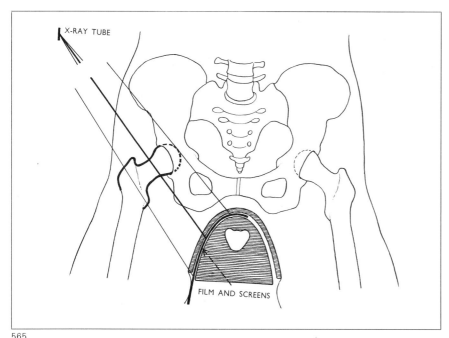

565

Lateral (4)

In the X-ray department both antero-posterior and lateral radiographs may be taken with the patient sitting on the couch. The patient leans against a backrest placed at an angle of 60° to the couch. The legs are allowed to flex over the side and under the couch with each foot supported on a stool (566, 567).

The radiographs (568a, b) show a clearly defined joint space.

For the antero-posterior projection, the cassette is placed in a Potter-Bucky diaphragm, or a stationary grid may be used (566). Because the patient is leaning back the tube can be centred over the hip joint (566, 568a, 569a).

Without moving the patient, the film and stationary grid are placed vertically adjacent to the thigh and parallel to the neck of the femur for the lateral projection. The cassette is held in position with sandbags. Centre to the medial aspect of the thigh at right angles to the neck of the femur and the cassette using a horizontal ray (567, 568b, 569b).

kVp	mAS	FFD	Film ILFORD	Screens ILFORD	Grid
75	80	100 cm (40″)	RAPID R	FT	Stat

Fracture Radiographs

The two radiographs (569) show the soft tissue shadows of a pendulous abdomen overlying the bone and obscuring bone detail when using the sitting method of examination. A hip prosthesis has been inserted which has a plastic head articulating with the acetabulum; only the retaining pin in the neck of the femur being visible.

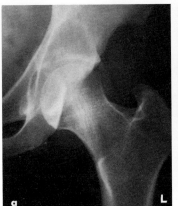
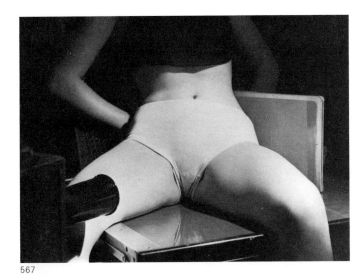

566

567

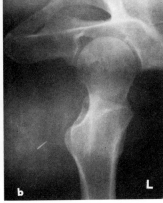
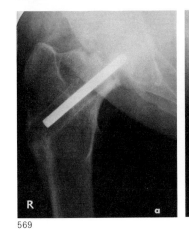
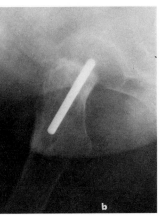

568

569

Note—A much higher kilovoltage is required for this projection which gives a true lateral view of the pelvis and acetabulum.

Medio-Lateral

The patient is turned on to the affected side in the lateral position with the knees flexed (570), however, when the symphysis pubis is to be shown the limbs are straight (571). Non-opaque pads are placed between the knees and ankles, and sandbags above and below the pelvis to maintain the patient in position. For thin patients a small non-opaque pad should be placed between the greater trochanter and the table top for comfort. Alternatively, when the patient cannot be moved into the lateral position a satisfactory projection can be produced by leaving the patient supine, using a horizontal ray, and a vertical Bucky or stationary grid (572).

■ Centre to the depression above the greater trochanter (570, 571 572).

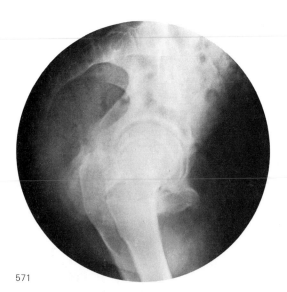

571

		Medio-Lateral			
kVp	mAS	FFD	Film ILFORD	Screens ILFORD	Grid
120	80	100 cm (40″)	RAPID	FT	Grid

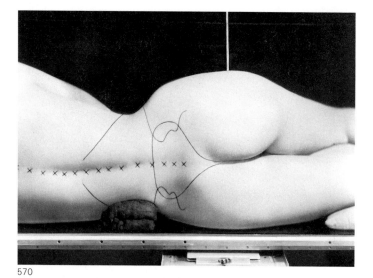

570

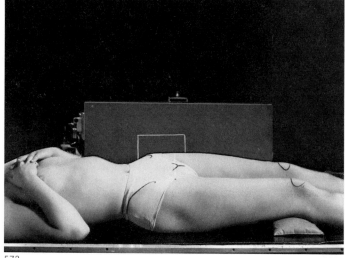

572

Arthrography

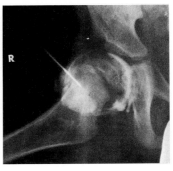
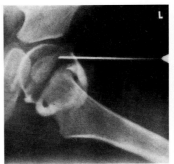

To show the internal structures of the hip joint, an opaque medium is injected into the joint cavity. Using one of the water soluble organic iodine compounds, 6 ml of the opaque medium, mixed with 1 ml of a local anaesthetic such as 2% novocaine, is injected. A general anaesthetic is used for children. Radiographs are taken in antero-posterior and oblique positions.

Two antero-posterior arthrograms of right and left hip joints, exposed separately, show the contrast medium within the capsule of the joint (573).

Two arthrograms of a child (574a, b), show the contrast medium within the joint capsule both from antero-posterior and lateral aspects of the joints, the right and left hips having been exposed simultaneously for each projection.

Two further antero-posterior arthrograms (575a, b) were taken stereoscopically, for three dimensional viewing of the contrast medium in the joint.

573

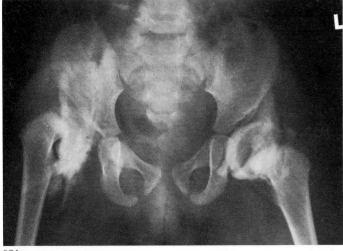

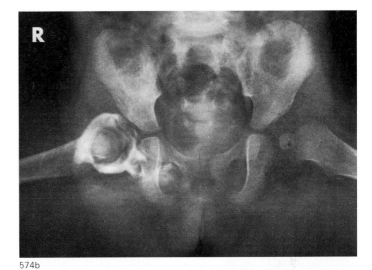

574a

574b

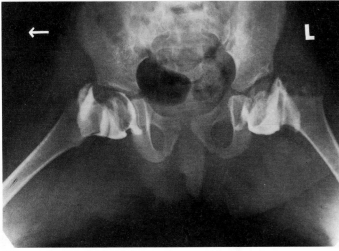

575a

575b

5

PELVIC GIRDLE

5 SECTION 5

PELVIC GIRDLE

The pelvis is formed by the innominate or hip bones and the sacrum providing a protective girdle for the pelvic organs at the base of the vertebral column. The innominate bones, consisting of the ilium, the ischium and pubis fuse laterally to form the acetabulum and articulate with the head of the femur at the hip joint. The pelvis supports the lower limbs. The innominate bones articulate anteriorly at the symphysis pubis and, posteriorly, the sacrum is wedged between the iliac bones to form the sacro-iliac joints.

The bony prominences in the pelvic region are important landmarks in radiography. These are, the symphysis pubis, particularly the upper border, the posterior superior iliac spines, the lower sacrum and coccyx, the ischial tuberosities, and the anterior superior iliac spines.

Radiographic Appearances
Lettered radiographs, antero-posterior (579) and lateral (580) of the pelvis will help the student to follow the anatomical references in the text.

Posture
When the subject is in the erect position the symphysis pubis and the anterior superior iliac spines are in the same vertical plane (576).

When the subject is in the sitting position the pelvic brim (symphysis to lumbo-sacral articulation) is approximately horizontal. Considerable movement of the vertebral column may occur without altering the position of the pelvis (577).

When the subject is supine (578), the pelvic brim is tilted dependent on the degree of angulation at the lumbo-sacral articulation, and this causes considerable variation in the radiographic appearance of the pelvis (581, 582).

Radiation Protection
Protection for the gonads, particularly in the female, cannot be used as in examining the hip joint, but depends on the region and condition being investigated. As an open field is desirable to include the whole pelvis on the one film, the only possible precautions are to use the minimum exposure with rare earth screens and only do essential projections.

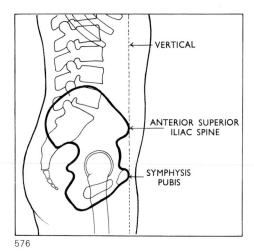

576

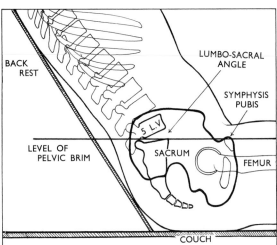

577

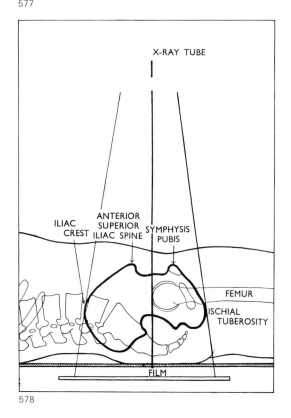

578

154

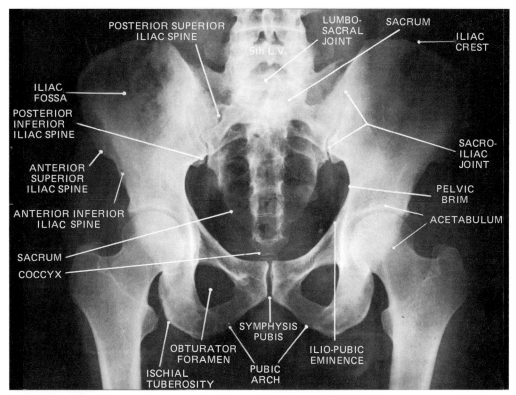

PELVIS
579

ANTERO-POSTERIOR

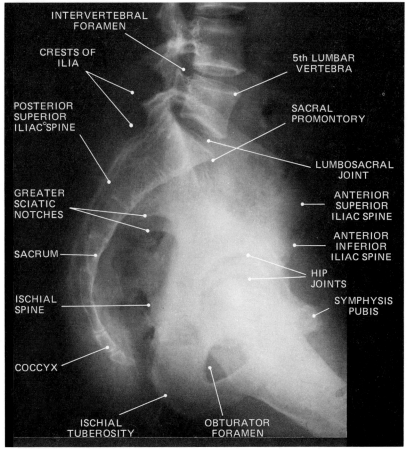

PELVIS
580

LATERAL

Pelvis

There is considerable variation in the size and shape of the pelvis which varies particularly with the sex of the individual. This is well shown on radiographs (581, 582). In positioning the typical female pelvis care must be taken to include its full width and in the typical male pelvis, full length.

To include the whole of the pelvis on the film, the centring point should be midway between the upper margin of the iliac crest and the lower margin of the ischial tuberosity (578), but it is not usually possible to use these landmarks. A common error is to centre between the iliac crest and the upper border of the symphysis pubis which projects the ischium below the lower border of the film.

Considerable distortion of the radiographic appearances can be caused by bad positioning as well as abnormality of the subject. A spirit level across the anterior superior iliac spines will show if any adjustment is needed when the pelvis is tilted from side to side. This tilting can be caused either by wasting of the muscles on one side or by a swelling. By inserting non-opaque pads under one side of the pelvis the asymmetrical appearance on the radiograph can be corrected. The pads should be adjusted to bring both sides of the pelvis equidistant from the film. The patient must also be central to grid and film and the tube centred correctly; (583) shows bad positioning which has been corrected in (584).

A clean colon free of faecal and gas shadows which may obscure bony detail, will give the best radiograph of the pelvis but suitable bowel preparation is not normally possible when dealing with accident and emergency patients.

The optimum focus-film distance for the antero-posterior projection is 100 cm (40 ins). This distance may be altered but must be kept within the specification of the grid in the Potter-Bucky diaphragm to avoid fading or grid cut off.

The exposure factors given refer to an average adult subject.

Basic positions
To avoid confusion initial routine projections are referred to as (Basic).

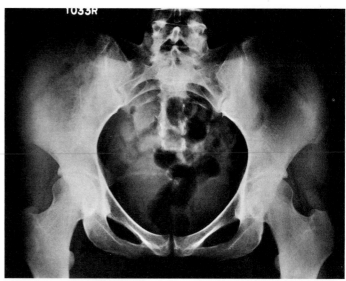

581

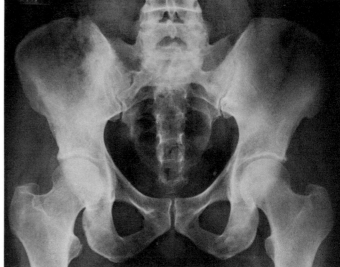

582

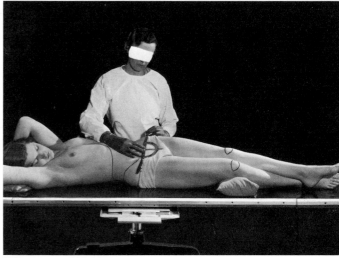

583

Antero-posterior (basic)

The patient is supine, with the pelvis symmetrical as for examination of the hip joints; the knees are flexed over a small sandbag and a pressure pad is placed under the heels.

■ Centre in the mid-line, half-way between the level of the anterior superior iliac spines and the upper border of the symphysis pubis (584, 585)

AP					
kVp	mAS	FFD	Film ILFORD	Screens ILFORD	Grid
70	60	100 cm (40")	RAPID R	FT	Grid

The width of the pelvis may be critical in relation to the width of the film and fading may occur from side to side, due to the unsatisfactory direction of the grid slats in relation to the direction of the X-ray beam as in (586).

Fracture Radiograph

A fracture of the pelvis may well involve both right and left sides in a diagonal direction, as shown in radiograph (586) of an injury to the right ilium and to the left ischium and pubis. It is therefore unwise to take only the one side of the pelvis as shown in (587).

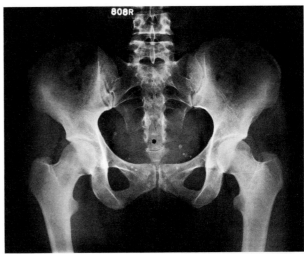

585

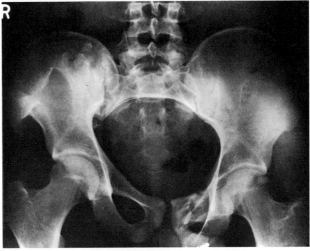

586

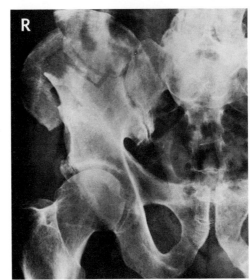

587

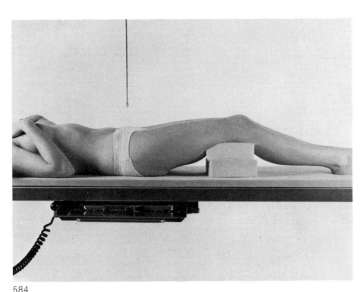

584

Lateral (basic)

The pelvis in the lateral projection is a very wide and a very dense area to examine needing a large radiographic exposure. Lateral radiographs may be taken in the supine position using a horizontal ray, in the erect position to assess posture or with the patient lying on the side. Radiographs in the erect position can be done using a vertical Potter-Bucky diaphragm.

Horizontal

The patient lies in the true lateral position with full extension at the hips; the position is maintained with sandbags at the front and back of trunk and thighs, above and below the pelvis. Small non-opaque pads are placed between knees and ankles for comfort, and a smaller pad between the greater trochanter and couch.

■ Centre above the depression over the greater trochanter on the lateral aspect of the thigh (588, 589)

| | | | Lat | | |
kVp	mAS	FFD	Film ILFORD	Screens ILFORD	Grid
120	100	100 cm	RAPID	FT	Grid
120	25	(40″)	R	RE	

Note—When the hips are flexed the symphysis pubis may be obscured by the femora.

Erect

In the erect lateral position the feet should be slightly separated so the patient is well balanced and the lateral aspect of the pelvis centred to the radiographic stand. To help immobilization the arm rests over the Bucky support. The vertebral column must be parallel to the film with the two hip joints at the same level. Radiograph (591) shows a pregnancy at full term taken in the erect lateral position.

■ Centre midway between front and back and between the anterior superior iliac spines and the border of the symphysis pubis (590, 591)

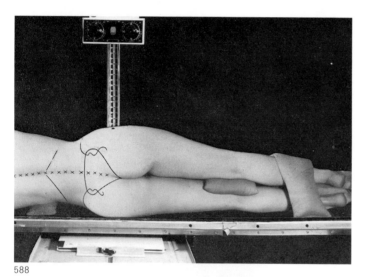

588

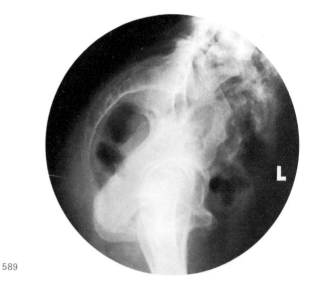

589

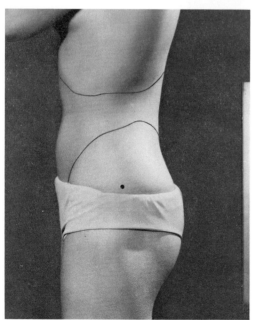

590

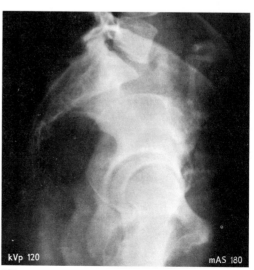

591

Antero-Posterior oblique (basic)

The oblique projection shows the iliac fossa, the ischium and the ischial spine but this projection should not be used in a patient with a fracture of the pelvis.

The patient is turned toward the side to be examined to bring the iliac fossa parallel to the film, the raised side of the pelvis is supported on a non-opaque pad with supporting sandbags above and below the pelvis. The knee and hip nearest to the film are slightly flexed but the other leg is kept in extension and supported.

■ Centre over the iliac fossa, halfway between the anterior superior iliac spine and the mid line (592, 593).

Antero-Posterior oblique

The affected side is raised until the pelvis is at angle of 45°. Maintain this position by supporting the raised side on non-opaque pads.

In this position, the posterior surface of the ilium on the raised side is in profile.

■ Centre 2·5 cm (1 in) behind the anterior superior iliac spine of the raised side (594, 595)

This position is used when a view of the posterior aspect of the ilium is required (595).

5

Ant-Post Oblique (Basic)

kVp	mAS	FFD	Film ILFORD	Screens ILFORD	Grid
70	50	100 cm (40")	RAPID R	FT	Grid

Ant-Post Oblique

kVp	mAS	FFD	Film ILFORD	Screens ILFORD	Grid
80	100	100 cm (40")	RAPID R	FT	Grid

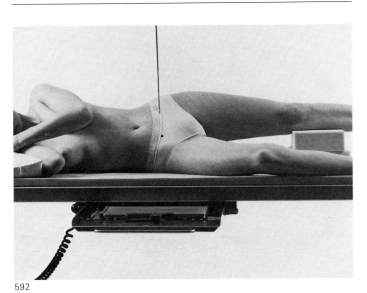

592

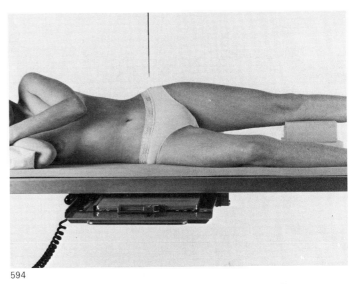

594

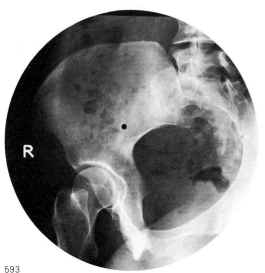

593

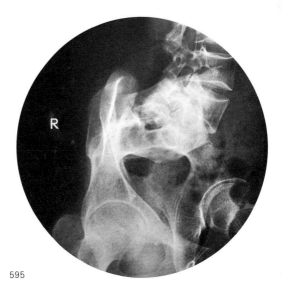

595

Acetabulum

The various views of the hip joint and pelvis show the acetabulum from different angles; both acetabulae being satisfactorily shown in the antero-posterior oblique projection (595). Oblique views of the acetabulum may be taken either antero-posterior or postero-anterior.

Posterior oblique

The patient lies in the postero-anterior oblique position for right and left sides in turn. From the lateral position the patient rotates forward on to 45° non-opaque pads placed above and below the hip joint and maintained in position with sandbags. In this position the rim of the acetabulum is approximately parallel to the film on the side nearest the couch. Both sides are taken separately using a small localizing cone (597, 598).

■ Centre 1 cm ($\frac{1}{2}$ in) distal to the coccyx with the tube angled 12° towards the head (596, 597, 598).

Note—Figure (596) shows the position of the patient for a view of the left acetabulum (597).

Acetabulum

kVp	mAS	FFD	Film ILFORD	Screens ILFORD	Grid
75	60	100 cm (40″)	RAPID R	FT	Grid

Pubic bones

The symphysis pubis and sacro-iliac joints may be examined for subluxation by comparing two radiographs taken in the erect position with the full weight of the trunk first on one foot and then on the other.

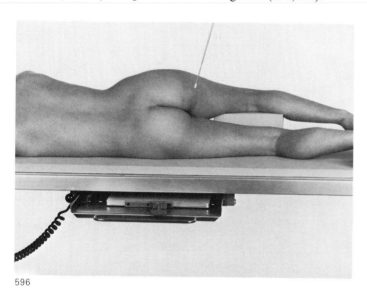

596

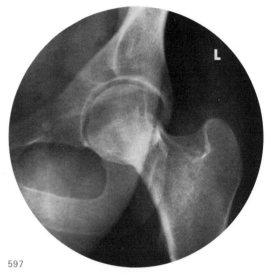

597

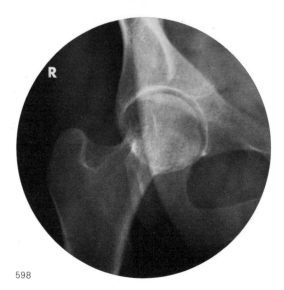

598

Subluxation of the Pubic Bones
(Postero-anterior)

The patient stands against the vertical Bucky with the mid point of the symphysis pubis central to the film. Two radiographs are taken in which the full weight of the body is allowed to fall on one foot and then the other.

■ Centre to the symphysis pubis with the central ray at right angles to the film.

Postero-anterior (599, 600) shows the posture of the patient with the corresponding radiograph (601). Radiograph (602) of a female pelvis with an os acetabulum at the right hip (arrow). Note tampon in vagina showing patient was examined in conformity with the ten day rule (crossed arrow). (603) shows assymetry at the symphysis pubis and (604) a prosthesis in the right hip.

Pubic Bones

kVp	mAS	FFD	Film ILFORD	Screens ILFORD	Grid
70	60	100 cm (40″)	RAPID R	FT	Grid

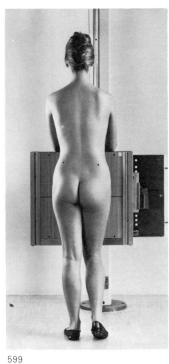

599

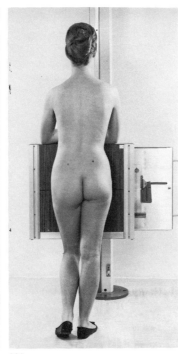

600

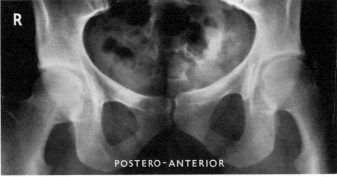

POSTERO-ANTERIOR

601

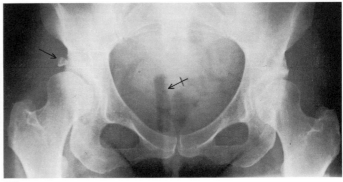

602

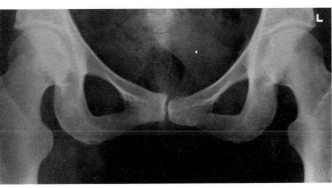

603

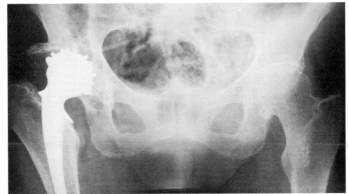

604

Sacro-Iliac Joints

The sacrum lies posteriorly between the two iliac bones, their adjacent surfaces form the sacro-iliac joints. The joint surfaces lie obliquely, sloping backwards, inwards and downwards. Tube angulation is required for a satisfactory demonstration of the joints (605, 606).

The degree of tube angulation for the antero-posterior projection varies from subject to subject according to type and sex as shown in radiographs (607) and (608). In the latter the sacro-iliac articulation lies almost horizontally.

In each radiograph a line has been drawn through the long axis of the first two sacral segments, with a second line at right angles to it to show the ideal direction of the X-ray beam. However, when this centring cannot be used (608) then the X-ray beam is centred along the broken line which results in some foreshortening of the joints in this type of subject.

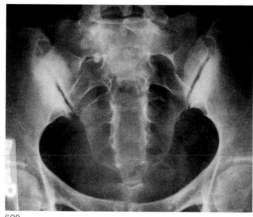
609

Bowel shadows frequently obscure the sacro-iliac region and patient preparation is essential. Radiograph (609) with an abnormality, osteitis condensans ilii, is taken after adequate preparation of the patient while the stereoscopic pair (617, 618) has a considerable amount of bowel gas obscuring the sacrum and sacro-iliac joints.

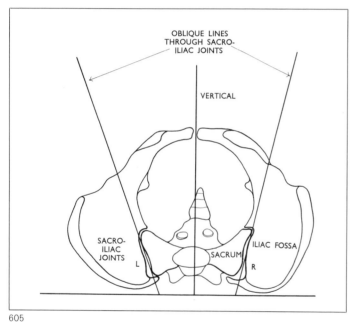
605

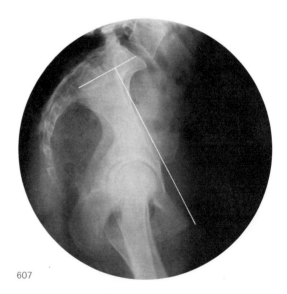
607

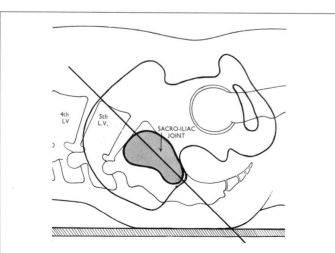
606

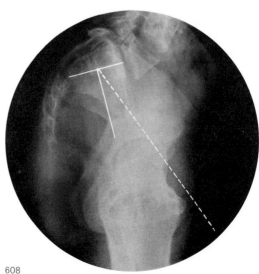
608

162

Antero-posterior (basic)

With the patient supine, the shoulders are raised to eliminate the lumbar arch, and the knees are flexed over a pad.

■ Centre above the upper border of the symphysis pubis with the tube angled 10°–25° towards the head depending upon the degree of lumbo-sacral angulation (610, 613, 612).

Postero-anterior

The patient is placed in the prone position, with a pad under the ankles.

■ Centre in the mid line between the dimples over the posterior superior iliac spines and the tube angled 5°–15° towards the feet as required (611, 614).

Note—Radiographs taken in this position show the anterior borders of the sacro-iliac articulation clearly defined. Postero-anterior projection (614) should be compared with the antero-posterior projection (613), both in the same subject.

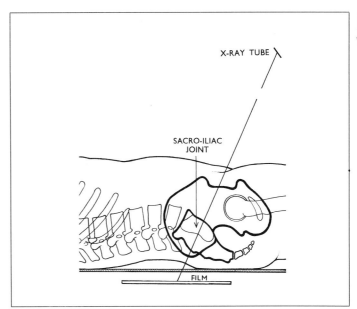

612

SI Jts AP

kVp	mAS	FFD	Film ILFORD	Screens ILFORD	Grid
70	70	100 cm (40″)	RAPID R	FT	Grid

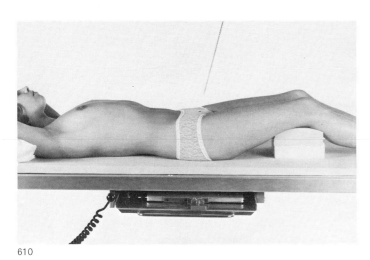

610

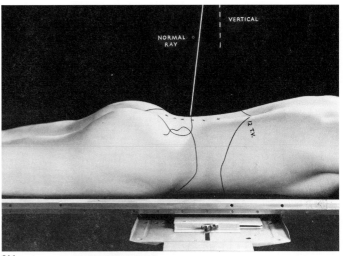

611

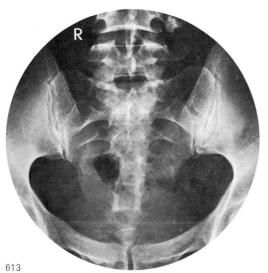

613

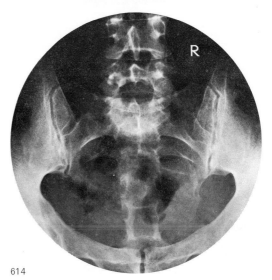

614

Antero-posterior—Erect

The sacro-iliac joint can also be examined in the erect position. The patient stands against the vertical Potter-Bucky diaphragm facing the X-ray tube; the feet are separated to assist balance and immobilization. The direction of the lumbo-sacral angle should be noted to determine the tube angulation as compared with the horizontal position.

■ Centre above the upper border of the symphysis pubis with the tube angled 15°–30° towards the joints (615, 616).

Note—Comparing the two radiographs of the one subject (616)—erect and supine, with the same tube angulation of 15°, it will be seen that, in the erect position, the pelvic brim is foreshortened indicating a change in relationship of the pelvis to the film. To obtain a comparable view in the erect position 10° less angulation should be used.

Stereography

Stereo-radiographs (617, 618) were taken in the horizontal position. The direction of the tube shift for each exposure is shown by the arrow.

A pair of stereoscopic binoculars are needed for effective viewing of these two radiographs and overcomes to some extent the effect of the bowel gas shadows.

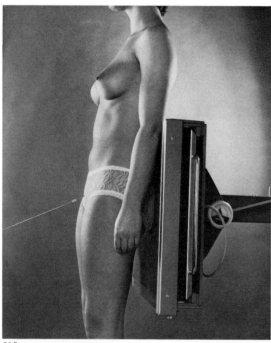

615

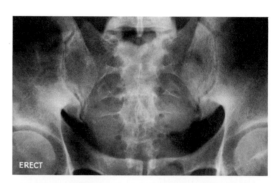

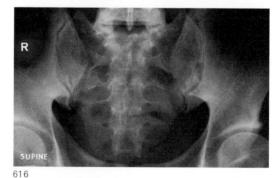

616

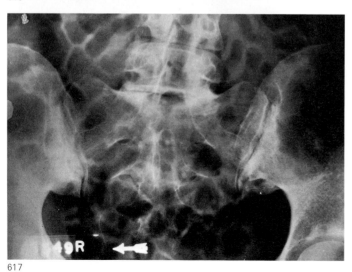

617

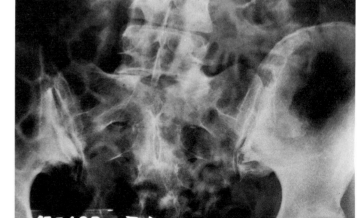

618

Subluxation of the Sacro-Iliac joints
Antero-posterior

The patient stands against the vertical Potter-Bucky diaphragm. With the patient taking her full weight on the right and then the left leg in turn two radiographs are taken.

■ Centre to the upper border of the symphysis pubis with the tube angled 15°–20° to the head.

The cassette should be displaced upwards to allow for tube angulation (619,620).

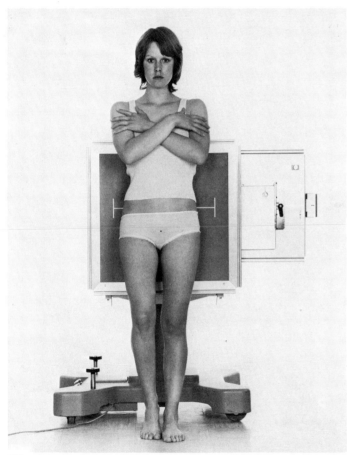

619

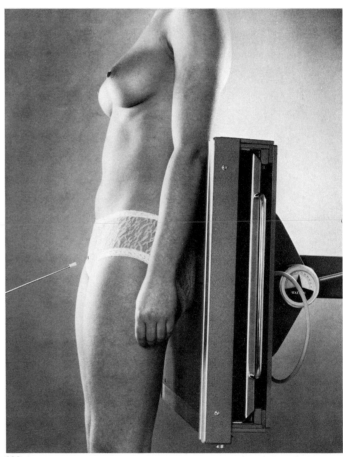

620

kVp	mAS	FFD	Film ILFORD	Screens ILFORD	Grid
70	75	100 cm (40″)	RAPID R	FT	Grid

R and L Antero-posterior oblique

From the supine position the patient is raised on one side until the antero-posterior plane of the pelvis is at an angle of 15°–20° to the horizontal; the pelvis is supported on non-opaque pads, with sandbags under the trunk and thigh. Using a small localizing cone both sides are examined in turn for comparison.

■ Centre 2 cm (1 in) medial to the anterior superior iliac spine on the raised side which is directly through the joint. To prevent foreshortening of the joint the central ray should be at a point 2 cm (1 in) medial to and 4 cm (2 ins) below the anterior superior iliac spine with the tube angled 15° towards the head. This is particularly useful for the lower part of the joint (621, 622, 623, 624).

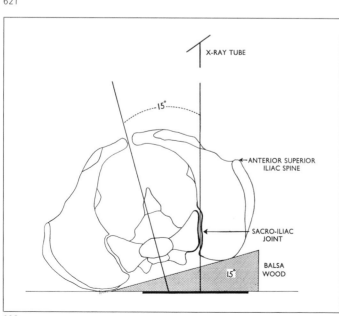

621

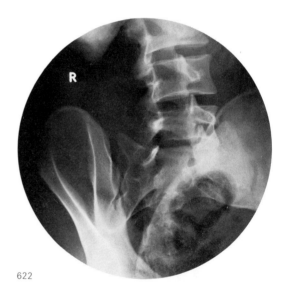

622

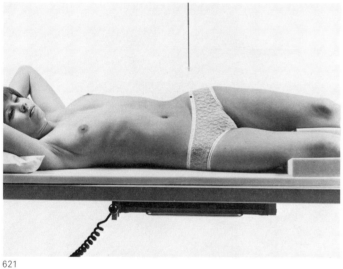

623

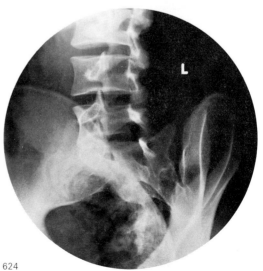

624

166

6

VERTEBRAL COLUMN

6 SECTION 6

VERTEBRAL COLUMN

The vertebral column forms the central bony framework of the body, it supports the head and protects the spinal cord. The ribs articulate with the dorsal vertebrae and the pelvis is attached to the sacrum. Large muscle groups are also attached to the spine and rib cage which, in turn, supports the shoulder girdle and the upper limbs. Similarly, there are large muscle attachments to the lower spine and pelvis for the lower limbs which articulate with the pelvis.

There are 33 articulated bones in the vertebral column to maintain an erect posture and permit the various movements required—flexion, extension, lateral bending and some rotation. The bodies of the vertebrae are separated one from the other by fibro-cartilaginous intervertebral discs.

Injuries to vertebrae can cause pressure on the spinal cord and produce sensory or motor effects; when severe total paralysis (paraplegia) can occur.

Radiographic Appearances

Individual bones of the vertebral column should be studied as well as their radiographs to help the student appreciate the radiographic anatomy of this region. Radiographs of a series of dry bones of each of the five sections of the vertebral column—cervical, thoracic, lumbar, sacral (fused together to form the sacrum), coccygeal (fused together to form the coccyx)—and an additional series of the cervical region for the atlas and axis are shown on pages 169, 171 and 172. These should be studied carefully and compared with radiographs of the live subject: cervical (625a, b, c); thoracic (627a), page 170; lumbar (628b), page 170; sacrum and coccyx, dry bones (630), page 171; living subject (629), page 170.

On page 169, vertebrae are shown in frontal view in the first column, then in axial view (from above downwards), and then in the lateral view. The vertebrae shown are (a) first and second cervical; (b) fourth and fifth cervical; (c) sixth and seventh thoracic; (d) third and fourth lumbar (626).

These illustrations are numbered and lettered to indicate the various regions of the individual vertebrae. The features common to many of the vertebrae are numbered from 1 to 12.

For first and second cervical vertebrae, the special features are lettered for the Atlas in small letters a to h and for the Axis in capital letters A to C.

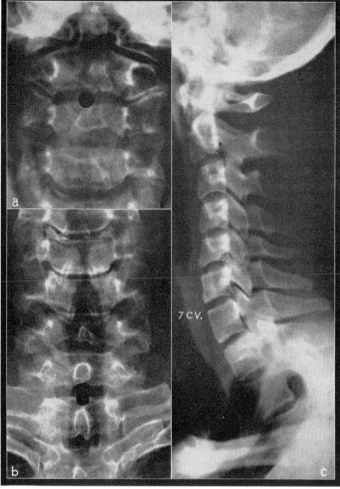

625

General (626)

1 Body
2 Pedicle
3 Lamina
4 Spinous process
5 Transverse process
6 Superior articular process
7 Inferior articular process
8 Spinal Canal
9 Intervertebral foramen formed by adjacent vertebrae
10 Demi-facet for head of rib
11 Facet for tubercle of rib
12 Foramen transversarium

Atlas (626)

a Lateral mass
b Anterior arch
c Posterior arch
d Anterior tubercle
e Posterior tubercle
f Facet for odontoid process
g Tubercle of transverse ligament
h Groove for vertebral artery

Axis (626)

A Odontoid process
B Articular surface for lateral mass of atlas
C Large spinous process

On page 171 the sacrum is numbered and the coccyx is lettered to show the individual vertebrae and also the more general features.

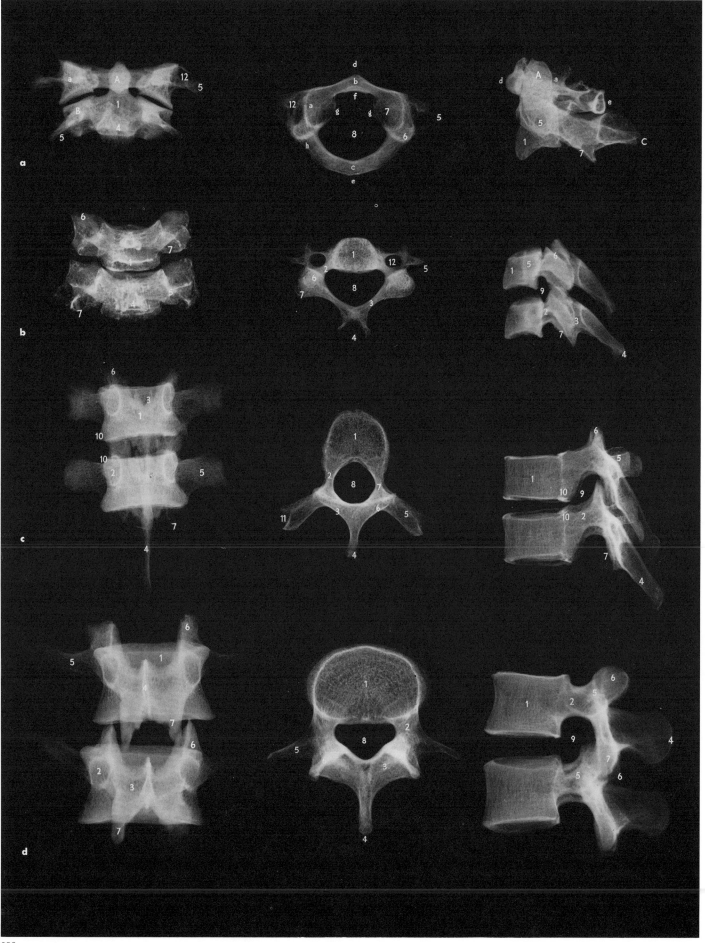

The radiographs of the dry bones of the sacrum taken from three aspects (a) antero-posterior, (b) supero-inferior, (d) lateral are numbered from 1 to 21.

In (c) and (d) the coccyx is shown attached to the sacrum; the radiograph of the dry bones of the sacrum and coccyx in (c) has been taken supero-inferior with a slight tube tilt towards the spine and centred over the coccyx.

Sacrum (630)

1 Body of first segment
2 Costal process
3 Transverse process
4 Sacral promontory
5 Superior articulated process of first segment
6 Sacral canal
7 Pedicle
8 Spinous tubercle
9 Articular tubercle
10 Transverse tubercle
11 Anterior sacral foramen
12 Posterior sacral foramen
13 Inferior lateral angle
14 Sacral cornu
15 Sacral hiatus
16 Lateral mass
17 Articular surface for sacro-iliac joint
18 Lamina
19 Anterior surface
20 Posterior surface
21 Sacro-coccygeal joint

Coccyx (630)

a Rudimentary transverse process
b Cornu
c Base of first segment

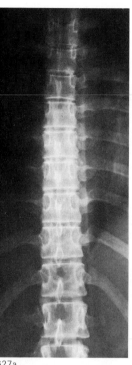

627a

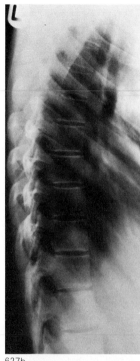

627b

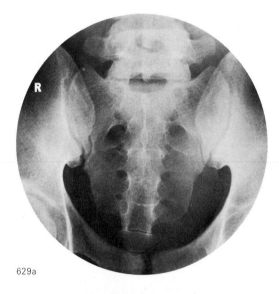

629a

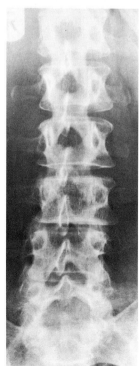

628a

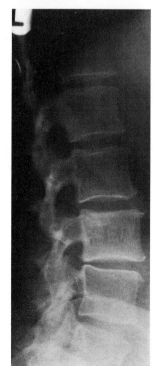

628b

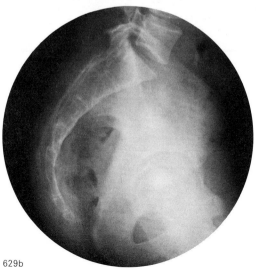

629b

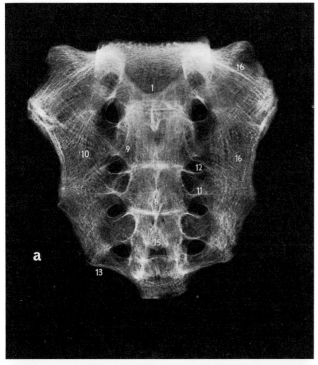

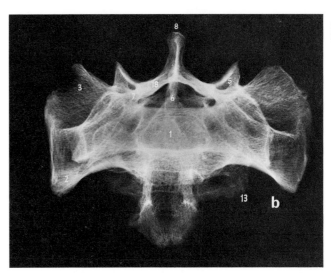

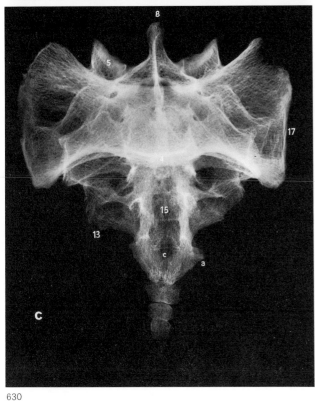

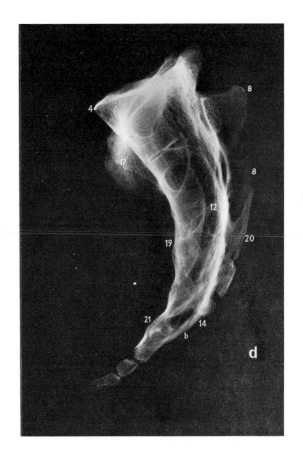

6 Vertebral column

Curves, Postures, Levels

After the student has studied the individual vertebrae of the skeleton and the radiographs shown on pages 168, 169, 170, the appearances of the various parts of the vertebral column should be familiar.

The vertebrae vary in size and shape from region to region, and are modified for the particular function of each region. The cervical vertebrae are smaller and have a proportionally larger spinal canal, the thoracic vertebrae have markedly downward sloping spinous processes and articular facets for the ribs, the lumbar vertebrae are the largest with a relatively small spinal canal and horizontal spinous processes. However, when the individual vertebrae are articulated with each other as in the living subject, the spine has a series of curves extending from the base of the skull to the sacro-coccygeal region.

In the neutral position the cervical spine is slightly convex anteriorly while the thoracic region is concave. At the lumbar region the curve is once more convex towards the front giving place to a marked concavity in the sacral region and is well shown on the lateral view of the skeleton (631a). In the frontal view the spine is normally straight and in the mid line (631b).

Scoliosis is the term for an abnormal lateral curve in the coronal plane; kyphosis refers to an increased curve, concave forwards of the spine in the sagittal plane bringing the cervical spine forwards; whereas a lordosis is an increase in the lumbar curve, convex forwards, bringing the dorsal spine backwards.

Because of the normal curve of the spine in various regions the intervertebral spaces will be radially directed. For a true frontal view of an individual vertebra the central ray must be suitably modified to allow for the natural curve of the spine.

In the routine frontal and lateral views adjacent bones may be superimposed in certain areas. The lower jaw overlies the upper cervical vertebrae in the frontal view, the shoulders overlie the lower cervical and upper dorsal vertebrae in the lateral view, the oblique line of the ribs overlies the dorsal vertebrae in the lateral view. For each of these areas suitable modification to the basic views will be needed. In a similar way an upward tilt to the tube will be required to show the sacrum in frontal view because of the tilt of the pelvis.

Photographs of the skeleton (631a,b,c) from the lateral, anterior, and posterior aspects help to make these points clear; the corresponding photographs of a model are shown on the facing page (632a,b,c).

While it is quite easy on a skeleton to see the position of the various regions of the spine, in the living subject anatomical reference points are needed. The full length figure (633) gives the levels of important landmarks in the left lateral, anterior, posterior, and right lateral positions in the standing subject (633). These relative positions will change somewhat when supine or prone radiographs are taken especially if the patient has thick-set shoulders, a pronounced lumbo-sacral angle or well developed buttocks.

A further guide for these levels can be obtained from the diagram (634) on page 173.

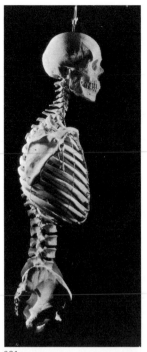
631a

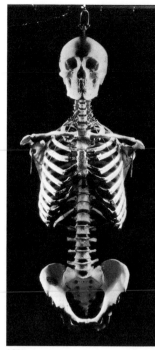
631b

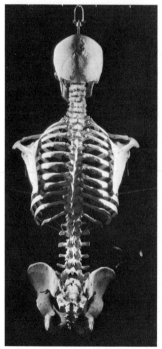
631c

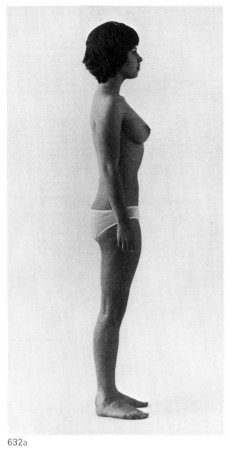

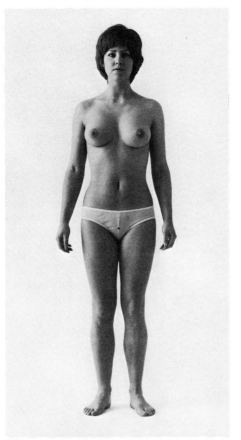

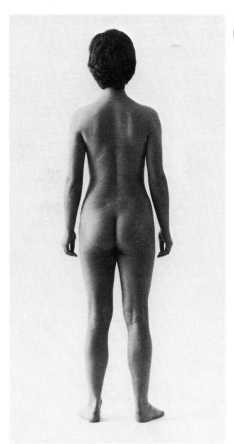

632a

632b

632c

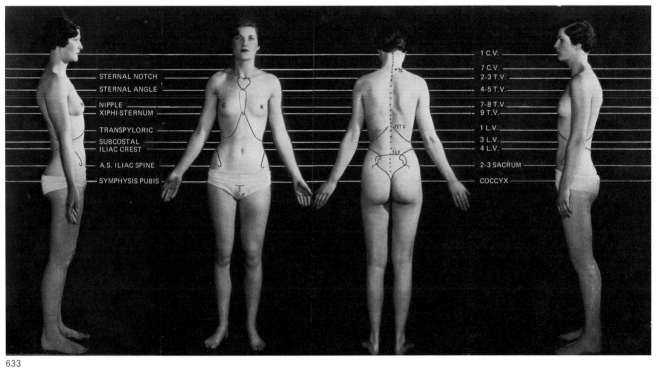

STERNAL NOTCH	1 C.V.
STERNAL ANGLE	7 C.V.
	2-3 T.V.
	4-5 T.V.
NIPPLE	7-8 T.V.
XIPHI-STERNUM	9 T.V.
TRANSPYLORIC	1 L.V.
SUBCOSTAL	3 L.V.
ILIAC CREST	4 L.V.
A.S. ILIAC SPINE	2-3 SACRUM
SYMPHYSIS PUBIS	COCCYX

633

6

173

6 Vertebral column

Summary of projections

The basic projections for the vertebral column are the antero-posterior and lateral; not infrequently the oblique and postero-anterior projections may also be required. The cervical spine is usually done erect, the rest of the spine with the patient horizontal. To obtain a clear picture of the intervertebral articulations the tube angulation must be adjusted to correspond with the curve of the spine for both the antero-posterior and lateral views.

A large length of spine may be radiographed on one film or a coned view may be done on a smaller film which will give greater detail. Occasionally the spine may be radiographed to show postural changes, with flexion or extension views may being carried out in either the frontal or lateral planes.

For the spine a Potter-Bucky diaphragm is required apart from the lateral view of the cervical vertebrae.

The parts to be examined vary in radiographic density as well as in their anatomy. The positioning technique will be considered in the following order:

Cervical

Antlanto-occipital articulation	Antero-posterior
	Postero-anterior or Oblique
	Lateral
Cervical vertebrae:	Antero-posterior, 1–3
	Antero-posterior, 2–7
	Lateral, 1–7
	Oblique, 1–7

Thoraco-Lumbar

Upper thoracic:	Antero-posterior
	Lateral or Oblique
Thoracic vertebrae:	Antero-posterior
	Lateral
	Oblique
Lumbar vertebrae:	Antero-posterior
	Postero-anterior
	Lateral
	Oblique

Lumbo-sacral

articulation:	Antero-posterior or Oblique
	Postero-anterior
	Lateral
Sacrum:	Antero-posterior
	Lateral
Coccyx:	Antero-posterior
	Lateral

When necessary add flexion, extension and lateral bending views as applicable.

Tomography is important when the detail of bone structures is to be shown whether for infective conditions, such as abscess formation, or for possible bone destruction by tumours. Stereography is sometimes required.

In cases of injury to the vertebral column the patient must be radiographed on a Casualty trolley unless otherwise stated. If lateral radiographs are needed they should be taken with a horizontal ray without moving the patient. Special radiographic trollies, readily adjustable X-ray tubes and a vertical Potter-Bucky diaphragm are essential for an adequate examination of a badly injured patient. If such equipment is not at the disposal of the radiographer a mobile unit may be used with a stationary grid.

The exposure factors in this section refer to an adult male of average physique.

Radiation Protection

Radiation to the patient is reduced to a minimum by examining only the appropriate region, limiting the area of exposure, and using suitable exposure factors to avoid repeat examinations. For the lower vertebrae gonad protection is required as already considered for the pelvis and lower femora; but in the female gonad protection cannot be used for views of the sacrum and coccyx.

Basic positions

The basic positions for each region are indicated and will be discussed at the beginning of each section.

6

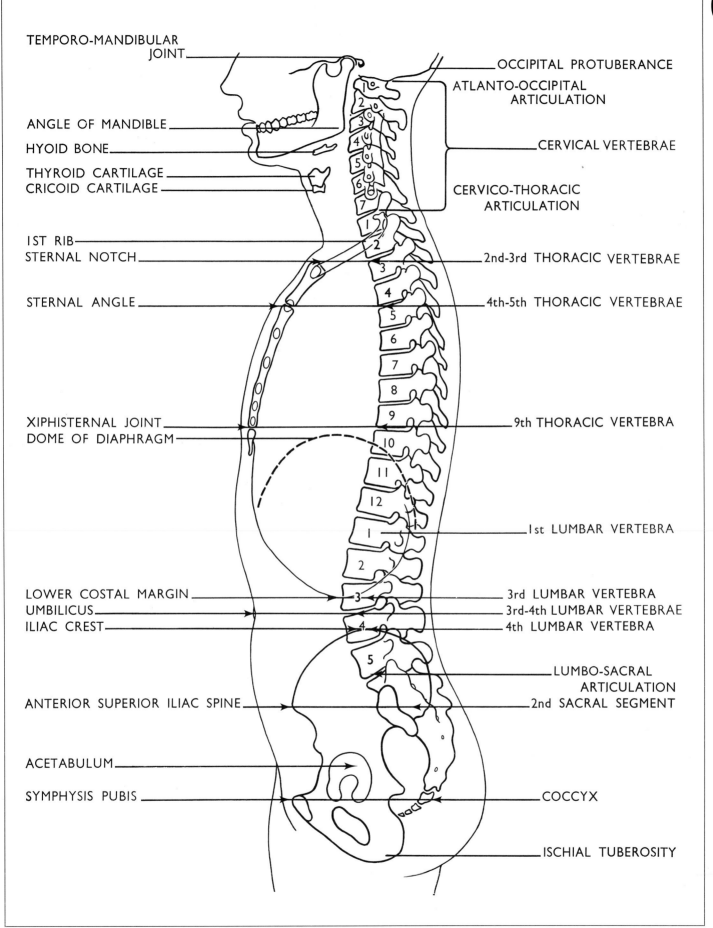

TEMPORO-MANDIBULAR JOINT

OCCIPITAL PROTUBERANCE

ATLANTO-OCCIPITAL ARTICULATION

ANGLE OF MANDIBLE

HYOID BONE

CERVICAL VERTEBRAE

THYROID CARTILAGE

CRICOID CARTILAGE

CERVICO-THORACIC ARTICULATION

1ST RIB

STERNAL NOTCH

2nd-3rd THORACIC VERTEBRAE

STERNAL ANGLE

4th-5th THORACIC VERTEBRAE

XIPHISTERNAL JOINT

DOME OF DIAPHRAGM

9th THORACIC VERTEBRA

1st LUMBAR VERTEBRA

LOWER COSTAL MARGIN

UMBILICUS

ILIAC CREST

3rd LUMBAR VERTEBRA

3rd-4th LUMBAR VERTEBRAE

4th LUMBAR VERTEBRA

LUMBO-SACRAL ARTICULATION

ANTERIOR SUPERIOR ILIAC SPINE

2nd SACRAL SEGMENT

ACETABULUM

SYMPHYSIS PUBIS

COCCYX

ISCHIAL TUBEROSITY

Cervical

Atlanto-Occipital articulation

The lateral masses of the atlas have shallow depressions for the occipital condyles which lie obliquely with their long axes forwards and inwards. From the antero-posterior aspect, the upper teeth (and the alveolar margin even in edentulous subjects), are superimposed on these articulations. In order to demonstrate this area a view with the mouth open must be done.

In the lateral position the mastoid processes overlie the upper cervical vertebrae but with accurate centring and suitable exposure factors the joint line is clearly defined.

For accurate positioning in examinations of the skull and upper cervical region a reference line is obviously required. The line used is known as the radiographic base line and is drawn from the outer canthus of the eye to the upper margin of the external auditory meatus (EAM). This is also known as the orbito-meatal base line (OMBL) (635a).

Before the radiographic examination is started all artificial "opacities" must be removed including dentures, hair pins and ear rings.

The basic views of this region are the lateral position (635a) and either antero-posterior (637) or antero-posterior obliques right and left (639).

Lateral

The patient may be seated (635a), or lying on the couch (635b), with the head and neck in the lateral position. The medial sagittal plane must be parallel to the plane of the cassette. The film is supported in contact with the head and neck.

■ Centre 2·5 cm (1 in) below and behind the external auditory meatus (EAM) perpendicular to the film using a small localizing cone (635a,b,636).

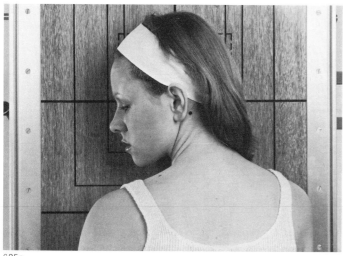

635a

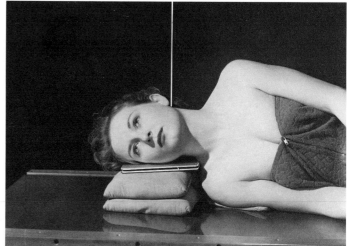

635b

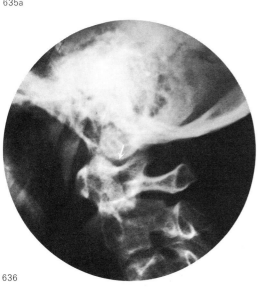

636

Antero-posterior

The patient may be seated or lying on the couch in the supine position, the chin is slightly raised to elevate the radiographic baseline 10° above the perpendicular (637,638).

■ This view is taken with the mouth open centring in the mid line through the open mouth with the tube angled 5° towards the head.

When the mouth is open it is essential to check whether the position of the baseline has been altered.

Antero-posterior oblique

With the patient facing the tube, the head is positioned with the base-line perpendicular to the film.

■ Centre between the orbits, then rotate the head so that the central ray is over the right and left orbit in turn, making an exposure in each position for comparison (639,640,641).

In this position the atlanto-occipital articulations are well demonstrated; they can also be shown in tomography of the odontoid region (655), page 181.

kVp			mAS				Film	Screens	
AP	Obl	Lat	AP	Obl	Lat	FFD	ILFORD	ILFORD	Grid
70	70	70	30	25	16	100 cm (40″)	RAPID R	FT	Grid

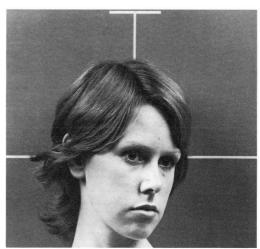

639

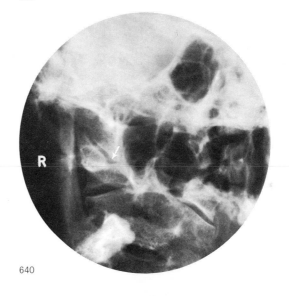

640

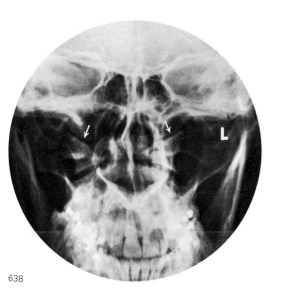

637

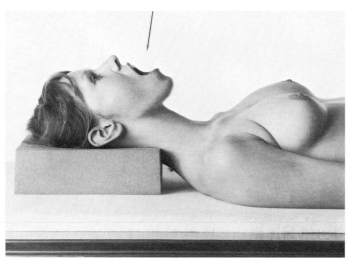

638

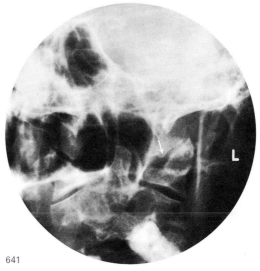

641

Vertebral column

Cervical

Before the examination all opacities such as artificial dentures, ear rings, hair pins, clips and neck ornaments must be removed. The patient is undressed to the level of the axillae. Standard intensifying screens are used and all projections may be taken with or without a grid, in the erect or horizontal position.

Antero-posterior—General
Whether the projection is through the open mouth for the first to third cervical vertebrae or below the jaw for the third to seventh cervical vertebrae, the radiographic baseline (OMBL) must be used as the reference line for tube angulation whenever adjusting the head and neck by flexion or extension.

In examining the cervical spine in the antero-posterior position the limiting density posteriorly is the lower level of the occipital bone and, anteriorly, the upper incisor teeth (642) and the lower margin of the mandible respectively (643).

To obtain maximum coverage of the vertebrae, the shadows of the anterior and posterior basal skull densities must coincide. After noting the initial tube to base line angle, adjustment can be made for the correct position.

The position of the bones should be carefully palpated before the first exposure. The seventh cervical vertebra and its prominent spinous process can be felt up to the third or second cervical vertebrae allowing for an accurate estimate of the cervical level from the lateral aspect of the neck. The level of the angle of the jaw will be found to coincide with the second to third cervical vertebrae in the neutral position.

In the open mouth view the shadows of the upper teeth and the lower occipital margin should coincide so as to show the first and second cervical vertebrae (644); in the edentulous subject the fourth may be included (645), while the vertebrae immediately below this level are obscured by the mandible.

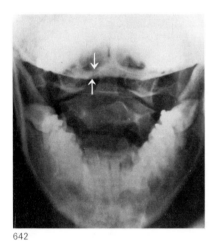

642

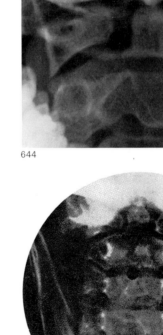

644

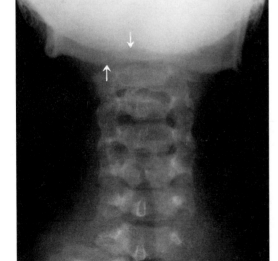

643

645

Antero-posterior
First to Third Vertebrae (basic)

The patient can be examined in the supine position. As the neck is flexed or extended the base line to film angle changes, necessitating adjustment of the tube direction through the open mouth. With the patient facing the X-ray tube, the base line should be at an angle of 20° to the normal tube direction bringing the first and second cervical vertebrae opposite the open mouth. The head should be immobilized in this position.

Movement of the mandible does not alter the relationship between upper jaw and vertebrae, so that having immobilized the head the patient need not be kept with the mouth open during final positioning. The largest bite block that can be used without discomfort is placed between the jaws to prevent the mouth from gradually closing during the exposure.

■ Centre through the open mouth with the tube in line with the upper three vertebrae so the normal ray is at an angle of 20° to the base line (646, 647).

Note—This view can equally well be taken in the erect position.

If the patient has a stiff neck with the head flexed or extended, the tube can be adjusted accordingly so that it is at an angle of 20° to 25° to the base line; with the tube angled towards the head when the neck is flexed (647) or towards the feet when the neck is extended (649).

6

AP C 1–3

kVp	mAS	FFD	Film ILFORD	Screens ILFORD	Grid
65	30	100 cm (40″)	RAPID R	FT	Grid

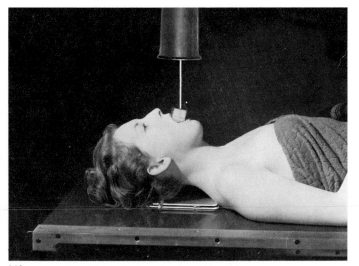

646

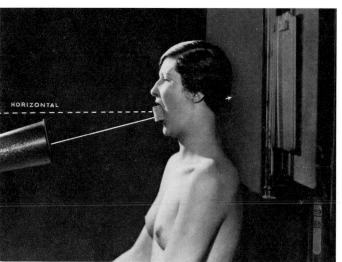

647

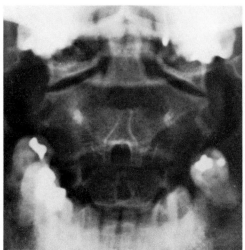

648

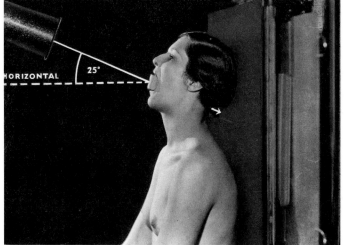

649

Odontoid process

When overshadowing densities of the jaw or skull cannot be avoided, a view which shows the odontoid peg through the occipital bone can be done, this gives almost a plan projection of the atlas.

Another way of obtaining a view of the odontoid peg is to use a dental machine with the end of the extension cone positioned in the mouth and directed toward the odontoid peg. This view should not be used routinely as the radiation dose is somewhat higher than for the basic views.

Axial, supine

With the patient supine, the neck is extended to bring the base line of the skull to an angle of 45° to the couch; the cassette is displaced upward because of the obliquity of the central ray.

■ Centre with the tube angled 35° toward the head in the mid line between the external auditory meatuses, use a small localizing cone (650, 652).

			Odontoid		
kVp	mAS	FFD	Film ILFORD	Screens ILFORD	Grid
80	40	100 cm (40")	RAPID R	FT	Grid

30° Vertico-Mental
Axial prone

The previous view can also be obtained in the prone position but this is not so convenient for the patient. Again the head must be extended so that the base line is at an angle of 45°.

■ Centre with the tube angled 30° towards the feet in the mid line between the external auditory meatuses, use a small localizing cone (651, 653).

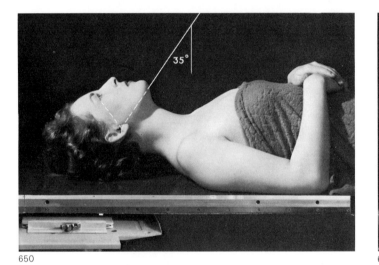

650

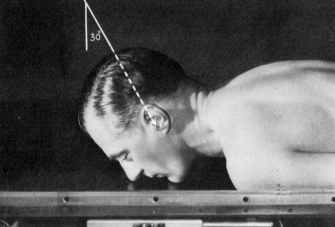

651

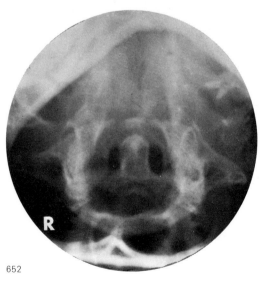

652

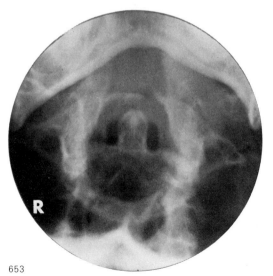

653

Fracture Radiographs

Radiograph (654) was taken for a suspected fracture of the odontoid peg, but, due to difficulty in adjusting the head, the bone injury is obscured by the mandible. Because of the suspected injury flexion and extension of the neck is contra-indicated; an antero-posterior view of the odontoid peg can be obtained by using tomography which blurs out the overlying shadow of the mandible and shows the fracture (655).

Lateral
First to fifth vertebrae

Commonly the lateral projection is taken to show all seven cervical vertebrae and their adjacent articulations, however, when the investigation is only for the upper five vertebrae, the patient can be examined with the cassette in contact with the neck.

The examination can be made with the patient seated or in the horizontal position (656) with the cassette supported to fit into the neck above the shoulder.

■ Centre to the third cervical vertebra (656, 657)

kVp	mAS	FFD	Film ILFORD	Screens ILFORD	Grid
65	8	100 cm (40")	RAPID R	FT	—

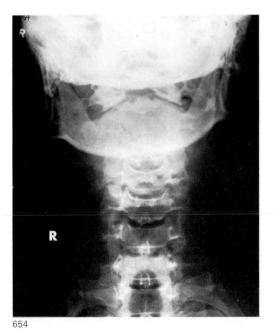

654

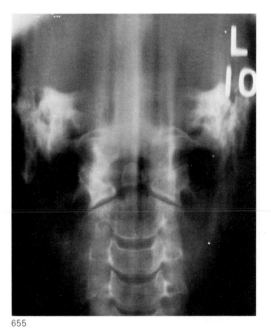

655

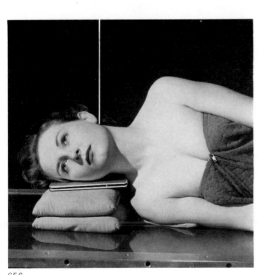

656

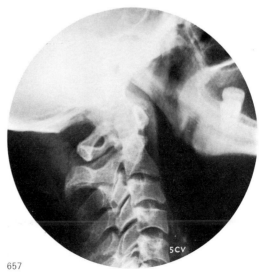

657

Antero-posterior
Third to seventh vertebrae (basic)

With the patient supine the neck is extended so that the base line is at an angle of 20° to the vertical. By using a 10° tube angulation the lower border of the mandible will be superimposed on the lower margin of the occipital bone, giving a clear view of the third to seventh cervical vertebrae.

■ Centre in the mid line at the level of the fourth cervical vertebra with the tube angled 10° towards the head (658, 660, 661a)

			Film	Screens	
kVp	mAS	ILFORD	ILFORD		Grid
80	40	100 cm (40")	RAPID R	FT	Grid

AP C 3–7

The direction of the beam provides the maximum intervertebral joint spaces and the maximum area of vertebrae free from superimposition. The line on radiograph (659) shows the effect of angulation toward the head; the lower mandible is projected over the occipital bone leaving the vertebral bodies below C.3 free of overlying shadow.

A Potter-Bucky is used to obtain a good quality radiograph.

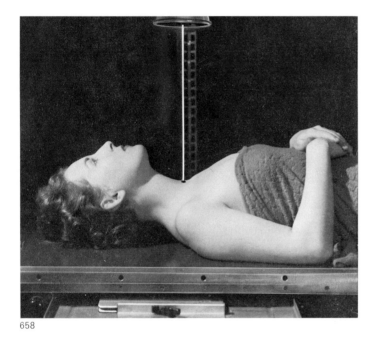

658

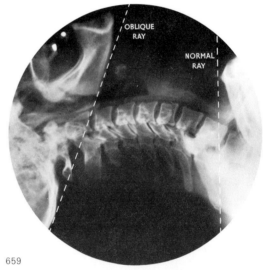

659

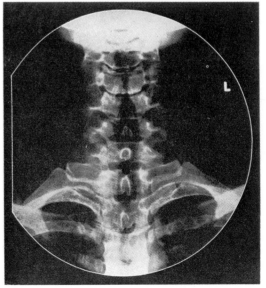

660

Antero-posterior
Second to seventh vertebrae

It is not always possible for a patient to extend or flex the head to bring the base line to 20° to the vertical, but then a 10° cephalad tube angulation projects the lower jaw to a position of maximum clearance and the intervertebral joint spaces are well shown (661a, 662).

When the chin cannot be raised to bring the base line to 20° to the vertical the tube can be angled to compensate; this improves coverage of third to seventh cervical area and clarity of the intervertebral joint spaces (661b, 663).

Less frequently, when there is hyper-extension of the cervical spine, a reverse tube angulation with a caudal tilt may be needed (661c, 664).

The degree of angulation required can be assessed after viewing the lateral film which should be taken first in this type of case.

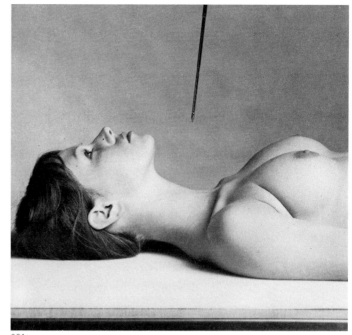

661a

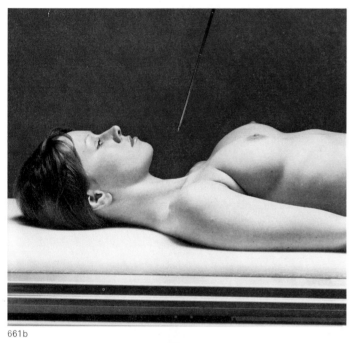

661b

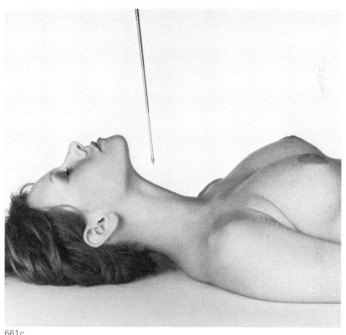

661c

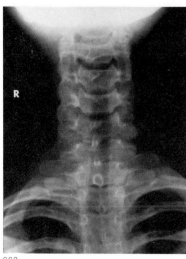

662

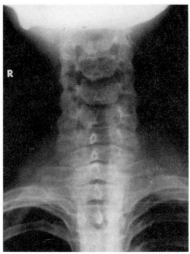

663

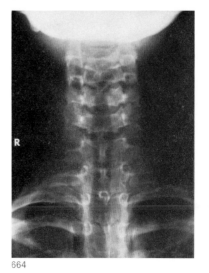

664

Diffusion Technique

By immobilizing the head and allowing the mouth to open and close continuously during the exposure there will be diffusion of the overlying shadow of the mandible and all the cervical vertebrae can then be seen using a single exposure with a long exposure time; the exposure time needs to be in the region of eight seconds (665). Alternatively, tomography may be used (666).

Lateral (basic)—General

The patient is seated or standing with the neck in the neutral position and the jaw slightly raised so that the angles of the mandible are clear of the cervical vertebral bodies, the shoulders are depressed so that their densities are projected below the level of the seventh cervical vertebra and the medial plane of the head is parallel to the film (669).

When the lateral aspect of the shoulder is against the vertical support, the cassette is a considerable distance from the vertebrae. To compensate for the large object/film distance which can cause considerable loss of definition particularly with a broad focus tube, the focus film distance is increased to a minimum of 150 cm (60 ins). However, with a fine focus tube definition may be satisfactory at a shorter distance.

Immobilization with a head clamp in the erect position or carefully placed sandbags in the supine position can be used for those patients who cannot remain still.

Lat Cerv. (Basic)

kVp	mAS	FFD	Film ILFORD	Screens ILFORD	Grid
65	40	180 cm (6')	RAPID R	FT	—

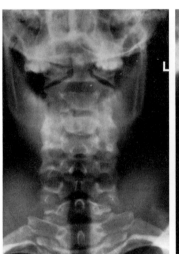 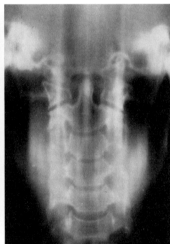

665/666

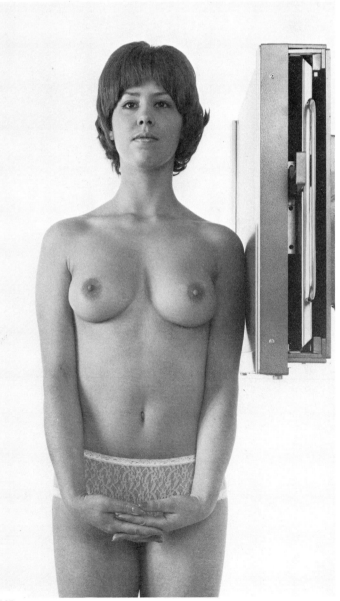

667

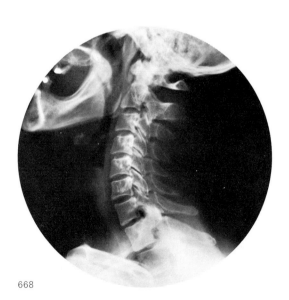

668

Figures (670, 671) show the difference between the levels of the shoulders when the arms are allowed to hang loosely as compared with the shoulders being deliberately depressed. When the shoulders are deliberately depressed they drop free of the lower cervical region showing the whole of the body of the seventh cervical vertebra on the radiograph.

Pathological radiographs

In severe ankylosing spondylitis (672) the patient will have an immobile cervical spine. There may be no difficulty in taking (a) the lateral view but to show the cervical vertebrae in the antero-posterior view two projections will be needed (b) a view through the open mouth for the upper cervical spine and (c) an angled view from below the jaw for the lower vertebrae.

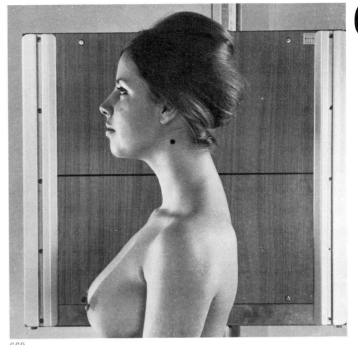

669

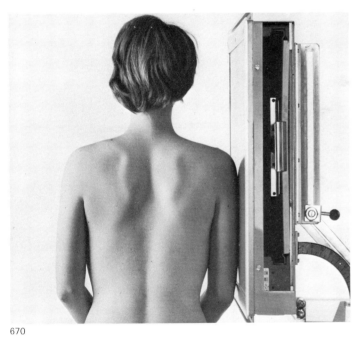

670

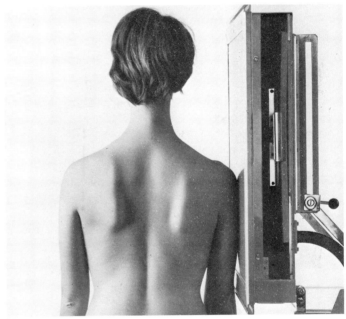

671

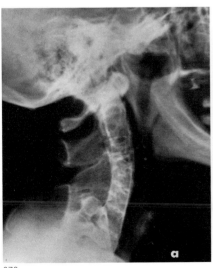

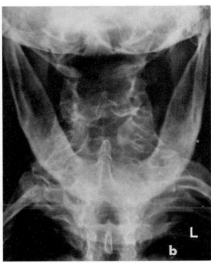

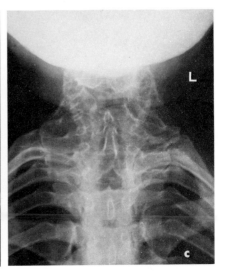

672

185

Stretcher patients

When the patient is sent to the X-ray department for exclusion of a fracture in the cervical region, the patient must not be moved from the casualty trolley. The lateral radiograph must be seen before proceeding with the antero-posterior projection.

For the lateral view the patient is in the horizontal supine position, the film is supported vertically at shoulder level, and the X-ray beam is directed horizontally using a focus film distance of 150–180 cm (45–60 in) (673,674).

If a definite fracture is seen on the lateral radiograph, place the film under the trolley surface to avoid moving the patient's head. If there is any doubt about whether the patient's head may have to be moved to place the cassette in position consult the Casualty officer before proceeding with the examination.

Fracture radiographs

Two radiographs (675a,b) show a fracture of the body of the seventh cervical vertebra.

A fracture dislocation of the fifth cervical vertebra is shown in the two radiographs (676) which were taken with the patient in the supine position.

Flexion and Extension

For the assessment of spinal movement and change in vertebral body relationships the views in flexion and extension are required.

These can be taken with the patient supine (677,678) but are much more conveniently done in the erect position (679,680).

The series of radiographs (681) were taken in the erect position (a) normal, (b) on flexion and (c) on extension.

Radiographs (682,683) show the results of an old whiplash injury with narrowing of the disc space at the level of C.4/5. Radiographs (683) were taken following a wiring operation to stabilize the vertebrae.

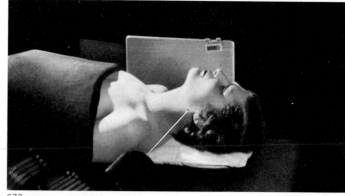

673

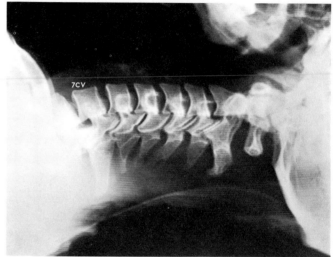

674

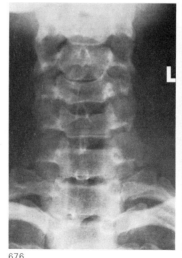

675

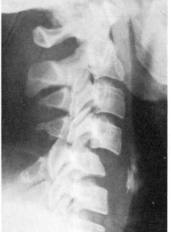

676

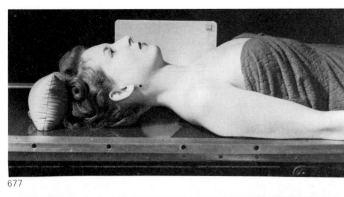

677

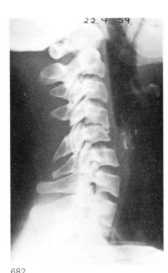

22.9.59.

682

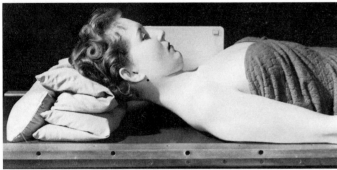

678

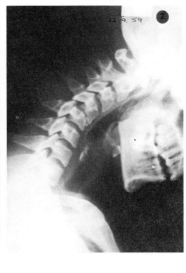

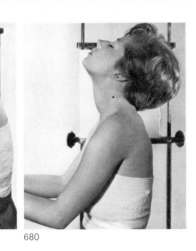

679

680

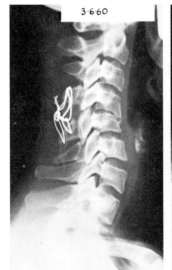

3.6.60

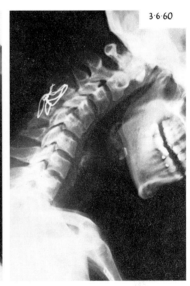

3.6.60

683

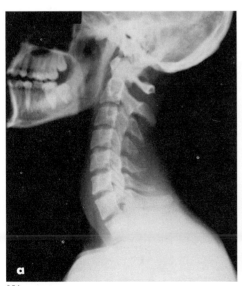

a

681

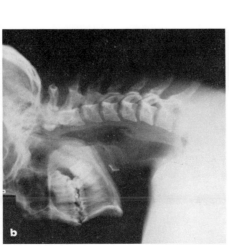

b

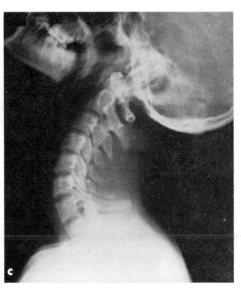

c

Oblique

Oblique projections of the cervical vertebrae are used to demonstrate the arches and the intervertebral foramina and are of particular interest for such conditions as a tumour of the posterior nerve ganglion.

Oblique views can be done with the patient either in antero-posterior or postero-anterior oblique positions; the antero-posterior oblique position is usually more convenient. The radiographic appearances are essentially similar. The angle of the mandible is usually superimposed on the anterior aspects of the upper two vertebral bodies. The foramina disclosed are of the side nearest the tube for the antero-posterior oblique projections (684,685,686a) and of the side nearest the film for the postero-anterior oblique projections (687,688,689a). These views are usually taken with the patient in the erect position but they may also be done with the patient horizontal.

Cervical spine erect
Right and left antero-posterior oblique

The patient is turned from the antero-posterior position through 45° for left and right sides in turn. The chin is slightly depressed. Initially the head is in a forward position (684) but is then turned approximately parallel with the film to avoid superimposition of the rami over the spine (685).

■ Centre to the mid neck at the level of C.4 with the tube angled 15° towards the head. This is in direct line with the foramina of each side in turn (685,686b).

Right and left postero-anterior oblique

With the patient facing the film, the right and left side of the patient is moved in turn 45° away from the film. The chin is slightly depressed and the head turned approximately parallel with the film to avoid superimposition of the rami over the spine.

■ Centre to the mid neck at the level of C.4 with the tube angled 15° towards the feet (687,688,689a)

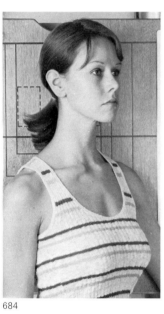

684

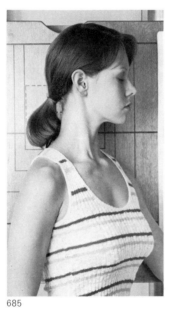

685

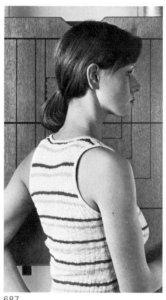

687

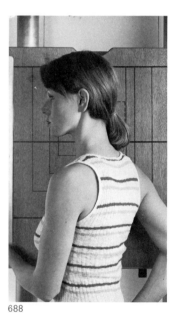

688

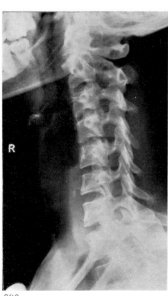

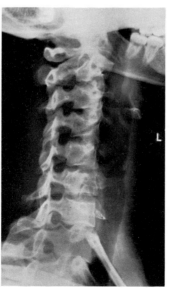

686a

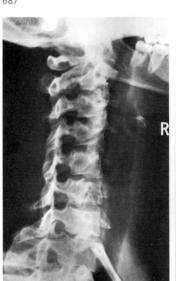

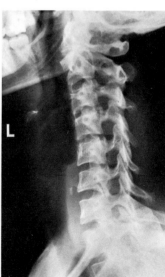

689a

Note—Turning the head does not interfere with the 45° oblique position of the cervical spine.

The four comparative oblique radiographs, antero-posterior (686) and postero-anterior oblique (689) have been included to show the difference between results obtained when the tube is straight (a) and angled (b).

Oblique—Supine anterior

If the patient cannot be turned into the correct position similar radiographic appearances may be obtained by angulation of the tube with the patient supine and the head straight. The tube is angled to right and left sides in turn (690) to produce results similar to those shown in the erect position (686).

The chin is raised to bring the radiographic base line 20° to the perpendicular.

■ Centre to the mid neck at the level of C.4 with the tube angled 45° thus directly through the intervertebral foramina, taking right and left sides in turn with appropriate film adjustment. Longitudinal angling of the tube by 15° towards the head may be necessary depending on the observed curviture of the spine in relation to the film (690a, b)

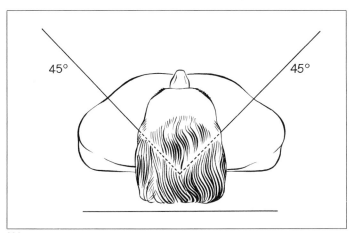

690

Cern Obl					
kVp	mAS	FFD	Film ILFORD	Screens ILFORD	Grid
70	40	180 cm (6')	RAPID R	FT	—

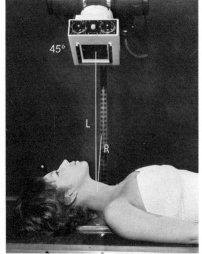

690a

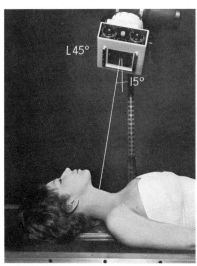

690b

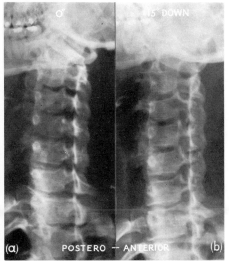

(a) POSTERO — ANTERIOR (b)

686b

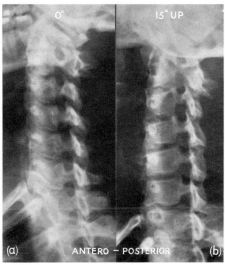

(a) ANTERO — POSTERIOR (b)

689b

Cervico-Thoracic region

Cervico-Thoracic AP					
kVp	mAS	FFD	Film ILFORD	Screens ILFORD	Grid
70	25	100 cm (40″)	RAPID R	FT	Grid

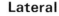

Cervico-Thoracic region
It is difficult to radiograph the region of the fifth cervical to fourth thoracic vertebrae in the lateral position as the spine is obscured by the density of the shoulders.

Antero-posterior (basic)
Positioning is similar to that used for the antero-posterior (basic) projection of the third to seventh cervical region. The film is positioned to include from the fourth cervical to the fourth thoracic vertebrae. The air-filled trachea is superimposed on this region of the spine.
■ Centre at the level of the sternal notch in the midline (691, 691a)

Lateral
The vertebrae may be shown above the shoulders (692), behind the shoulders (694), between the shoulders from side to side (693) and between the shoulders from above downward (696).

Lateral (1)
Use a similar technique as for the lateral cervical vertebrae (basic) but depress the shoulders to the lowest possible level.
■ Centre laterally to the sixth cervical vertebra (692, 692a)

Increase the lateral cervical exposure by 5 kilovolts. For a long neck the first, second and sometimes third thoracic vertebral bodies are shown.

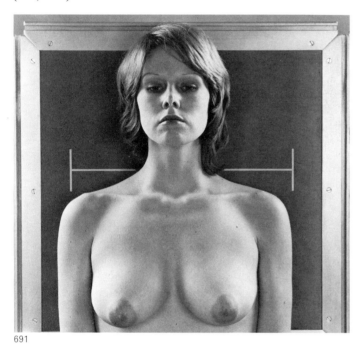

691

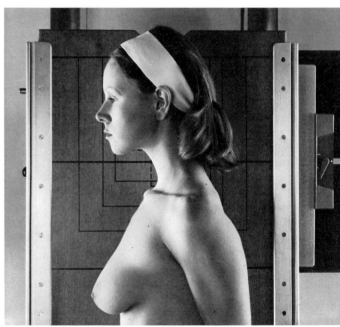

692

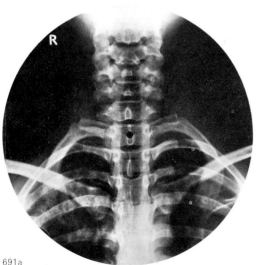

691a

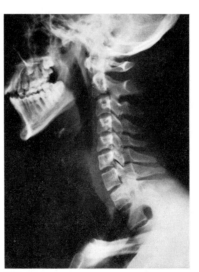

692a

Lateral (2) (between the shoulders)

From the lateral position the patient is turned through approximately 20° with the arm nearest to the film brought forward and the other arm moved backward to remove the densities of the shoulders from the spine.

In this position the spine is seen between the shoulders (693a) but with little effect on the lateral appearance of the vertebrae. The head is kept in the same direction as the trunk.

■ Centre to the level of the sternal notch, below the mid-point of the clavicle remote from the film (693, 693a, 693b)

			OBL		
kVp	mAS	FFD	Film ILFORD	Screens ILFORD	Grid
70	40	100 cm (40")	RAPID R	FT	Grid

The fracture radiographs (693b) show the value of the oblique projection. The routine lateral projection shown in (a) suggests a fracture of the seventh cervical vertebrae but this is not well shown. However, on the oblique projection the seventh cervical vertebra is well seen as well as the upper thoracic vertebrae. The third radiograph in this series shows a lateral oblique projection after a plaster cast has been applied.

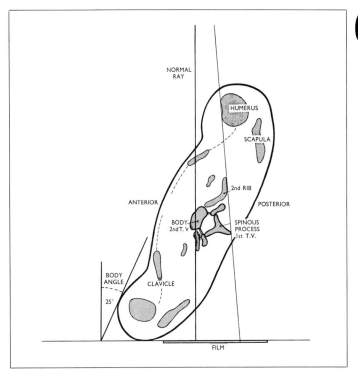

693a

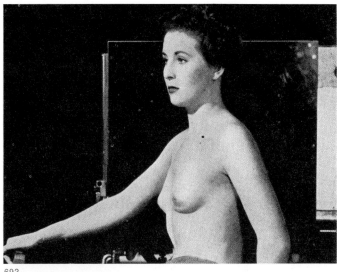

693

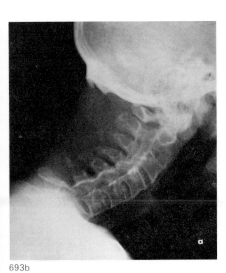

693b

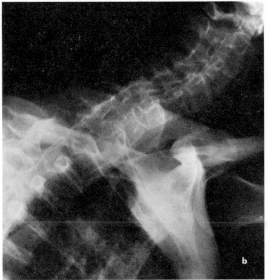

a

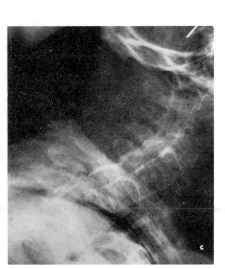

b

c

191

6

Lateral (3) and Spinous processes

With the patient in the lateral (basic) position, the arms are brought forward and the neck flexed to rest the chin on the upper chest, in this position the shoulders are well forward in front of the vertebral bodies.

■ Centre between the shoulders at the level of the first thoracic vertebra (694, 694a)

To show the whole length of the spinous process the exposure should be reduced by 50%.

When the patient is sufficiently mobile for this position to be used, the vertebral bodies are well demonstrated, as well as the spinous processes which are elevated on flexion. In this position there is maximum separation of the vertebral bodies and the rib shadows.

			Lat (2)		
kVp	mAS	FFD	Film ILFORD	Screens ILFORD	Grid
90	40	100 cm (40″)	RAPID R	FT	Grid

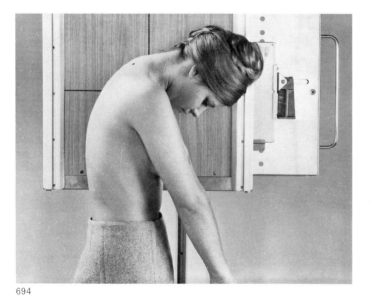

694

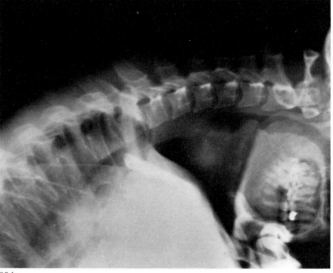

694a

Lateral (4)

The patient is placed laterally against the vertical Bucky with the arm of that side folded over the head and with the trunk bending a little laterally at the waist towards the tube. In this position the film is adjacent to the axilla and upper arm, and the beam is directed between the vertically separated shoulders which are at different levels.

■ Centre above the shoulder remote from the tube toward the axilla adjacent to the film with the tube angled 10°–15° to the head (695, 695a, 696, 697).

			Film ILFORD	Screens ILFORD	
kVp	mAS	FFD			Grid
120	32	100 cm (40″)	RAPID R	FT	Grid

Lat (3)

The cervico-thoracic region is well shown without undue distortion. Radiograph (695a) covers the general projection and (697) the localized region concerned.

The photograph (696) shows the posture of the patient from the anterior aspect, and (695) the relationship from the lateral aspect.

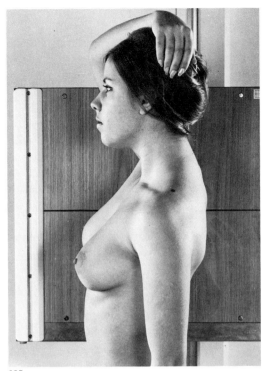

695

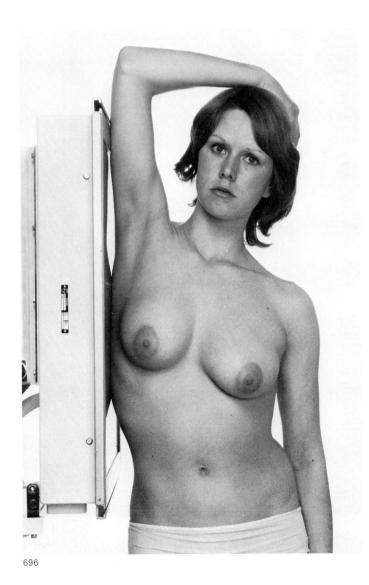

696

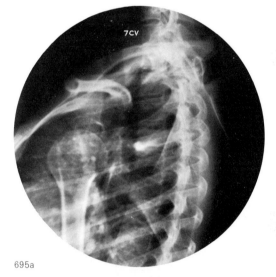

695a

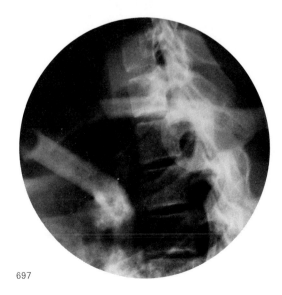

697

Thoracic

Radiographic density in the thoracic region varies considerably. In the antero-posterior view upper thoracic vertebrae are more radiolucent because of the overlying air-filled trachea; whereas the lower thoracic vertebral region is much denser due to overlying heart, aorta, dome of diaphragm and liver. The lower thoracic vertebrae are also larger than the upper vertebrae.

To compensate for the overlying dense shadows on the lower two-thirds of the thoracic vertebrae (700a, 700b) the exposure technique must be adjusted if both the lower and the upper vertebrae are to be shown on one film (700c). As increasing the kilovoltage may not be sufficient to overcome this difficulty a wedge filter may be used to obtain a satisfactory radiograph; the thicker part of the wedge must be placed over the upper thoracic region.

Antero-posterior (basic)

The patient is supine, in the middle of the table and centralized to the Potter-Bucky with the arms beside the trunk. A low pillow under the head maintains the spinal curve and pads are placed under the knee and ankle joints for the patient's comfort.
■ Centre in the mid line mid-way between the cricoid cartilage and the xiphoid process of the sternum, approximately 2·5 cm (1 in) below the sternal angle (699, 700c).

Thoracic AP					
kVp	mAS	FFD	Film ILFORD	Screens ILFORD	Grid
80	40	100 cm (40″)	RAPID R	FT	Grid

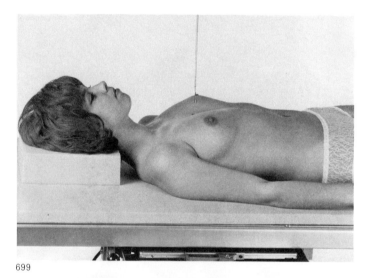

699

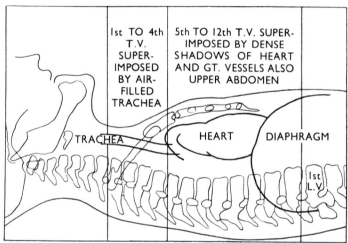

698

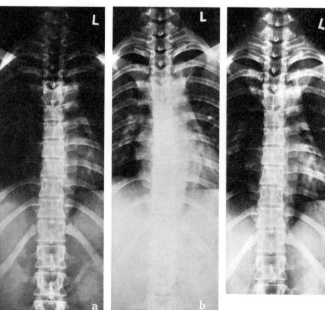

700

The importance of correct positioning and centring is shown in the antero-posterior radiographs (702)—two exposures of the one subject—(a) correct, with joint spaces clearly seen, and (b) incorrect with joint spaces overshadowed by adjacent bodies. Similarly there is loss of the joint spaces in the lateral view (703).

When taking the antero-posterior (basic) projection of the thoracic spine, errors can occur in placing the film so that the upper three thoracic vertebrae are excluded; errors can also occur in centring. The ribs lie obliquely across the spine. The sternal angle and adjacent second costal cartilage are at the level of the disc between the fourth and fifth thoracic vertebrae; the seventh cervical vertebra can be palpated because of its prominent spinous process.

Separation of the vertebral bodies is obtained when the X-ray beam is directed at right angles to the arc of the curve formed by the vertebrae. This varies with the individual, and is judged more easily with the patient in the erect position (701).

After a large film of the thoracic vertebrae has been taken an abnormality may be better demonstrated by taking a localized view (704); close the diaphragms to the appropriate size or use a localizing cone (711).

6

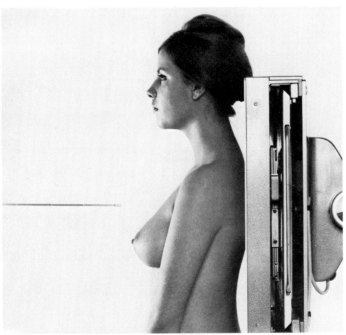

701

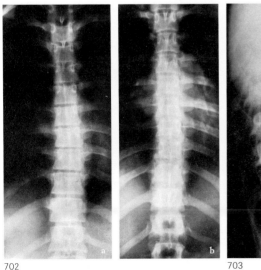

702

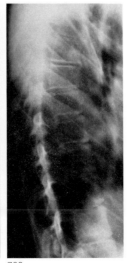

703

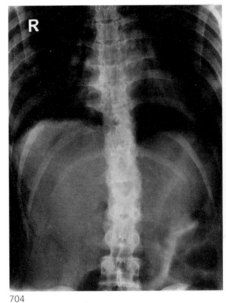
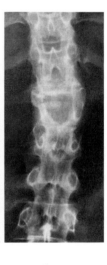

704

Lateral (basic)

The patient is turned on to one side, with the head on a pillow so that the whole of the spine is parallel to the table top, the hips and knees are flexed with a pad between the knees for support as shown from above in (705) and posteriorly in (706).

Both arms may be folded over the head or, with the uppermost arm at a right angle to the trunk, the hand may grip the side of the table (705) to help immobilization. Stretching the uppermost arm above the head helps to bring the spine parallel to the table top.

The obliquity of the long axis of the spine will vary from subject to subject and the position of each individual should be adjusted accordingly. To compensate for sagging of the vertebral column in the thoraco-lumbar region angle the tube towards the head, so that the central ray bisects the long axis of the vertebrae at right angles.

Alternatively, place a non-opaque pad under the thoraco-lumbar region to bring the long axis of the thoracic region parallel to the film. The tube is positioned with the axial ray vertical and at right angles to the vertebral column and film (706).

Whenever it is possible to align the patient with the spine parallel to the film this should be done in preference to angling the tube.

■ Centre through the axilla at the level of the sixth thoracic vertebra, and at right angles to the long axis of the thoracic region (705, 706, 707).

When using the Potter-Bucky compression band to immobilize the vertebral column, the patient is allowed to breathe gently during a long exposure at low milliamperage to produce, by movement, diffusion of the lung and rib shadows over the vertebrae.

In (708) the projection has been slightly modified which is particularly useful for the upper thoracic vertebrae. In this position the lower arm is brought well forward and the upper arm backward away from the body. The spine is then slightly oblique to the true lateral position but the appearances are hardly distinguishable from the true lateral (basic). There is however much less overlying shadowing.

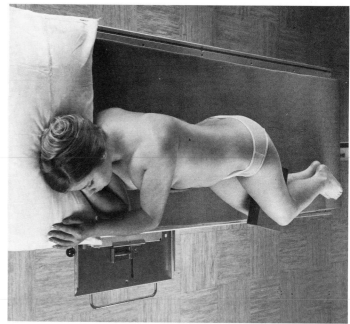

705

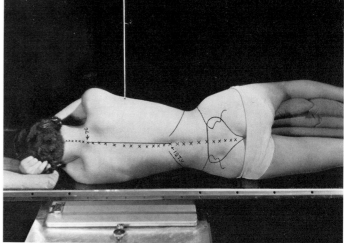

706

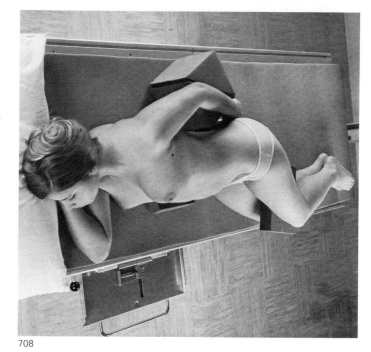

708

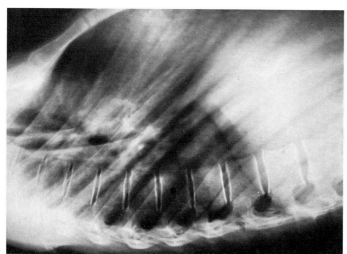

707

196

Erect

The patient stands in the lateral position, and is adjusted to bring the long axis of the vertebral column parallel to the film, with the arms brought forward and externally rotated so that the back of the hands touch. Alternatively, the arms may be folded forward over the head. This view may be taken standing or seated.

■ Centre below the inferior angle of the scapula, at the level of the sixth to seventh thoracic vertebrae (709, 710)

Pathological radiographs

Coned views of the upper thoracic region are shown in radiograph (711).

(712) shows a widening of the soft tissues around the mid thoracic region due to a para-vertebral abscess. Because of the overlying soft tissue shadowing a radiograph with an increased exposure may be required to show the bone detail. The lateral projection is also shown (712b) with compression of the intervertebral disc.

6

			Lat (Basic)		
kVp	mAS	FFD	Film ILFORD	Screens ILFORD	Grid
70	60	100 cm (40″)	RAPID R	FT	Grid

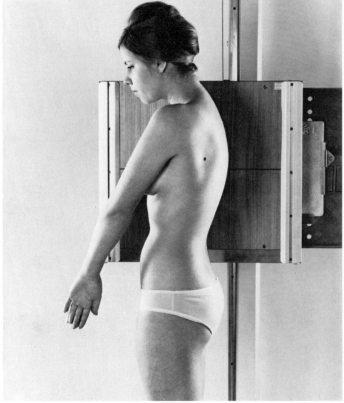

709

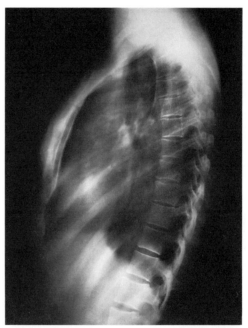

710

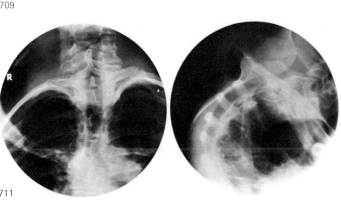

711

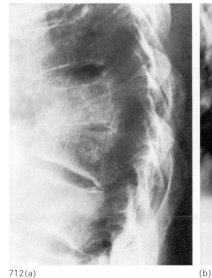
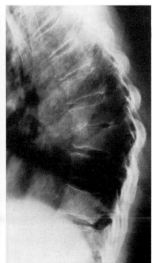

712(a)   (b)

197

Right or Left posterior oblique

From the antero-posterior position, supine or erect, the patient is rotated through 45° to right and left sides in turn, and when supine, supported in position with non-opaque pads. The arms may be placed beside the trunk with one arm slightly forward and the other slightly backward.

■ Centre to the mid clavicular line 2·5 cm (1 in) below the level of the sternal notch on the side of the thorax nearest the tube (713, 714)

			Oblique		
kVp	mAS	FFD	Film ILFORD	Screens ILFORD	Grid
70	40	100 cm (40″)	RAPID R	FT	Grid

As will be seen in radiographs (714), the rib articulations of the side next to the film are well demonstrated and also the intervertebral articulations of the opposite side.

For the left oblique projection, an increase of 5 kilovolts is required to allow for the overshadowing density of the heart.

The oblique projections (715) are regarded as useful additions to the routine projections (716), antero-posterior and lateral, which show the condition of hemi-vertebrae.

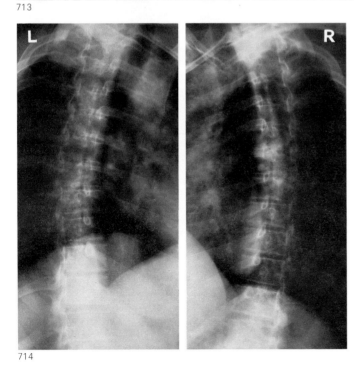

713

714

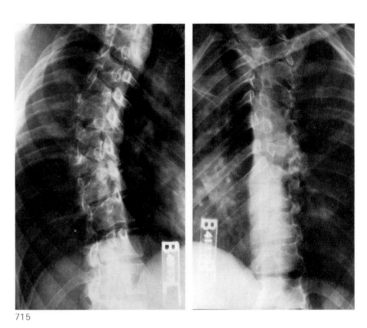

715

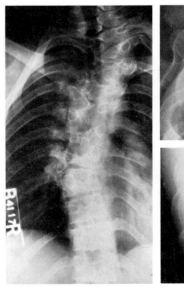

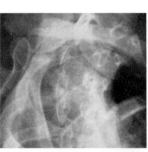

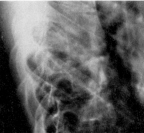

716

Pathological Radiographs

Three radiographs (717, 718, 719) show a tuberculous lesion in a child and are typical of the results using a small cone to localize the area following the initial general exploratory examination.

The lateral projections (718, 719) show the difference in the appearance of the lesion on using short and long exposure times; (718) was exposed for 0·8 seconds at 100 milliamperes during arrested respiration and (719) for 4 seconds at 20 milliamperes during gentle respiration, both taken without the Potter-Bucky diaphragm at a focus-film distance of 150 cm.

Tomography is also valuable in giving a clearer view of the lesion; in (720) a tuberculous bone abscess is shown in a thoracic vertebra on lateral tomography.

Intervertebral Discs

To demonstrate intervertebral discs care must be taken to have the central ray at right angles to the long axis of the spine. The exact angulation of the central ray will depend upon the spinal curve which must be adjusted to each individual.

Disc protrusions may be recognized on myelography, an examination in which contrast medium is injected into the subarachnoid space of the spinal canal.

6

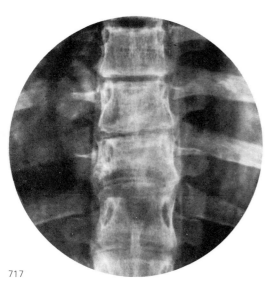

717

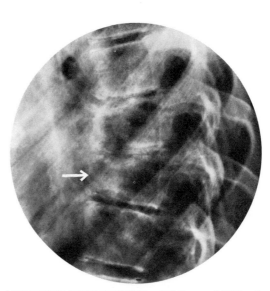

ARRESTED RESPIRATION   4/5 Second 100 mA
718

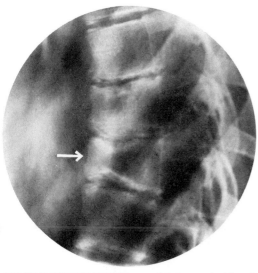

GENTLE RESPIRATION   10 Seconds 10 mA
719

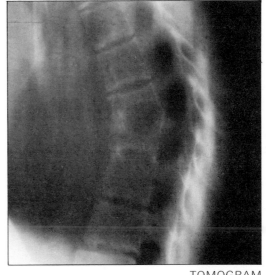

TOMOGRAM

720

199

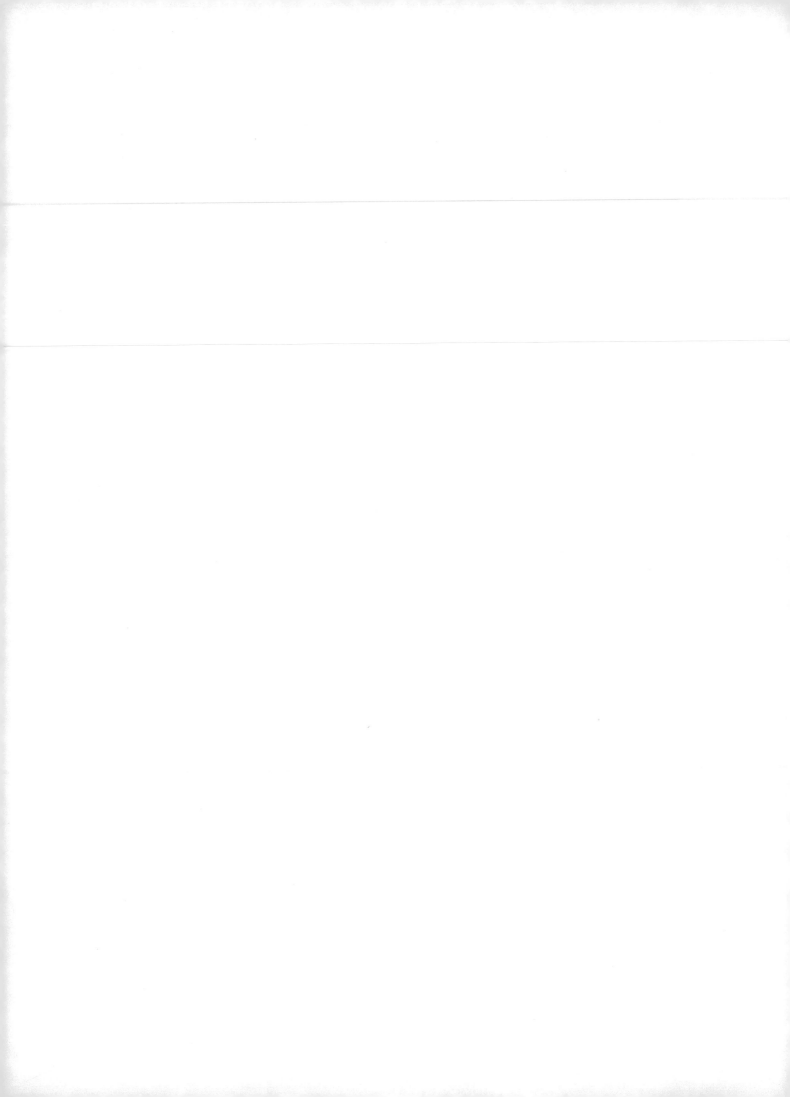

7

VERTEBRAL COLUMN

7 SECTION 7

VERTEBRAL COLUMN

Radiation Protection

Radiation to the genital organs must always be minimized by careful choice of exposure factors, the use of fast film/screen combinations, by limiting the number of exposures, adequate collimation and by local shielding with lead rubber.

Lumbar

Correct positioning is also important in the lumbar region to prevent the vertebral bodies from not overshadowing the intervertebral spaces in either the antero-posterior or lateral projections.

Because the lumbar curve is convex anteriorly with a space of 5·0–7·5 cm (2–3 ins) between the apex of the curve and the couch, the convexity should be reduced wherever possible, before taking the antero-posterior radiographs.

With the patient horizontal this can be done in two ways. In (721) the patient is supine and in the natural position showing a well marked lumbar arch which is reduced in (722) by flexing the hip and knee joints thus straightening the back. Alternatively, the shoulders may be raised as in (723) with a small sandbag placed under the knees which brings the dorsal aspect of the trunk into contact with the couch.

The diagram (724) shows the varying relationships of the vertebral bodies and the film depending on the position of the trunk. Tracings were made from two pairs of lateral radiographs taken of the same subject to show soft tissue and bone structures. The exposures were made as previously described on this page, the patient was (a) in a relaxed position (721), to show the maximum lumbar curve and (b) with the back straight (722) or (723) to reduce the lumbar curve.

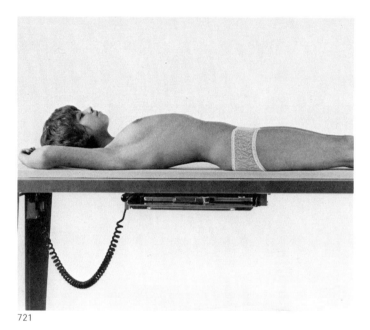

721

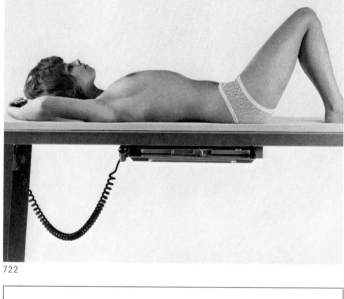

722

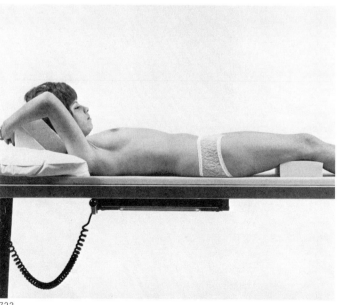

723

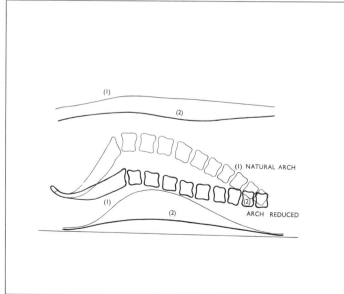

724

In (725) the patient is standing naturally and shows a normal curve in the lumbar region. The lumbar arch can be reduced by bringing the shoulders forward, as in (726).

The fifth lumbar vertebra is not always clearly demonstrated in the general antero-posterior projection, its appearance depending on the angle at the lumbo-sacral articulation. In (729) on page 204 the fifth lumbar vertebra is clearly shown because the articulation is almost horizontal and should be compared with (730), where it is foreshortened with the lumbo-sacral articulation obscured because of a well marked angle. It is therefore, often necessary to take a separate radiograph for the fifth lumbar vertebra, as described for the lumbo-sacral articulation, page 214.

In antero-posterior radiographs a psoas muscle is seen on each side of the vertebral column from the level of the twelfth thoracic vertebra to the iliac crest (729). The psoas muscles are inserted into the lesser trochanters of the femora but are obscured by the bone density over the region of the pelvis.

There is a marked advantage in using compression whenever possible for large subjects; (727), (a) having been exposed without compression and (b) with compression. The broad Potter-Bucky compression band is a good method for applying widespread even compression to improve the definition and clarity of a radiograph.

The exposure factors in this section refer to an adult subject of average physique.

It is essential to include the thoraco-lumbar and the lumbo-sacral articulations when a 24×30 cm $(10 \times 12$ ins) film is used (729), and the lower thoracic and sacral regions may also be included on a 30×40 cm $(12 \times 15$ ins) film (730).

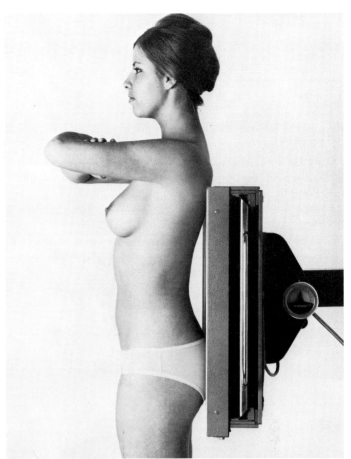

725

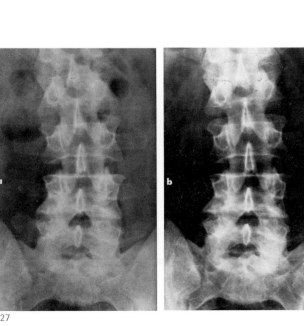

727

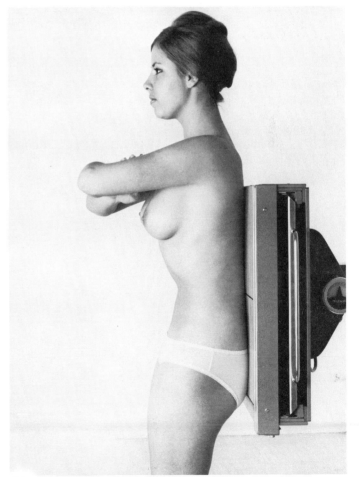

726

Antero-posterior (basic)

Radiographs are taken from the antero-posterior aspect after reducing the lumbar arch as discussed previously. A focus-film distance of 100 cm (40 ins) may be used.

With the patient horizontal (728), the knees are raised to reduce the lumbar arch and a sandbag placed across the feet to maintain the limbs in position. The patient is adjusted to the middle of the couch to be central to the grid and tube.

■ Centre to the mid line between the lower costal margins, at the level of the third lumbar vertebra (728, 729, 730)

There is a strong tendency when taking this projection to centre at too low a level and the radiograph then includes too much of the sacrum while omitting the upper two lumbar vertebrae.

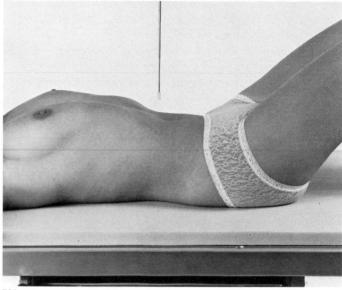
728

Lumbar AP

kVp	mAS	FFD	Film ILFORD	Screens ILFORD	Grid
70	80	100 cm (40″)	RAPID R	FT	Grid

Transverse processes

The transverse processes are often over-penetrated with the conventional kilovoltage for the spine. If detail of the transverse processes is required particularly to exclude a fracture, further radiographs should be taken using a reduction of 5–7 kilovolts.

When gas and faeces in the colon obscure the spine a long exposure technique can be used. The patient is instructed to continue quiet breathing and with the milliamperes suitably adjusted an exposure of 3–5 seconds is made. This technique is similar to that used for the dorsal region to eliminate the shadowing of the overlying ribs. (719) page 199.

In the lumbar region the effect of breathing is to reduce the colon density by diffusing it over a greater area.

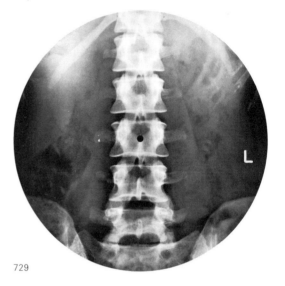
729

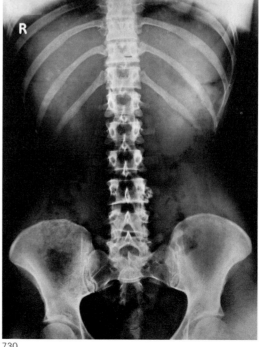
730

Posterior-anterior (prone)

Radiographs of the lumbar spine may also be taken in the postero-anterior position but then the lumbar curve is in the opposite direction. To prevent over-shadowing of the vertebral bodies onto the intervertebral spaces the tube angulation must be reversed with the tube angled cranially. In some patients it be possible to straighten the curve by placing pads under the abdomen.

In thin subjects the vertebral bodies are brought nearer to the film in the prone position (733) as compared with the supine position.

■ Centre in the midline over the third lumbar vertebra at the level of the lower costal margin with a tube angulation of 10° towards the head to compensate for the lumbar curve.

Radiographs were taken of the same subject (732) in the prone position and (734) in the supine position. There is little difference in definition in the two positions, but the most marked variation is in the appearance of the sacro-iliac joints which are elongated and more clearly defined with the patient prone.

In diagram (733) line drawings of lateral radiographs of the lumbar spine are compared in the prone (1) and supine (2) positions; the changing relationships of the soft tissues as well as the bone is shown.

Postero-anterior—Erect

With the patient facing the film, the shoulders and hips are pressed firmly against the film support, with the head turned to one side and the feet separated.

■ Centre in the mid line over the third lumbar vertebra at the level of the lower costal margin.

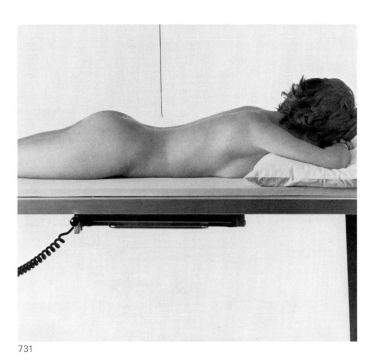

731

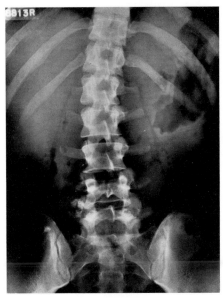

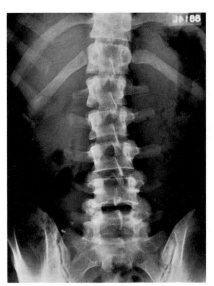

PRONE
732

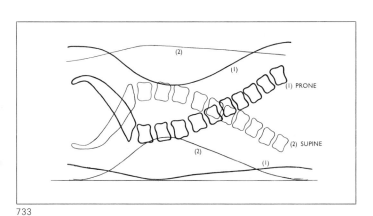

733

SUPINE
734

Lateral—horizontal (basic)

Whenever possible the patient is moved into the lateral position, with the knees and hips flexed and the uppermost leg supported at the hip level (735). The arm nearest the couch is placed under the head to bring the elbow away from the vertebrae, and the uppermost arm brought forward to grasp the side of the couch to steady the trunk in position. The uppermost arm can also be stretched over the head which helps to bring the spine parallel to the table top. A non-opaque pad between the hip joint and the couch adds to the patient's comfort.

The long axis of the lumbar region tends to lie obliquely from the first to the fifth lumbar level, as the body sags at the waist towards the film (735) and is more marked in women who have wider pelves. In male subjects with narrower pelves, the vertebral line tends to be more horizontal.

To bring the long axis of the spine parallel to the film, a non-opaque sponge roll should be placed under the thoraco-lumbar

region (736). Alternatively, the tube may be angled towards the feet, so that the central ray bisects the long axis of the vertebrae at right angles (735). Without this adjustment there will be overlapping of vertebral bodies on the radiograph obscuring the intervertebral disc spaces occupied by fibro-cartilage. The radiograph (738) shows a correctly aligned central ray which is at right angles to the spine compared with (739) where there is some overlapping of the vertebral bodies on the intervertebral disc spaces. Under suitable conditions the focus-film distance may be increased to 120 cm (48 ins) to reduce magnification and loss of definition due to the long object-film distance, although a fine focus tube may help to compensate for subject film displacement.

■ Centre 10 cm (4 ins) in front of the third lumbar spinous process at the level of the lower costal margin (735, 736, 737)

Lat (Basic)

kVp	mAS	FFD	Film ILFORD	Screens ILFORD	Grid
90	100	100 cm (40″)	RAPID R	FT	Grid

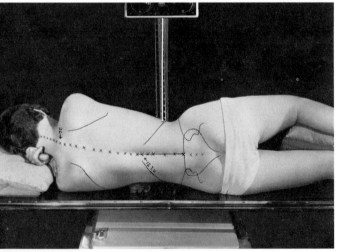

735

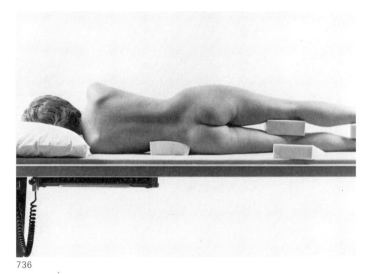

736

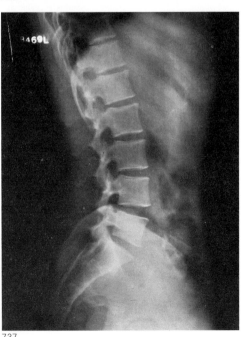

737

Because, on the lateral view, the fifth lumbar vertebra is overshadowed by the iliac crest, the overlying radiographic density is markedly increased, even more so in the broad subject. Thus the exposure factors required will be the same as for the lumbo-sacral articulation, page 214.

This point is illustrated in (738/739). In (739) the exposure factors were increased to show the fifth lumbar vertebra while in (738) the fifth lumbar vertebra is under-penetrated due to the density of the iliac crests. There is another difference between radiographs (738) and (739). In (728) the long axis of the lumbar region is parallel to the film and the intervertebral disc spaces are clearly shown, whereas in (739), because of the lateral curve in the lumbar region when the tube angle is not corrected, the vertebral bodies overlap the intervertebral disc spaces.

To visualize the spinous processes the exposure is reduced by half because, in the lateral (basic) projection of the lumbar region the spinous processes are grossly over-exposed. The spinous processes can also be shown if a high kilovoltage is used which reduces the contrast and evens out the difference in density between the spinous processes and the vertebral bodies.

Lateral—erect
The patient stands in the lateral position with the long axis of the lumbar vertebrae parallel to the film. The feet are slightly separated to give balance, and the arms folded and allowed to rest on the film support.

■ Centring point and exposure factors are the same as for lateral horizontal (basic) (740, 741)

High kilovoltage technique
To overcome the large differences in radiographic density of adjacent structures such as spinous processes and vertebral bodies higher kilovoltages, which are available on the majority of radiographic units, can be used. Using 120 kilovolts with an X-ray tube of suitable rating and an efficient grid the whole of the lumbar and lumbo-sacral regions may be adequately demonstrated.

Grid efficiency
Two radiographs (741) show the difference between (a) an efficient grid and (b) a less efficient grid. The excessive scattered radiation in (b) reduces the contrast considerably in the radiograph of a large subject exposed at 100 kilovolts.

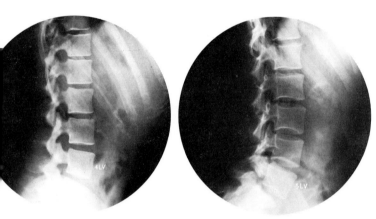

738/739

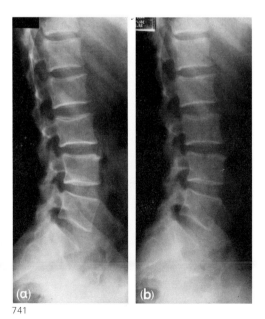

(a) (b)

741

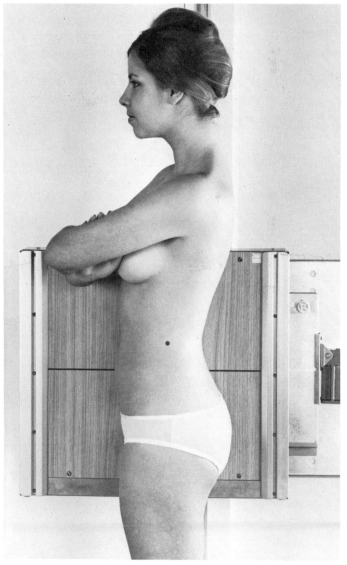

740

Oblique

Oblique views can be taken either from the antero-posterior or from the postero-anterior aspect with rotation to the right and left sides in turn.

With careful coning and the appropriate degree of rotation small lesions can be clearly shown which may be difficult to detect in other projections.

Four radiographs (744, 747) show the apophyseal joints between the articular processes as well as the laminae and pedicles. The narrow area between upper and lower apophyseal joints (the neck of the Scottie dog) is known as the pars interarticularis and most clearly seen with oblique projections, overlying the vertebral bodies.

When there is a marked lordosis the tube must be angled 10°–15°, usually towards the head but sometimes towards the feet, to show the intervertebral disc spaces clearly.

Posterior—oblique (basic)

The patient is supine and rotated 45° to the right and left sides in turn using non-opaque pads under the lower thorax and pelvis for support as is shown in (742) and illustrated diagramatically in (743).

■ Centre in turn in the mid-clavicular line on the raised side at the level of the lower costal margin (742, 743, 745)

Diagram (743) shows a cross-section of the trunk at the level of the fifth lumbar vertebra.

Note—When the oblique projections are being used to show only the fifth lumbar vertebra in heavy subjects, the centring point should be adjusted to the level of the anterior superior iliac spine.

The transverse axial radiograph of a dry bone viewed from below which is in the left antero-posterior oblique position with the tube centred through the point nearest to the film (745a), is shown next to the corresponding radiograph of two dry lumbar vertebrae (745b). This corresponds to (744L).

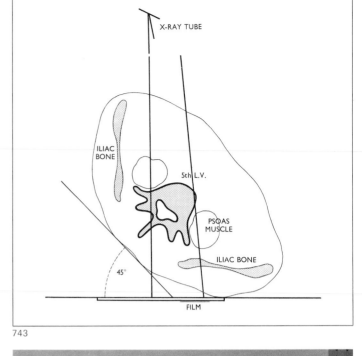

743

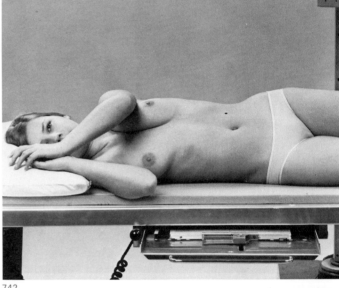

742

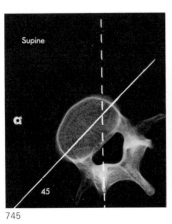
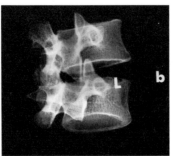

745

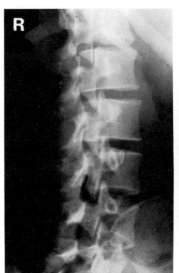
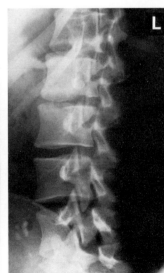

744

Postero-anterior—oblique

From the lateral position, the patient is rotated forward on to 45° non-opaque pads for right and left sides in turn.

■ Centre mid-way between the spinous processes and the axillary line at the level of the lower costal margin (746, 747)

			AP Oblique			
kVp	mAS	FFD	Film ILFORD	Screens ILFORD	Grid	
75	80	100 cm (40″)	RAPID R	FT		Grid

A transverse axial radiograph of a dry bone viewed from below shows the centring point through the pars interarticularis. In the prone position the central ray passes through the joint remote from the film and the corresponding view is shown in (748b) which is similar to (747R).

Injuries (749b)

In spite of gas shadows in the colon the radiograph taken in the right antero-posterior oblique position (b) taken in 1958 shows a fracture of the pars interarticularis (arrowed). In 1959 the antero-posterior radiograph (c) and the lateral radiograph (d) show a metal plate acting as a splint in the lumbar region. In 1960 the condition has been stabilized with the metal plate broken, disc space narrowing and an anterior osteophyte at L.3/4. This series of radiographs done over a period of years records treatment and progress of the injury.

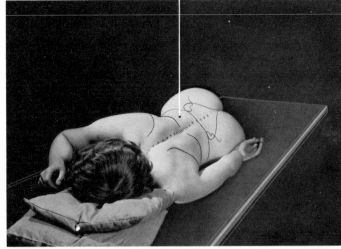

746

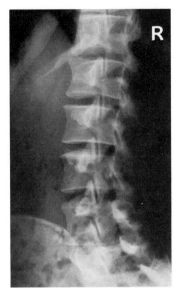
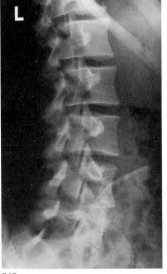

747

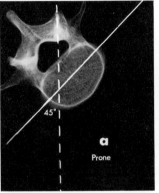
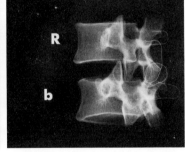
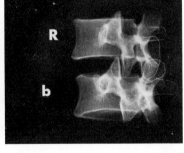

748

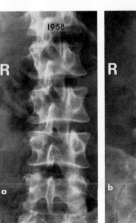
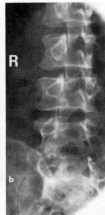
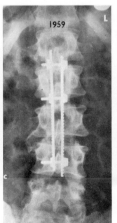
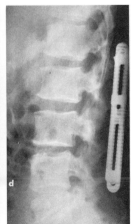
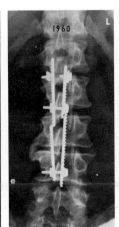
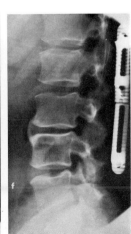

749

Stretcher Patients
Lateral (prone)

Seriously injured patients brought to the X-ray department in the prone position as shown in (750), should be radiographed in this position from both lateral and postero-anterior aspects.

Clothing containing metallic objects should be removed from the region concerned and the patient covered with blankets throughout the examination.

For the lateral projection the film cassette is vertical and supported adjacent to the lateral aspect of the trunk; a horizontal ray is used.

Stretcher

kVp		mAS			Film	Screens	
PA	Lat	PA	Lat	FFD			Grid
65	85	60	80	100 cm (40")	RAPID R	FT	Stat

■ Centre 7·5 cm (3 ins) anterior to the third lumbar spinous process, at the level of the lower costal margin (750, 751a).

Postero-anterior (prone)

Using a pedestal type Potter-Bucky diaphragm the film is placed in the Bucky tray to avoid moving the patient.
■ Centre in the mid line over the third lumbar spinous process, at the level of the lower costal margin (752, 751b).

Injury

Radiograph (753) shows a spondylolisthesis at L.4/5 with a large defect in the pars interarticularis; there is a forward slip of L.4 on L.5.

With an adjustable Potter-Bucky diaphragm and a special X-ray trolley the complete examination can be carried out without moving the patient with the additional advantage that a moving grid can be used for the postero-anterior projection.

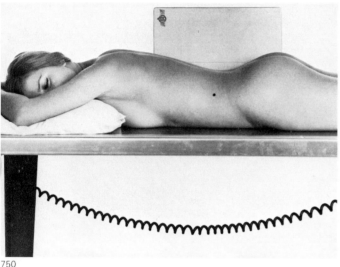

750

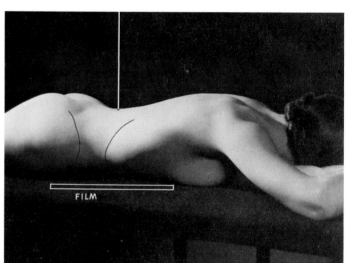

752

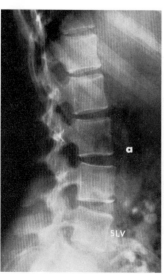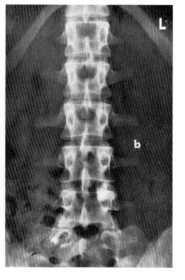

751

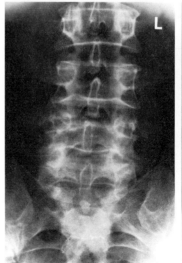

753

On the other hand, with modern highly efficient fine line stationary grids excellent results can be produced particularly where the grid is incorporated in the film cassette, greatly simplifying mobile examinations (750).

With badly injured patients who will obviously be admitted to the ward following an X-ray examination special radiographic trolleys should be used in the Accident and Emergency department. These trolleys have a suitable transradient surface which can be placed over the pedestal Potter-Bucky diaphragm in the horizontal position and can be raised to be closely aligned with the patient. The trolley can easily be moved over the Bucky to examine several areas in frontal projection in turn. For the lateral projection a grid cassette can be used as in (754) or the trolley can be moved away from the Bucky which is then swivelled into the vertical position against the side of the patient and the tube lowered for horizontal projection (755). In this way a complete X-ray examination for any part of the body is done smoothly and efficiently in a minimum of time without disturbing the patient who is taken direct to the ward on the same trolley (756).

Pathological conditions

Two further lateral radiographs taken with the patient supine show calcification of the aorta anterior to the vertebral body in (757) and a marked pathological compression fracture of the vertebral body in (758).

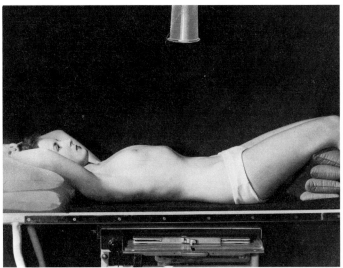

754

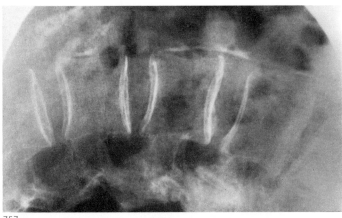

757

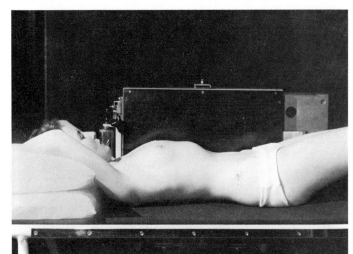

755

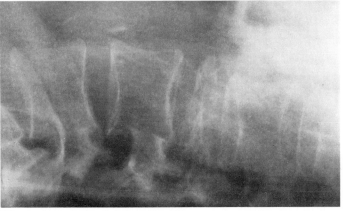

758

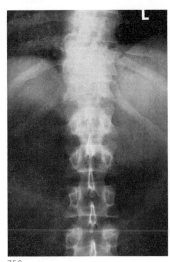

756

Children

In children it is usually possible to cover the spine from the cervico-thoracic region to the coccyx in frontal and lateral projections on four films (759). Subsequently localized views with suitable exposures if required will give maximum detail.

Post-operative Radiography

Radiograph (760) shows a bone graft in the interspinous region of L3/4 in frontal and lateral projections; if further detail of the graft is necessary particularly in the lateral projection, tomography can be used.

Radiograph (761) shows a compression fracture of the body of L.1 treated with metal plates; acute angulation of the spine is present centred on a wedged-shaped vertebra.

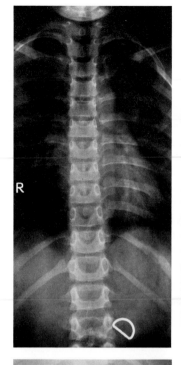
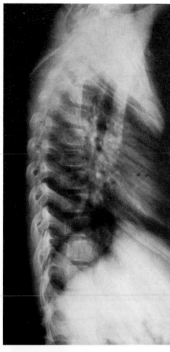
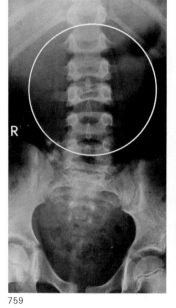
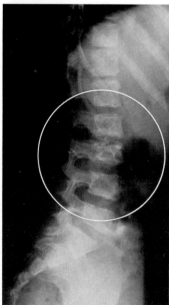

759

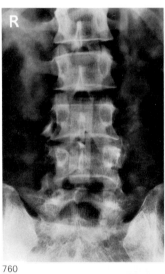
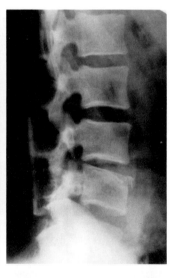

760

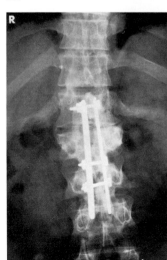
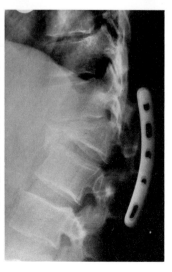

761

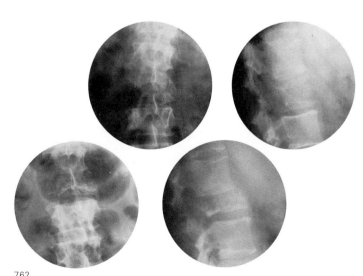

762

Pathology

In adults metastases to bone from carcinoma, particularly from the breast and prostate, are not uncommon. In radiographs (762) metastases are shown in antero-posterior and lateral projections. Where the bones have become rarefied due to osteolytic metastases over-exposed radiographs must be avoided by lowering the mAs. Prostatic metastes are frequently dense which are well shown with a conventional technique, but a normal exposure for an A-P view in a patient with an angular kyphosis will be under exposed (763).

Psoas Muscles

The psoas muscles are seen as triangular shadows running from the twelfth dorsal vertebra towards the iliac crest (764, 765), but where the psoas muscles pass over the iliac crest to insert into the lesser trochanters, their soft tissue shadowing is lost over the bone (765).

On occasion part of the psoas muscle can be seen across the iliac crest particularly in children (766).

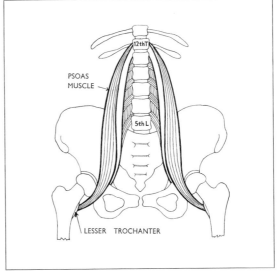

764

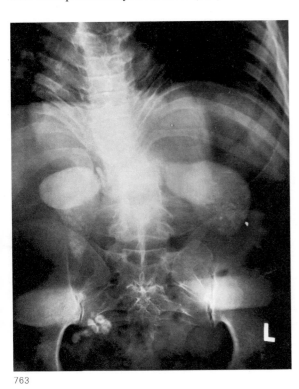

763

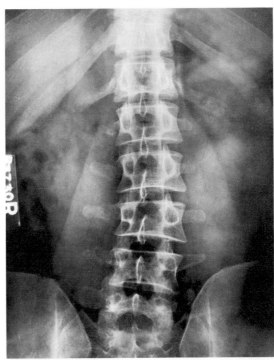

765

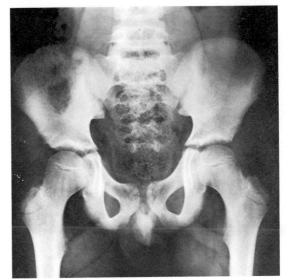

766

Lumbo-Sacral Articulation

In the general antero-posterior projection of the lumbar vertebrae the vertebral bodies obscure the disc space at the lumbo-sacral articulation because it lies obliquely. A special projection with tube angulation is therefore needed to show the L.5/S.1 disc space in the frontal view.

Radiographs can also be taken of this area in the lateral projection in both flexion and extension to study the relative movement of spine and pelvis. However, because of the greater radiographic density of this region in the lateral projection the exposure must be increased.

Antero-posterior (basic)
With the patient supine centred correctly on the X-ray couch, the film is displaced toward the head to allow for the obliquity of the X-ray beam.

■ Centre in the midline at the level of the anterior superior iliac spines, with the tube angled 5°–15° toward the head. The degree of angulation can be judged from the lateral view and will vary according to the type and sex of the subject (767, 768, 769).

Note—In the lateral radiograph (768) the direction of the X-ray beam through the joint space for the antero-posterior projection is indicated by the solid line.

Lumbo Sacral AP					
kVp	mAS	FFD	Film ILFORD	Screens ILFORD	Gr
75	80	100 cm (40")	RAPID R	FT	Gr

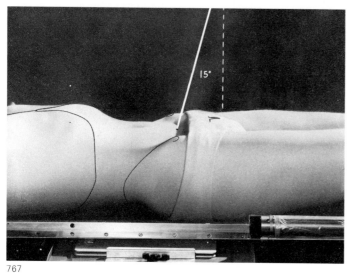

767

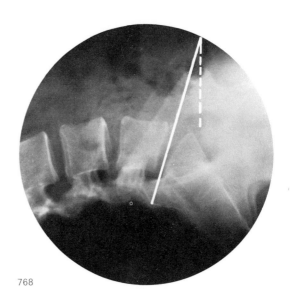

768

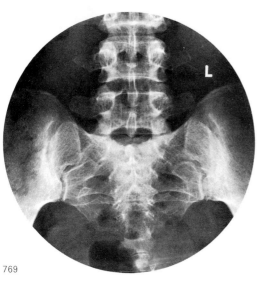

769

Lateral (basic)

Lateral radiographs taken in the erect and horizontal positions have different appearances because of the variation in the alignment of the lumbo-sacral region. Similarly there are differences in alignment when the patient is lying with full extension at the hips or in flexion, as shown in diagram (783), page 218.

In the true lateral position the mid line of the lumbo-sacral region must be parallel to the film. With the patient horizontal a non-opaque pad under the mid lumbar region will prevent the lumbar spine from sagging, and for the comfort of the patient a small pad should be placed between the hip and the couch. Flexion of hips and knees, with the raised limb supported on sandbags, is essential for immobilization.

In the erect position the shoulder rests against the film support, the feet being placed apart for better balance.

■ Centre 7·5 cm (3 ins) forward from and at the level of the fifth lumbar spinous process (770, 771).

Note—When a high powered X-ray unit is available the focus-film distance may be increased to compensate for the large object-film distance of this region. However, if a localizing cone and fast screens are used at a focus-film distance of 100 cm (40 ins) satisfactory radiographs can be obtained.

Radiograph (771) shows a high kilovoltage technique (120 kVp, 30 mAs) and should be compared with (772) which was done at a lower kilovoltage (85 kVp 120 mAs).

For larger subjects, a high kilovoltage is essential for this region but this produces increase in scattered radiation which can be corrected by the use of a higher ratio grid. Alternatively radiographs can be taken at 100 kVp which is a reasonable compromise.

Radiograph (773) shows disc degeneration at L5/S1 with a forward slip of L5 on S1. A lateral radiograph is essential for its demonstration.

Lateral Basic

kVp	mAS	FFD	Film ILFORD	Screens ILFORD	Grid
105	100	100 cm (40")	RAPID R	FT	Grid

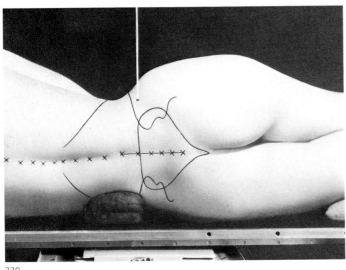

770

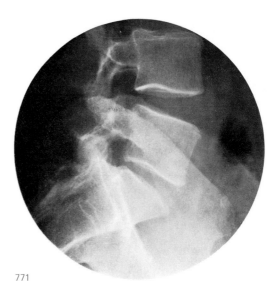

771

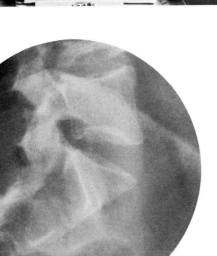

772

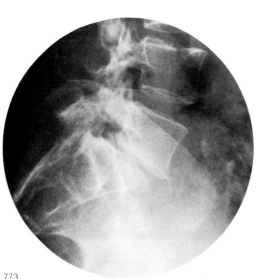

773

Postero-anterior

Because the lumbo-sacral articulation is sufficiently anterior (provided the patient is not too large) a satisfactory projection without undue magnification can be obtained with the patient prone. It is also easier to estimate the direction of the intervertebral disc space from the posterior aspect and thus to gauge the correct tube angulation.

The patient is placed symmetrically in the prone position, central to the couch and grid. The film is displaced in a caudal direction to allow for the obliquity of the X-ray beam.
■ Centre to the fifth lumbar spinous process, with the tube angled from 5°–15° toward the feet (774,775,776).

The lateral radiograph (775) shows the position of the vertebrae with the patient prone (774) and indicates the tube angulation required for (776).

Axial

An axial projection of the sacrum is shown in (777). The patient sits at the end of the couch leaning forward with the arms supported on the back of a chair and the feet resting on a stool.
■ Centre over the fifth lumbar spinous process (777,778)

Radiograph (778) shows a bullet lodged in the sacrum, positioning as in (777).

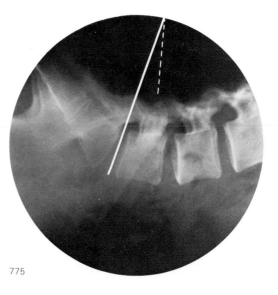

775

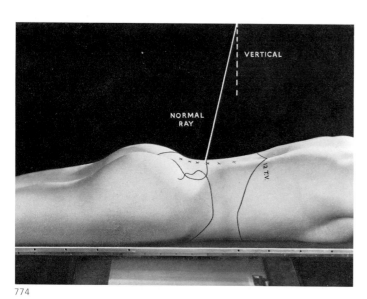

774

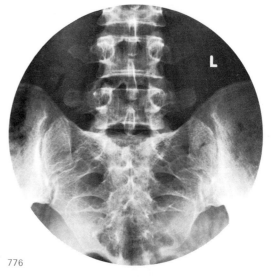

776

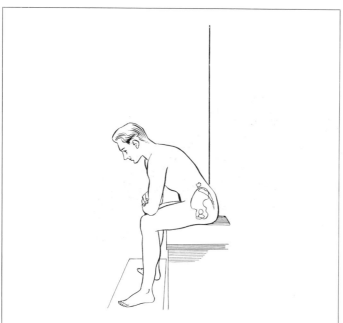

777

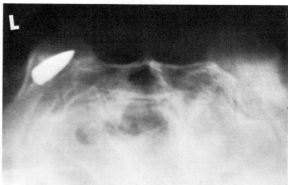

778

Antero-posterior oblique

For the antero-posterior oblique view the patient is rotated 45°
from the supine position and supported on non-opaque pads.
■ Centre approximately 7 cm (3 ins) medial to and 2 cm
(1 in) above the anterior superior iliac spine on the raised side
(779, 780)

			Post-Oblique		
kVp	mAS	FFD	Film ILFORD	Screens ILFORD	Grid
85	80	100 cm (40")	RAPID R	FT	Grid

Pathological Radiographs

Radiographs (781, 782) show a forward slip of L.5 on S.1
(spondylolisthesis). A satisfactory lateral projection is needed
to show this condition.

Note—Spondylolisthesis is caused by a defect in the pars
interarticularis leading to a forward slip of one vertebra upon
the other and usually occurs in the lumbo-sacral region.

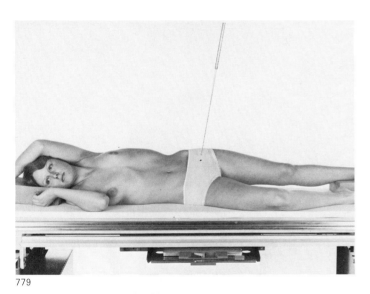

779

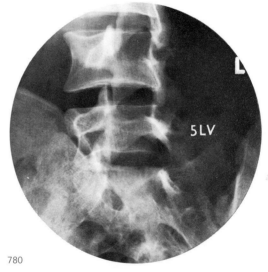

780

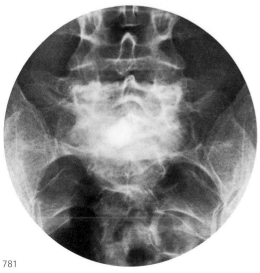

781

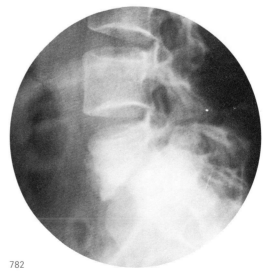

782

Movements at joint

The photographs and radiographs on page 219 show four lateral postures in the erect position (786) to (793).

The range of movement at the lumbo-sacral articulation is shown—(786,789) with the subject in the normal erect position; (787,790) with the subject leaning backward; (788,791) with the subject leaning forward with slight flexion; and (792,793) with the subject leaning forward with marked flexion. Both the photographs and the radiographs show the considerable movement which occurs in this region of the vertebral column. This is further illustrated in the line drawings of the subject in (a) erect and (b) flexed positions which have been superimposed to show the vertebrae to pelvis relationship.

The two radiographs (784,785) show radiographic appearances at the lumbo-sacral region in flexion and extension. In (784) the lumbo-sacral region is straightened by flexing the trunk on the hips—see diagram (783b) while in (785) the normal lumbar curve is present with the patient erect—see diagram (783a). Both radiographs were taken with the patient horizontal as illustrated in diagram (783).

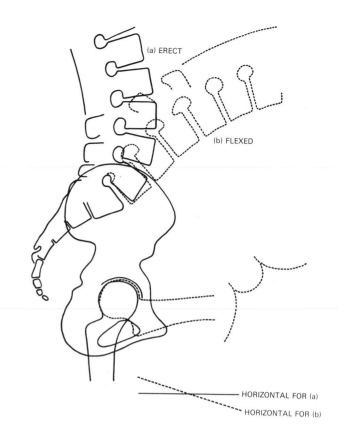

(a) ERECT

(b) FLEXED

HORIZONTAL FOR (a)

HORIZONTAL FOR (b)

783

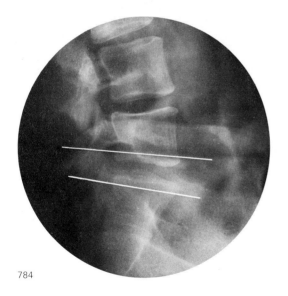

784

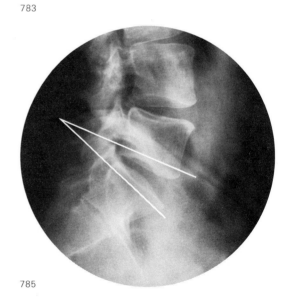

785

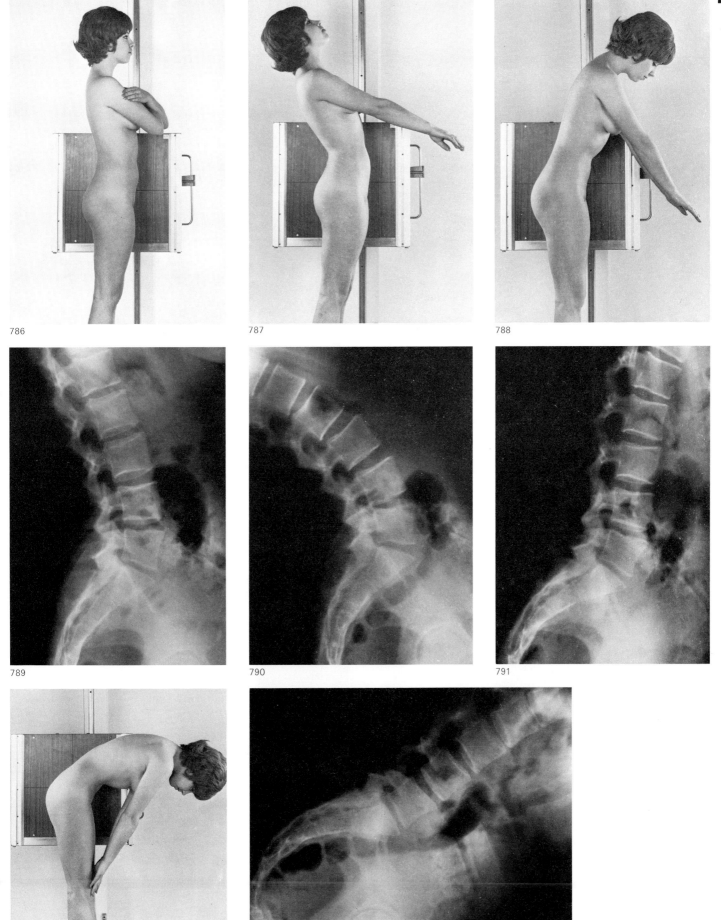

786

787

788

789

790

791

792

793

Sacrum

The five sacral vertebrae are fused together to form a triangular wedge lying between the iliac bones and completing the posterior part of the pelvic girdle. It lies obliquely sloping backward and downward forming an angle at the lower margin of the fifth lumbar vertebra. The obliquity differs in male and female subjects. In a typical male the lumbo-sacral angle is small and the long axis of the sacrum almost vertical, but in the female there is often a large lumbo-sacral angle which requires appropriate tube angulation for an undistorted antero-posterior projection of the sacrum.

The difference between male (794) and female (795) lumbo-sacral angles is shown in the two lateral radiographs; solid white lines indicate the direction of the X-ray beam for the antero-posterior projection to avoid overshadowing by the pubic bones. In subjects where there is marked angulation at the lumbo-sacral junction (795) there will always be some foreshortening in the antero-posterior projection. To overcome gas and faecal shadows which are frequently present in this region obscuring bone detail, the patient must be carefully prepared. The antero-posterior radiograph (796) and the lateral view (797) show gas and faeces in the colon with the lower part of the sacrum not visible in the frontal view.

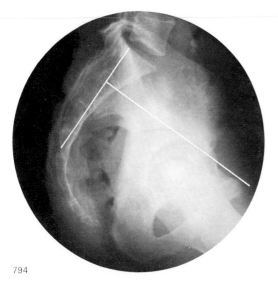

794

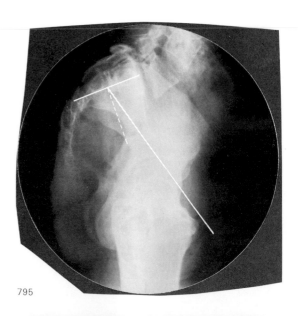

795

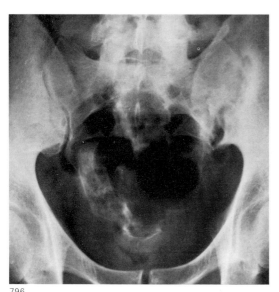

796

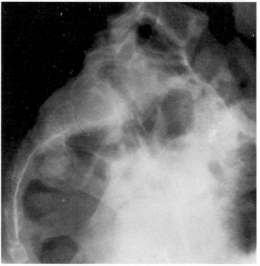

797

Radiographs (798, 799) of a male subject should be compared with (800, 801) of a female. The same centring point was used in each of the four radiographs, however, the tube was straight in (798, male) and (800, female), and show a little foreshortening in the male but gross foreshortening in the female sacrum which has the larger lumbo-sacral angle. In (799, male) and (801, female) the tube was angled 10° towards the head which produced over-angling in the male (799) with the lower sacrum over-shadowed by the pubic bones, but there was still a little fore-shortening of the female sacrum (801). The correct projection for a female with a large lumbo-sacral angle was finally produced by angling the tube 15° towards the head (802).

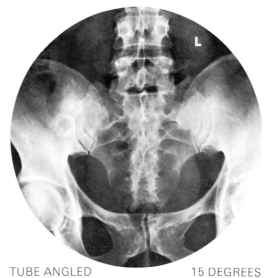

TUBE ANGLED   15 DEGREES
802

MALE

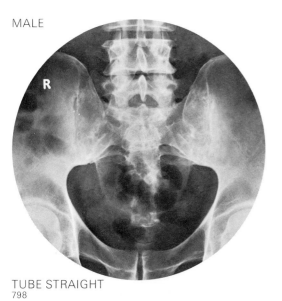

TUBE STRAIGHT
798

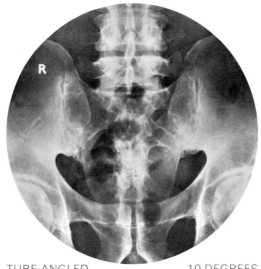

TUBE ANGLED   10 DEGREES
799

FEMALE

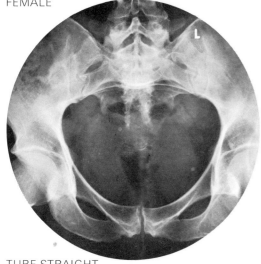

TUBE STRAIGHT
800

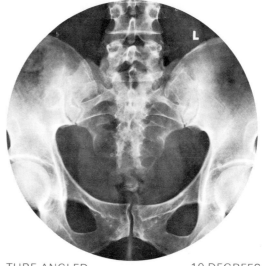

TUBE ANGLED   10 DEGREES
801

Antero-posterior (basic)

The patient lies supine, with the knees flexed over a small sandbag and the shoulders raised to reduce the lumbar arch.

■ Centre in the midline above the symphysis pubis with the tube angled 5°–15° towards the head. The degree of angulation will depend upon the angle of the sacrum in relation to the film (803, 804)

The central ray is directed as nearly as possible at right angles to the long axis of the sacrum, the position of the film being adjusted depending on the tube angulation. As was explained and illustrated on the previous page the tube angulation varies with the lumbo-sacral angle and differs in males and females and from subject to subject.

			Sacrum AP		
kVp	mAS	FFD	Film ILFORD	Screens ILFORD	Gri
75	80	100 cm (40″)	RAPID R	FT	Gri

Fracture Radiographs

Antero-posterior (805) and lateral (806) projections of the sacrum show a fracture of the lower segment which would have been hidden if there had been any gas or faeces overlying it.

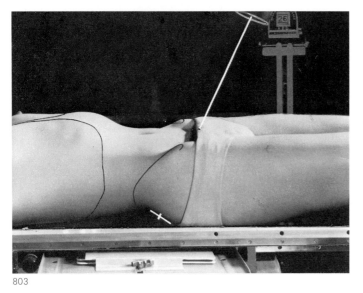

803

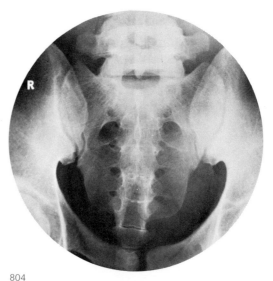

804

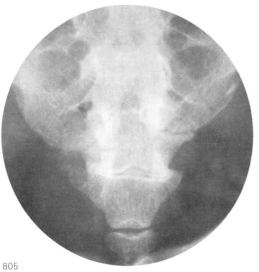

805

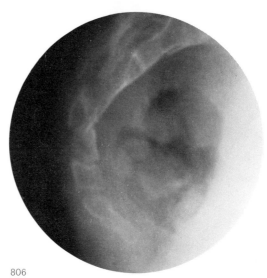

806

Lateral (basic)

With the patient in the lateral position and flexion at hips and knees the raised leg is supported at hip level in front of the lower limb. The patient will appreciate a soft pad placed between the hip and the couch.

A pad is placed under the mid lumbar region to obtain a true lateral position with the long axis of the sacrum parallel to the film (807). Alternatively, the tube should be positioned perpendicular to the long axis of the sacrum by angling it towards the feet (808).

■ Centre 7·5 cm (3 ins) anterior to and at the level of the posterior inferior iliac spine. The position of the iliac spine can be determined by following the line of the crest to the posterior aspect where iliac bone and sacrum meet to form the sacro-iliac joint (807, 808, 809). The positions of the posterior iliac spines are frequently marked by dimples.

Note—Radiograph (810), taken at 120 kilovolts, is included as an example of high kilovoltage radiography.

			Lateral		
kVp	mAS	FFD	Film ILFORD	Screens ILFORD	Grid
120	80	100 cm (40″)	RAPID R	FT	Grid

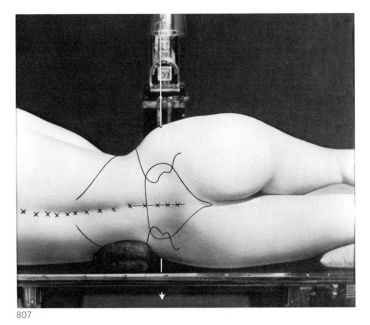

807

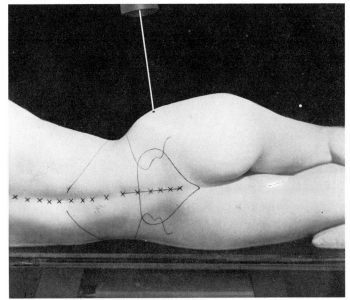

808

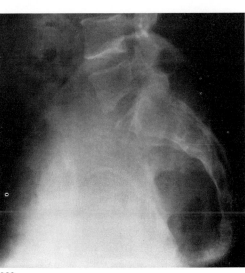

809

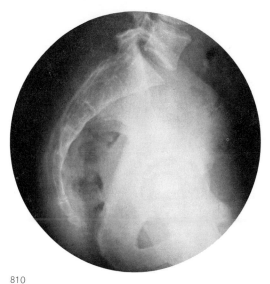

810

Coccyx

Coccyx							
kVp		mAS		Film	Screens		
AP	Lat	AP	Lat	FFD	ILFORD	ILFORD	Grid
65	75	60	60	100 cm (40")	RAPID R	FT	Grid

The coccyx consisting of four rudimentary vertebral segments fused together, lies at the end of the vertebral column and is quite superficial, curving downward and forward. The most satisfactory antero-posterior projection is usually obtained when the tube is angled toward the feet (811). Inevitably radiographs of the coccyx give a high radiation dose to the gonads particularly in females and the area of the coccyx is often obscured by gas and faeces in the colon. Radiographs of this area should only be done when absolutely necessary.

Antero-posterior (basic)

The patient is supine, being in the same position as for the antero-posterior projection of the sacrum (811,812).

■ Centre in the midline 3 cms (1¼ ins) above the superior margin of the symphysis pubis with the tube angled 5°–10° towards the feet.

Note—When bowel shadows obscure the coccyx, it can be helpful to make a second exposure with the tube angled towards the head as for the sacrum.

This differences in tube angulation may project unwanted shadows away from the sacrum and coccyx as in (813a), showing the downward angle and (813b) the reverse upward angle.

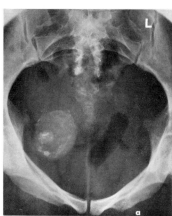

811

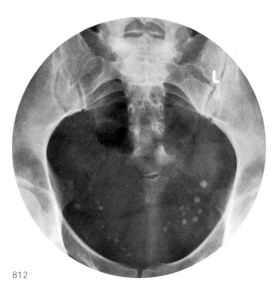

812

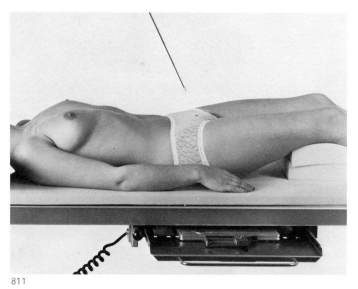
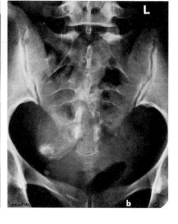

813

Lateral (basic)
The patient is placed in the same position as for the lateral sacrum, but with the coccyx over the middle of the couch.
■ Centre over the coccyx, which is readily felt between the buttocks (814,815)
For **Exposure Factors** see page 224

Note—Because the coccyx is very superficial the centring point lies more posterior than is often expected. Unless the central ray is directly over the coccyx, because of the large object to film distance, it will be projected obliquely, possibly beyond the edge of the film. It is therefore an advantage to increase the focus-film distance to improve the definition and to diminish the subject film displacement. The low contrast between the small bones of the coccyx and the surrounding soft tissues is thereby enhanced. Furthermore, a small localizing cone must be used to help to reduce scatter.

Normal Variation
Radiographs (815,816) show variations in the direction of the coccyx. In (816) the coccyx has an acute bend and lies more anteriorly.

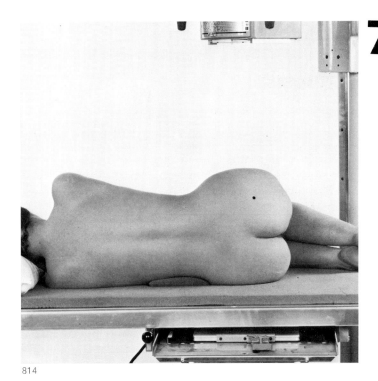

814

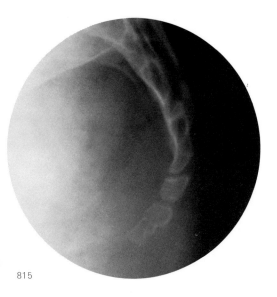

815

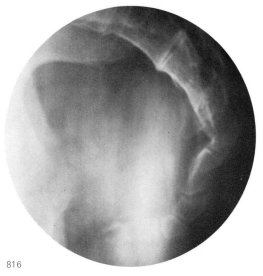

816

Scoliosis

Scoliosis is the term for lateral curvature of the spine and is associated with rotation being due to either postural or pathological causes. Usually the major part of the vertebral column is involved because the initial curve subsequently gives rise to additional compensatory curves, as shown in the antero-posterior radiograph (817).

To show the general alignment of the vertebral column in these cases, it is essential to include as large an area as possible on a single film (817). Should more than one exposure be necessary each film should include part of the adjoining area, so that with the overlap the two together reproduce the whole of the curve (818,819). The use of a narrow 18 × 42 cm (7 × 17 ins) film is not recommended, as variations shown in the adjacent ribs and pelvis which might be of importance, are excluded.

Radiographs (817), (819) show the use of a small protective triangle of lead rubber over the genital organs.

Projections may include antero-posterior with the patient seated (819), sometimes with one buttock raised on a 7·5 cm (3-ins) block, and with corrective splints (818,819).

The epiphyses of the iliac crest should be included in each examination because fusion of these epiphyses indicate the limiting age for effective treatment.

Except when the radiograph is required to show the posture of the subject, it is not possible to obtain a satisfactory lateral projection of the whole vertebral column with a single exposure (817). Each area will required compensatory tube angulation to demonstrate the vertebral bodies and disc spaces and is obtained by centring to the long axis of each part of the curve, taking each section in turn (828).

These lateral localizing projections are not necessary for every subject, as the general projection may be found to give all the information required (817).

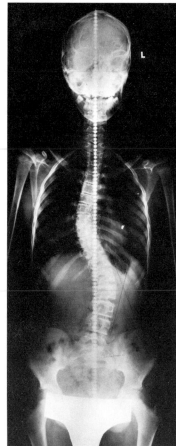 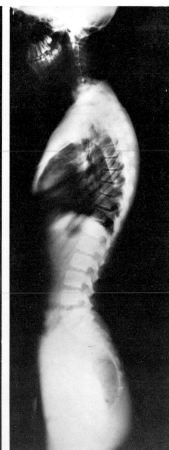

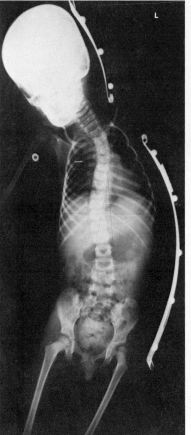 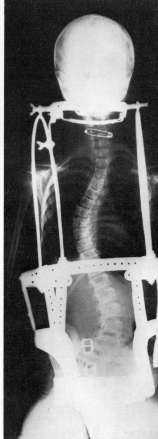

817
818
819

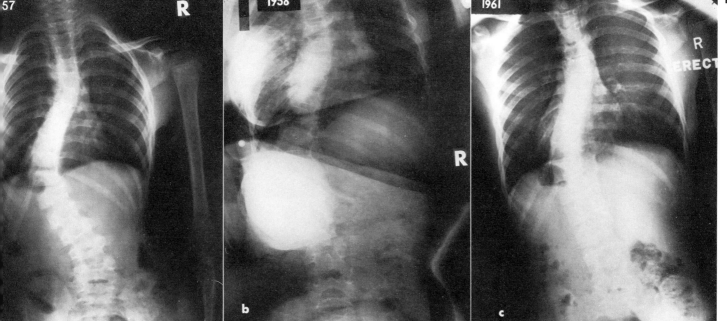

Radiographs (820) and (821) selected from the records of two patients show the difficulties encountered during the treatment of patients for scoliosis.

(820) (a) Taken 1957.

    (b) 1958, pre-operative correction in a plaster jacket by adjustable wedging of the plaster.

    (c) 1961, post-operative showing correction.

(821) (a) Taken in 1956.

    (b) 1960, patient in corrective post-operative splint.

    (c) 1961, post-operative showing correction.

Note—Pencil lines on these radiographs indicate the relative angles of adjacent curves on which surgical treatment is based.

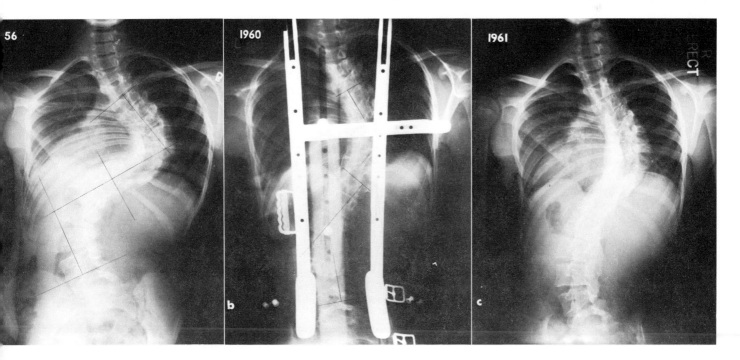

In both erect and supine positions, it is usually necessary to take radiographs with the patient bending towards right and left sides in turn, the more important bending position being toward the side of the convexity of the compensatory curve, (823, 826).

A group of radiographs (823) to (827) shows a part of the series involved in the radiographic examination for scoliosis, including both supine and erect positioning.

On the initial visit to hospital, the scoliosis patient is radiographed and photographed to commence a series of recordings of the condition, for comparative purposes, throughout the period of treatment. Photographs are taken in the erect position with the patient in a natural posture and bending to the right and left sides (822). Radiographs are taken in the same positions, antero-posterior erect (823) and included is the more important of the bending positions (824), when bending is toward the side of the convexity of the secondary curve. Radiographs are also taken in the supine position, with the subject straight, as in (825) and bending (826).

Every care must be taken in positioning these patients to ensure that the pelvis in symmetrical, that the iliac epiphyses are included in every exposure, that the maximum bending is obtained as applicable and that the fullest possible coverage is made within the limit of the size of film available. Bearing in mind the necessity for periodic repetition of these positions, there should be no difficulty in obtaining comparable results during the following years of treatment.

Radiographs erect (824) and supine (826) show a series of added pencil lines which intersect to form angles between one curve and another. From this evidence, the surgeon is able to decide on the degree of compensation suitable for each subject. The post-operative result for the subject concerned with radiographs (823) to (826) is shown in (827), which should be compared with straight radiographs (823, 825).

Note—As an alternative to full-length stationary or moving grids, two 14 × 17-ins stationary grids may be butted together end-on to cover the full length of the cassette. Only a thin dark line on the radiograph indicates the division between the grids. Similarly, when a full-length film is not available two 14 × 17 inch films are placed end-on in the 36-ins cassette.

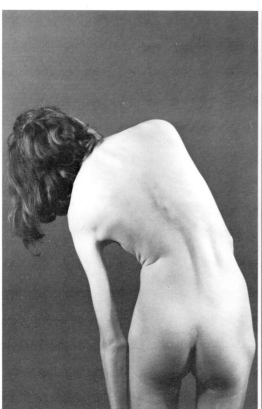
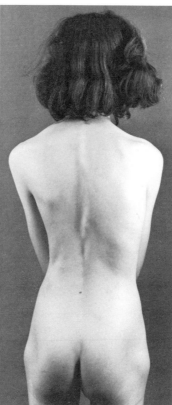
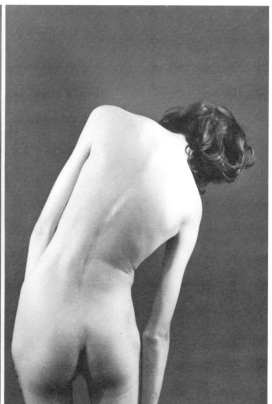

822

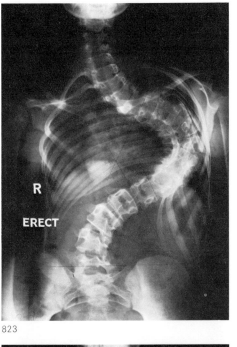

823

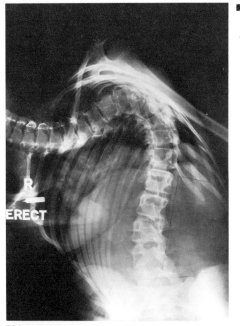

824

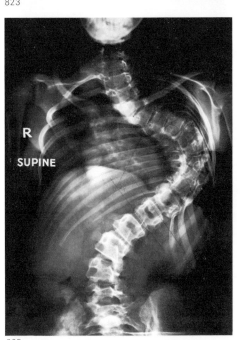

825

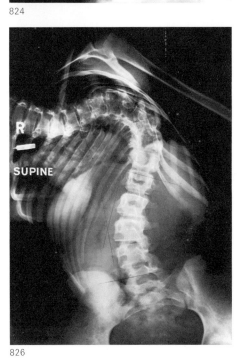

826

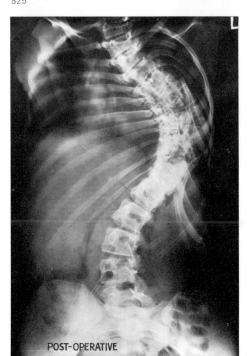

827

7

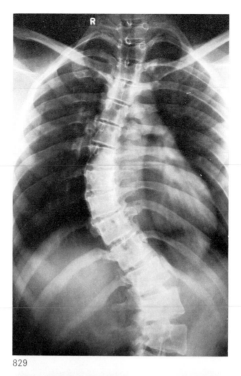

829

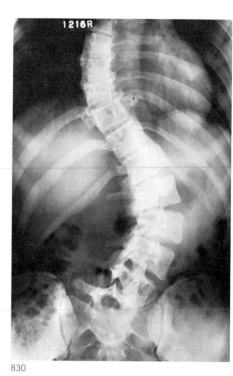

830

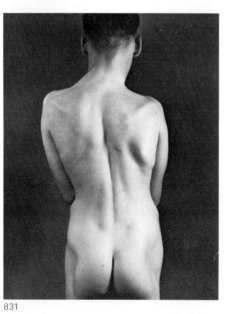

831

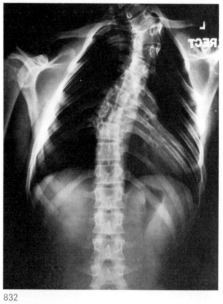

832

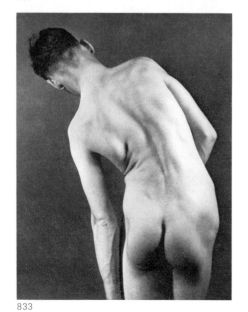

833

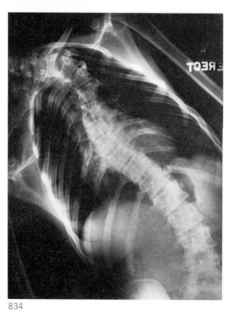

834

Re-examinations are often required at varying intervals to show improvement or otherwise in response to treatment, and it is essential to be able to repeat the general position of the patient adopted at the initial examination so that subsequent radiographs may facilitate close comparison. In the subject illustrated, the shoulders (829) and pelvis (830) were carefully adjusted to the true antero-posterior position, and this positioning was closely adhered to at subsequent examinations.

No two patients are alike, each presenting a new problem to be dealt with as circumstances permit.

Illustrations (831) to (834) show a primary curve high up in the thoracic region with compensatory curves below. The bending position (833) records in radiograph (834) the degree of mobility present in the vertebral column.

Kyphosis

Kyphosis of the vertebral column is an antero-posterior curvature which may affect any region of the spine, and is due to deformity or collapse of one or more vertebral bodies, producing sharp angulation in the early stages and, later, the rounded appearance of the typical hunch-back. There is sometimes a combined scoliosis and kyphosis.

Antero-posterior
When there is an advanced kyphosis, it is difficult to obtain a satisfactory antero-posterior projection.

These patients require careful manipulation to prevent painful pressure at the apex of the kyphosis. Plastic sponge blocks and firm sandbags are used to support the trunk, as shown in the illustration (835). In the early, acute stages of the disease the kyphosis is less marked, but if the patient is being treated in a plaster bed and is turned over into the prone position on removal from the cast, satisfactory projections may be taken from the postero-anterior aspect.

In suitable subjects the erect position is used and pressure thus avoided, the patient being maintained in position by the Potter-Bucky compression band.

■ Centre to the apex, bisecting the angle of the kyphosis (835, 836)

In a marked kyphosis it is necessary to increase the kilovoltage considerably and is usually in excess of that required for the lateral project of the same patient.

At an early stage, when films for comparison are taken more frequently, it is essential that each projection should be at the same angle. The patient should be closely adjusted to the same position for each examination. By noting the relationship to the film of shoulders or pelvis, a similar position can be adopted on each occasion.

These remarks may also be applied to the evidence required to show the variation in the size of an abscess surrounding the bone lesion. However the exposure factors for a pronounced kyphosis may result in over-exposure of the abscess, necessitating an additional soft tissue film. Tomography is employed to locate an abscess within the bone structure as shown in (720).

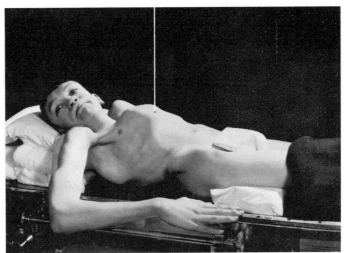
835

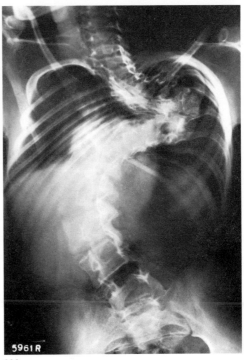
5961R
836

Lateral

This position is often of greater value than the antero-posterior projection as the condition of the collapsed vertebral bodies is clearly shown and the radiograph is also more readily obtained with less discomfort to the patient. Again, erect positioning may be preferred.

In a well-marked kyphosis the bones concerned may be quite clear of other structures requiring considerably less penetration and exposure than for the antero-posterior projection.

The position is similar to that required for the ordinary lateral projection of the vertebrae, but an additional lateral adjustment is necessary to place the whole diseased area within the range of the X-ray beam and film. Plastic sponge blocks and sandbags serve to steady the patient in position.

■ Centre within the apex of the curve of the kyphosis (837, 838)

The additional lateral projection (839) is included to show a typical lateral kyphosis of the spine without the complication of a scoliosis, as shown in the other kyphosis illustrations. The white line indicates the direction of the X-ray beam when centred to produce an antero-posterior projection.

Lateral radiographs may be required of a patient who is under treatment by hyperextension and encased in a plaster cast. It is therefore not always possible to use the Potter-Bucky diaphragm unless a vertical grid is available. It is sometimes possible, however, to place a flexible cassette with flexible intensifying screens, such as are used in industrial radiography, inside the plaster jacket, opposite to the vertebral bodies being examined, by which means useful radiographs are obtained.

Radiographs (840, 841) show the end result of treatment for kyphosis.

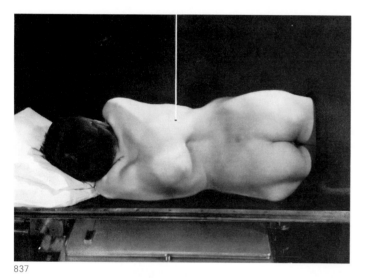

837

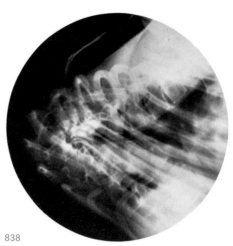

838

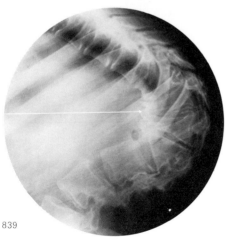

839

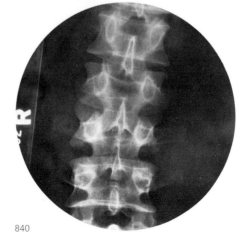

840

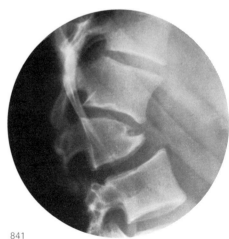

841

8

BONES OF THE THORAX

BONES OF THE THORAX

The bony thorax is formed by twelve pairs of ribs which articulate with the vertebrae posteriorly, the upper ten pairs articulating with the sternum anteriorly through the costal cartilages, forming a flexible cage enclosing the thoracic viscera (842). This section deals with the ribs and sternum; exposure factors refer to an adult of average physique. Basic positions are indicated as (Basic).

Sternum

The sternum or breast bone is divided into three parts, the manubrium, body and xiphoid process. It is thin, flat, elongated in shape and quite superficial, so that the chief regions of radiographic interest can be felt. These are the suprasternal notch, formed by the superior border of the manubrium, the sternal angle formed by the junction of the manubrium with the body at the level of the second costal cartilage, and the xiphoid process which varies considerably in shape and is often quite rudimentary. At its junction with the body it forms the xiphisternal joint.

In the postero-anterior projection the sternum is obscured by the third to the ninth thoracic vertebrae, necessitating an oblique projection for its demonstration which may be made from either the right or the left side. The projected shadow of the sternum should be parallel to that of the vertebral column (844).

There are two methods of making the oblique postero-anterior projection, either (a) with the trunk straight and the tube off-centre and angled towards the vertebrae, or (b) with the trunk rotated and the tube straight.

Although right and left sides are shown (845, 848) only one postero-anterior oblique projection is required for each examination.

If, during a 5 second exposure when prone the patient breathes quietly while otherwise immobilized, the sternum will show more clearly by diffusion of the superimposing lung shadows. The patient is usually horizontal when using this technique because immobilization is easier in this position.

kVp	mAS	FFD	Film ILFORD	Screens ILFORD	Grid
60	5mA 8sec	100 cm (40″)	RAPID R	Standard	Grid

Sternum

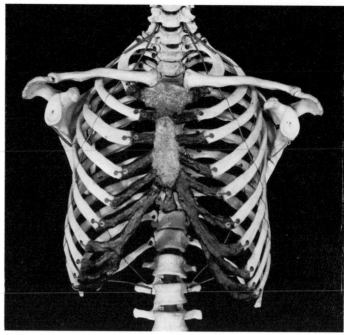

842

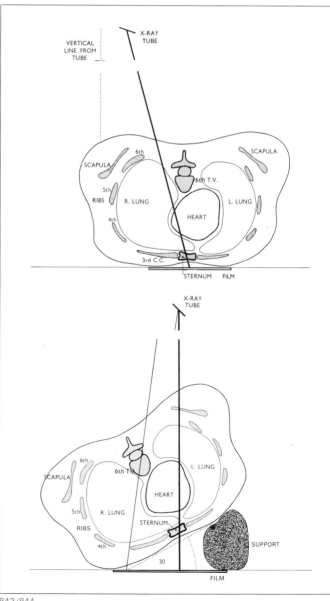

843/844

Positioning terminology

In oblique films it is at first difficult to relate the positions of sternum and spine relative to each other to correspond with a particular oblique projection. The two projections (845, 848) are explained in the following illustrations.

(845) In the right postero-anterior oblique position the left side of the chest appears considerably larger than the right which is markedly foreshortened with the sternum lying to the left of the spine.

Viewed from the front of the patient the sternum therefore overlies the left side of the chest, which is the larger side. (Diagram 846a)

(848) In the left postero-anterior oblique position the right side of the chest appears considerably larger than the left and now the left side of the chest is foreshortened with the sternum lying to the right of the spine.

Viewed from the front of the patient the sternum therefore overlies the right side of the chest which now appears to be the larger side (Diagram 847a).

Both the oblique views are shown in this explanation but, in practice only one oblique projection is required (846, 847)

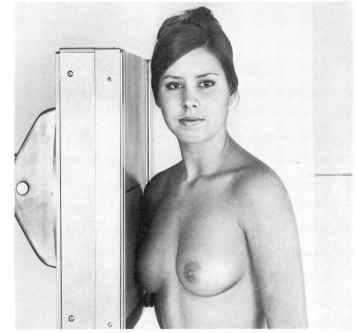

845

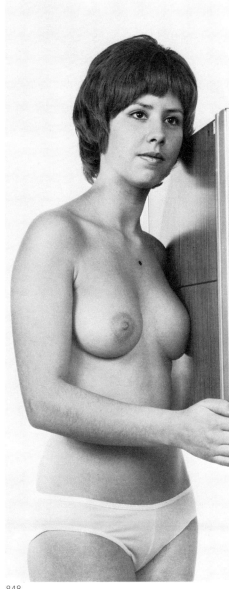

848

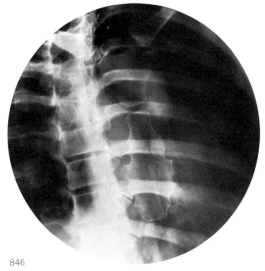

846

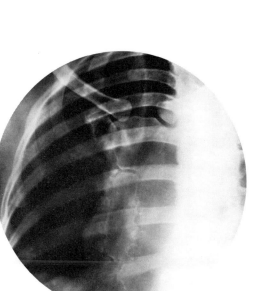

847

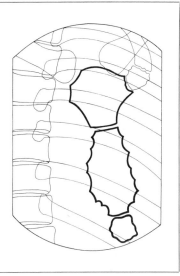

846a

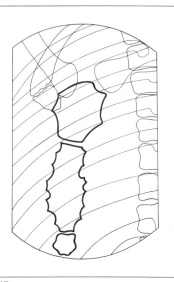

847a

8 Bones of the thorax
Sternum

Postero-anterior (1) (basic)
Trunk straight, Tube angled

The patient lies prone on the cassette with the chin over its upper border. It is often more comfortable for the patient if the top of the cassette is slightly raised on a block of wood and the chin supported on a small pad (849). The patient should be immobilized by using a compression band (852). To calculate the position of the tube the same method can be used as in examining the sterno-clavicular joints (see page 74).

Sternum Postero-Anterior

kVp	mAS	FFD	Film ILFORD	Screens ILFORD	Grid
60	40	100 cm (40")	RAPID R	Standard	Grid

■ Centre to the axilla at the level of the sternal angle and then angle the tube toward the sternum to enable the normal ray to pass approximately 7·5 cm (3 ins) to the tube side of the vertebrae. Exposure is made during quiet respiration (849, 850, 851, 852).

The projection is illustrated in the cross-sectional diagram (850). The vertebral body no longer overlies the sternum.

If a grid is used the slats must be in the direction of the tube tilt and will be transverse to the patient. With a moving grid, a stretcher trolley should be placed at right angles to the Bucky couch to enable the patient to be positioned transversely to the grid slats.

Note—In (852) a stationary grid was used because the patient is lying on the long axis of the couch.

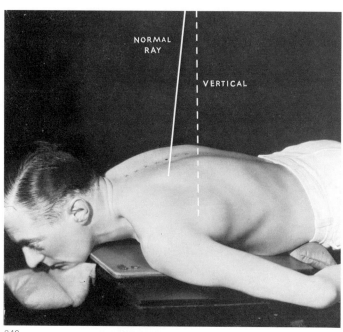

849

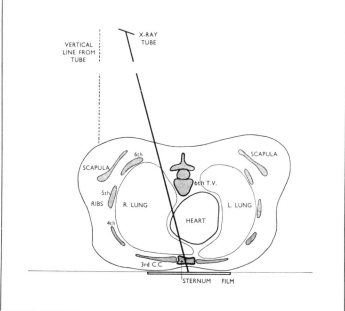

850

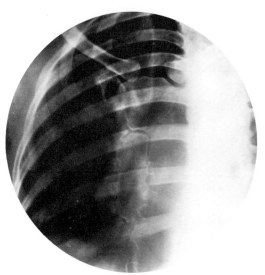

GENTLE RESPIRATION
851

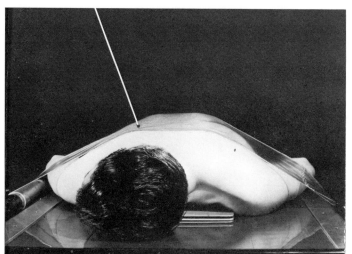

852

Right postero-anterior oblique
Trunk rotated, Tube straight (erect)

With the right side of the patient in contact with the film, the left side is rotated away from the cassette through an angle of 30°–40°.

■ Centre at the level of the fifth thoracic vertebra, 9 cm (4 ins) from the vertebra on the side nearest the tube with the axial ray passing through the sternum.

In the diagram (854) taken at the level of the sixth thoracic vertebra the method of projecting the sternum clear of the vertebral shadow when the trunk is angled and tube straight is shown. The diagram illustrates a right postero-anterior projection (853).

Note—This projection may be made with the trunk in either right or left postero-anterior oblique positions.

Right anterior-oblique
Trunk rotated, Tube straight (horizontal)

With the patient prone the left side is raised through an angle of 30°–40° degrees which throws the sternum clear of the overlying vertebral column (855–856).

With the central ray perpendicular to the film, centre at the level of the fifth thoracic vertebra 9 cm (4 ins) from the vertebra on the side nearest the tube.

Note—With the patient supported on non-opaque pads and using a compression band a 5 to 8 second exposure is made during quiet respiration.

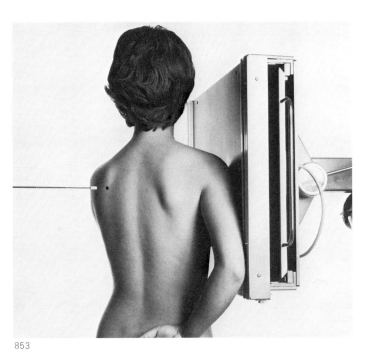

853

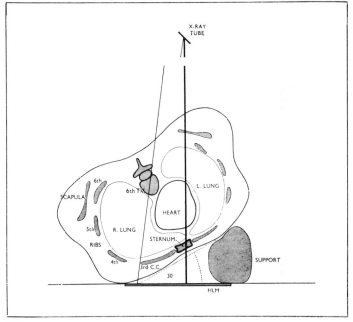

854

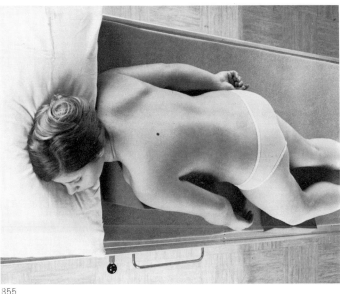

855

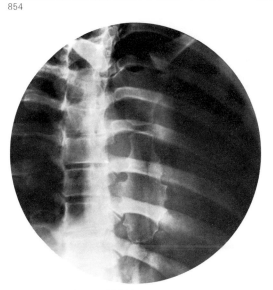

GENTLE RESPIRATION

856

237

Lateral (basic)

In the lateral position the broad plane of the sternum is at right angles to the film. The shoulders must be well back and the patient immobilized. When standing, patients should have their feet separated for better balance.

The film is taken on deep inspiration; use a lateral lung exposure with an increase of 5 kilovolts. For a lateral view the focus film distance is increased to 150 cm (5 ft) compared with the 100 cm (40 ins) focus film distance used in the oblique view because of the large object-film distance.

■ Centre to the sternal angle (857,858)

Sternum Lateral

kVp	mAS	FFD	Film ILFORD	Screens ILFORD	Grid
80	60	150 cm (60″)	RAPID R	Standard	Grid

Fracture Radiographs

A transverse fracture of the body of the sternum without displacement is shown in (859) but is not well seen in the lateral projection.

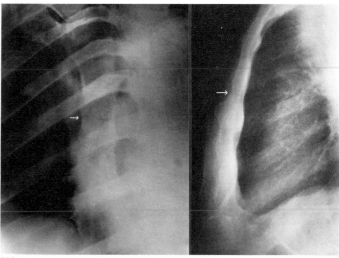

859

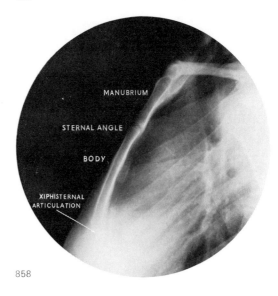

858

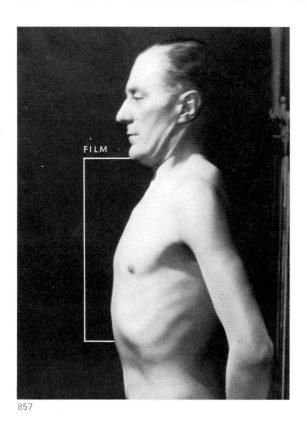

857

Ribs

The radiographic techniques must allow for the slope and curvature of the ribs, their relationship to each other and underlying viscera, and the effect of respiratory movements.

From the posterior costovertebral joints to their anterior ends ribs slope downwards and forwards to encircle the thoracic viscera. Anteriorly the ribs become cartilaginous and the top ten ribs join the sternum at the costo-chondral junctions. The lower two pairs of ribs are unattached laterally and are known as 'floating' ribs. The more horizontal posterior part of each rib is 7·5 to 12·5 cm (3–5 ins) above the anterior end (860).

The sloping anterior parts of the ribs change from bone to cartilage at the costo-chondral junctions and then join the sternum at the sterno-costal joints. The cartilaginous parts of the ribs increase in length from above downwards and are not usually visible on radiographs until, in middle age, they become partly calcified. Anteriorly the lower margins of the ribs form an inverted 'V'. These features are shown on the photograph (860) of a skeletal thorax. The fibro-muscular dome-shaped diaphragm separates the thorax from the abdomen and resembles an open umbrella. The diaphragm is attached at its periphery around the inner aspect of the rib cage forming the floor of the thorax and the roof of the abdomen. On a frontal radiograph the diaphragm overshadows the lower ribs and, with respiratory movements, varies in position by 2·5 to 5·0 cm (1–2 ins) as can be shown on the radiograph of a normal subject (861) with a double exposure on the one film, in inspiration and expiration. The dome of the diaphragm is higher anteriorly than posteriorly and can be projected above or below its usual level by changing the obliquity of the X-ray beam as represented diagrammatically in (873, 888).

In the frontal view the lower ribs cannot be correctly exposed along their whole length because of the difference in the radiographic density of the thorax and the abdomen, appearing over-exposed on thoracic films and under-exposed on abdominal films.

Because of the slope of the ribs, the light-beam diaphragm must be opened sufficiently to cover the whole length of a rib, bearing in mind that there can be as much as a 12·5 cm (5 ins) difference vertically between the back and front ends.

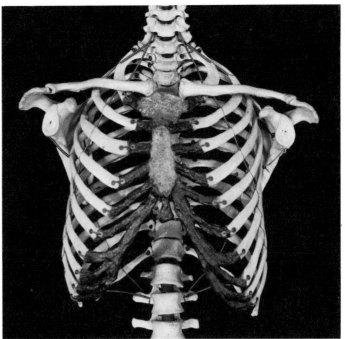

860

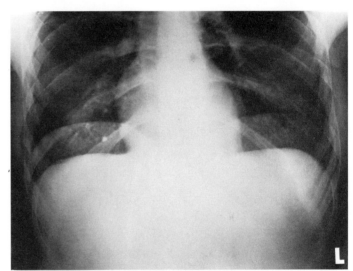

861

8 Bones of the thorax
Ribs

To show as many as possible of the upper ribs including the tenth rib the patient should be erect, the tube should be centred high preferably in the region of the third thoracic vertebra and the exposure made in deep inspiration. Alternatively to show the lower ribs it is best if the patient is horizontal and the tube centred low at the level of the second lumbar vertebra and the exposure made in full expiration. In this way, by using the obliquity of the rays a maximum area is covered.

Clothing must always be removed over the affected area to avoid over-lying shadows from artefacts. Most hospital gowns which are provided for patients in an X-ray department are radiolucent and will not produce artefacts. A clear understanding of the radiographic request will help to produce the best results and is especially true in Accident and Emergency departments where close cooperation between medical and radiographic staff is absolutely essential.

First and Second Ribs

To show the first and second ribs satisfactorily localized views with the necessary modification are needed particularly for the axial and oblique projections.

Antero-posterior
Postero-anterior

When the radiographs are taken in the erect position as for showing the lungs, the ribs will appear crowded due to overlapping particularly the first and second ribs (862). However, in this example cervical ribs are also present which accentuates the overlapping shadows.

In the horizontal position using the same projection as for the medial part of the clavicle, the appearances of the ribs differ when taken supine antero-posterior (863, 864) and prone postero-anterior (865, 866). The part of the rib closest to the film shows most clearly.

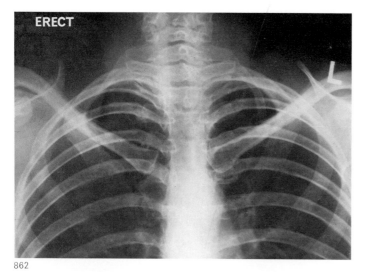

862

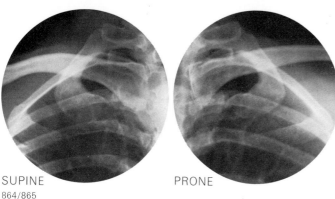

SUPINE   PRONE
864/865

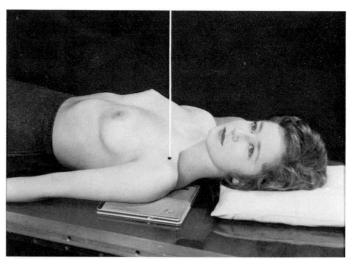

863

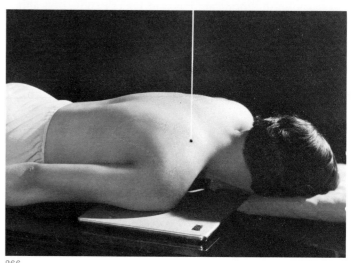

866

Antero-posterior oblique

In the horizontal position, for the whole length of the upper shorter ribs, the patient is rotated toward the side being examined, the arm being abducted to avoid over-shadowing of soft tissue structures (867).

In the alternative erect position, the patient faces the tube at an angle of approximately 45°.

■ Centre at the level of the seventh cervical vertebra above the mid-third of the clavicle (867, 868, 870)

Note—Radiographs (868) antero-posterior oblique and (869) antero-posterior are of the same subject.

Exposure factors in the oblique projections should be increased by 7 kVp over those shown for the antero-posterior projection.

Ribs Posterior Oblique

kVp	mAS	FFD	Film ILFORD	Screens ILFORD	Grid
65	20	100 cm (40″)	RAPID R	Standard	

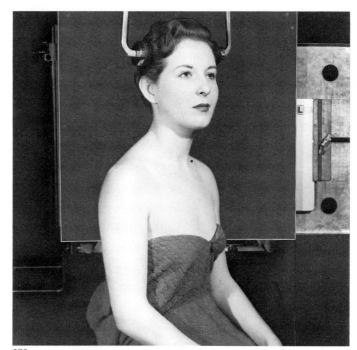

870

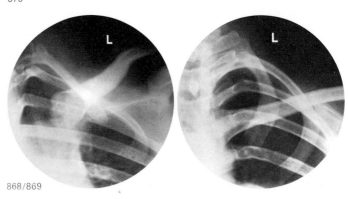

868/869

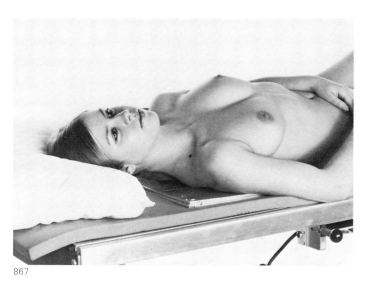

867

First to tenth Ribs
Antero-posterior (basic)

With the patient erect in the antero-posterior position the back of the chest is in contact with the cassette. The elbows are flexed, the hands are behind the hips and the shoulders brought forward so that the upper arms and scapulae do not obscure the rib shadows. This position is preferred when the posterior parts of the ribs are to be demonstrated; use a focus film distance of 100 cm (40 ins).

■ Centre to the sternal angle (871, 872)

Ribs 1–10 A–P

kVp	mAS	FFD	Film ILFORD	Screens ILFORD	Grid
75	50	100 cm (40″)	RAPID R	Standard	Grid

To include the maximum numbers of ribs above the diaphragm a high centring point is used and the exposure made on deep inspiration using a focus film distance of 100 cms (40 inches) (873). Compare diagram (888) for the projection for the lower ribs.

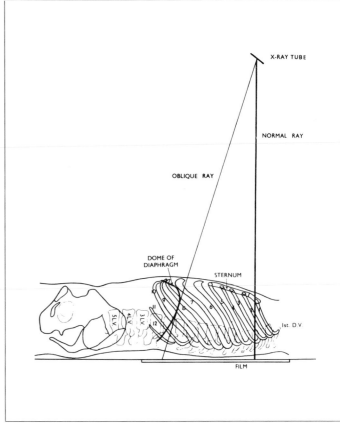

873

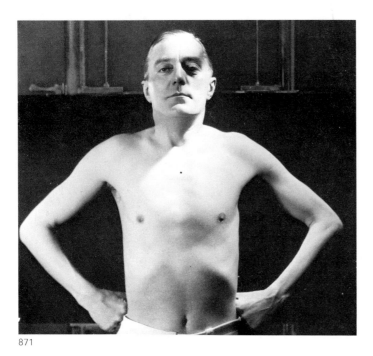

871

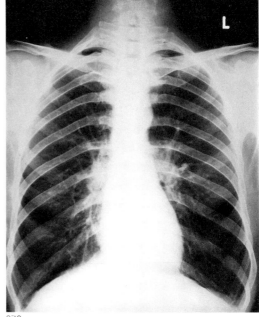

872

Postero-anterior (basic)

With the patient facing the cassette the arms are abducted and flexed at the elbows to encircle the film cassette; the chin rests on the top edge of the cassette. This position is preferred for demonstrating the anterior parts of the ribs; use a focus-film distance of 100 cm (40 ins). This is also the projection used for the postero-anterior chest radiograph but then the focus film distance is increased to 180 cm (72 ins).

■ Centre to the fourth thoracic vertebra

Two radiographs of the same subject (875,876) should be compared to show the difference in appearance between inspiration (875) and expiration (876). The diaphragm is lower on inspiration and the whole of the ninth rib becomes visible.

The difference in the appearance of the ribs between antero-posterior and postero-anterior projections is more marked when the shorter focus-film distance of 100 cm (40 ins) is used. Any advantage tends to be lost with the more usual focus-film distance of 180 cm (72 ins). However, at both the short and the long focus-film distance, in the antero-posterior projection the scapulae may overlie the lateral part of the upper ribs where as in the postero-anterior position the scapulae are moved away from the rib cage.

A higher kilovoltage which produces more even penetration but less contrast should be used and gives a better view of the ribs than a lower kilovoltage particularly for the ribs in the axillae and those which overlie heart and aortic shadows.

For the posterior ribs, where there is no movement during quiet respiration, a long exposure time with a low milliamperage may be used. Diffusion of the lung shadows shows the posterior ribs in greater detail.

8

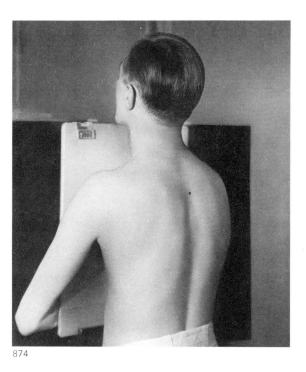

874

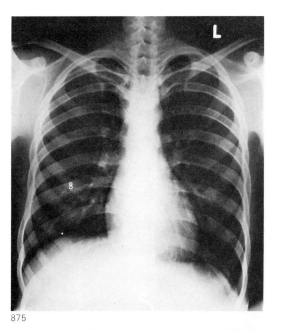

875

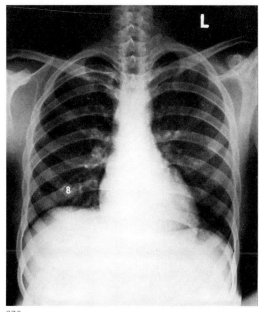

876

243

kVp	mAS	FFD	Film ILFORD	Screens ILFORD	Grid
75	60	100 cm (40")	RAPID R	Standard	Grid

Right antero-posterior oblique (basic)

The lateral parts of the ribs are poorly shown in the antero-posterior and postero-anterior projections but can be well demonstrated in the oblique position. Each side must be examined separately.

The patient is erect in the antero-posterior position and then rotated 45° towards the side to be examined with the posterior chest wall of affected side (in this instance the right side) against the vertical Bucky (877).

A 45° pad is used behind the patient to indicate the degree of rotation required (882).

Ideally the arms should be held above the shoulders with the hands clasped behind the head but, if the patient cannot manage this position then the arms must be moved out of the way of the trunk, the arm nearest the bucky forward and the other arm backward.

■ Centre on the sternal angle (877, 878)

For the left antero-posterior oblique projection exposure should be increased by 5 kVp because of the overlying heart shadow.

The focus film distance should not exceed 100 cm (40 ins) making full use of the oblique rays to allow for the complexity of the ribs.

Fracture Radiographs

In the antero-posterior position (879) a fracture of the rib in the right axillary line is barely visible, but with the patient in the right oblique position (880), with the axillary area parallel to the film, the fracture is clearly seen against the shadow of the lung.

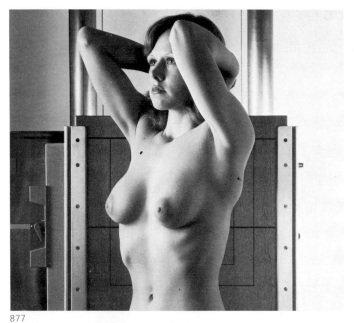

877

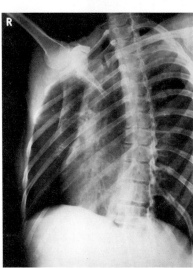

878

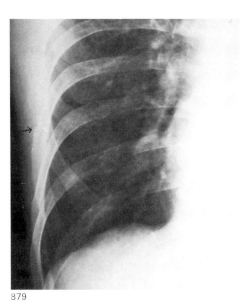

879

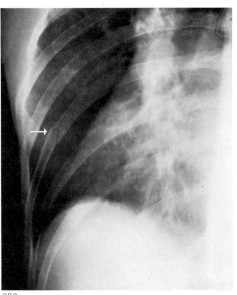

880

244

Left antero-posterior oblique (basic)

Using the technique described on the previous page but with the left side in contact with the vertical Bucky the patient is rotated 45° to show the left ribs.

■ Centre on the sternal angle (881, 882, 883)

The cross-sectional diagram (882) shows the relationship between ribs, film and tube when the patient is placed in the left posterior oblique position and corresponds to radiograph (883).

Fracture Radiographs

Radiograph (884) shows a fractured clavicle and fractured ribs. In (c) injury to the second rib is shown in profile.

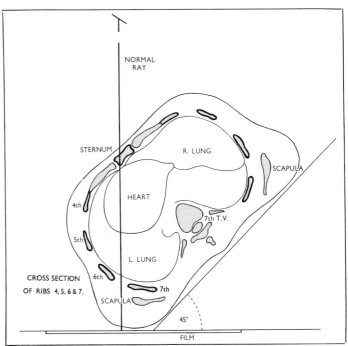

882

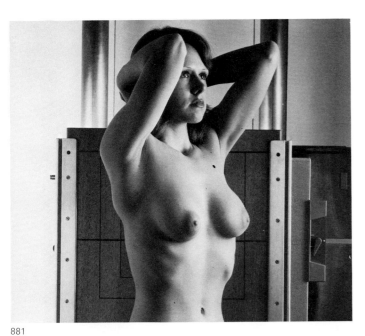

881

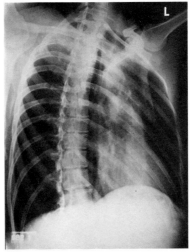

883

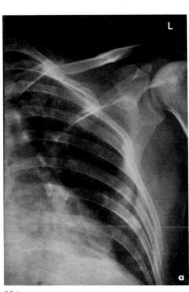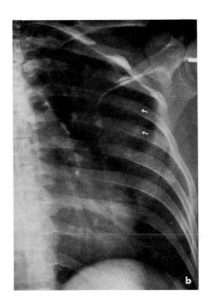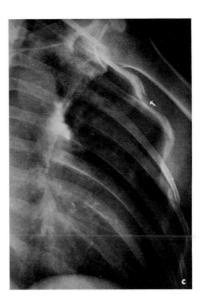

884

Ninth to twelfth

When the lower four pairs of ribs required examination the projection should be done showing them all below the level of the diaphragm. These ribs are always well shown in radiographs of the renal areas and lumbar vertebrae.

A similar centring point is used which is at the level of the lower costal margin. The difference in the radiographic appearances of the ribs and diaphragm depending on tube centring and respiratory movements is shown in the following illustrations:

(885), taken on expiration, with the tube centred over the lower costal margin, as in diagram (888), shows the dome of the diaphragm at the level of the eighth to ninth thoracic vertebrae but radiograph (886), taken on inspiration, with the tube centred at the level of the sternal angle as in diagram (873) shows the dome of the diaphragm at the level of the tenth to eleventh thoracic vertebrae.

In each radiograph (885, 886) a 100 cm (40 ins) focus-film distance was used, the same region covered in each film, namely, from the sixth thoracic to the third lumbar vertebra.

The diagram (888) shows how to project the diaphragm to overshadow the greatest number of ribs by using an oblique ray from a low centring point. The dome of the diaphragm is at its highest level on expiration.

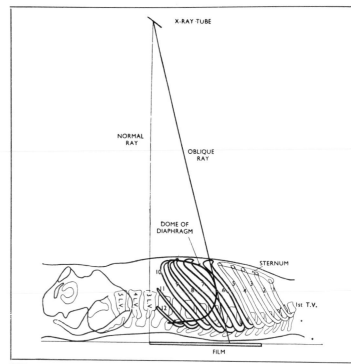

888

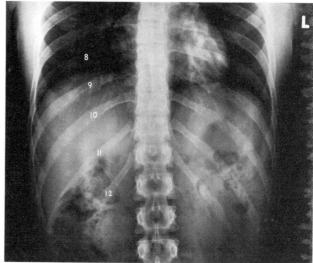

885

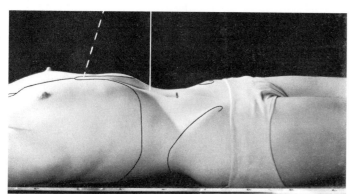

887

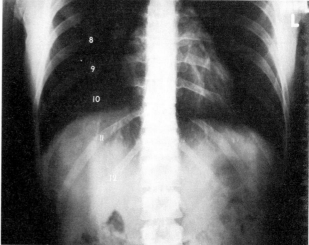

886

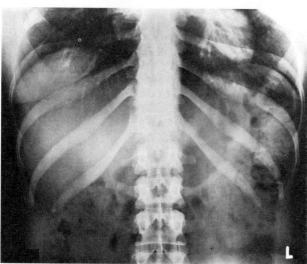

889

Antero-posterior (basic)

The patient lies supine (887) on the Potter-Bucky couch with a cassette placed transversely to include the whole of the right and left sides from the nipple line to the lower costal margin.

The floating ribs (11th, 12th) end at the lateral aspect of the trunk while the antero-medial part of the costal margin which is felt at the level of lumbar vertebrae 1–3, is usually cartilaginous and does not show on a radiograph.

■ Centre in the midline at the level of the lower costal margin. This is to the lower part and not to the middle of the film (887, 888, 889)

Ribs 9–10 Antero-Posterior

kVp		mAS			Film	Screens	
AP	OBL	AP	OBL	FFD	ILFORD	ILFORD	Grid
75	75	80	100	100 cm (40″)	RAPID R	Standard	Grid

The ribs will be shown to the best advantage if the overlying colon is free of gas and faeces.

Antero-posterior oblique (basic)

The patient is erect or supine in the antero-posterior position and then rotated 45° toward the side to be examined.

■ Centre in the midline at the level of the lower costal margin (890, 891)

The ribs are shown from the vertebral articulation to costo-chondral junctions. The oblique view (891) should be compared with the antero-posterior radiograph of the same subject shown in (892).

For the oblique projection increase the kilovoltage by 7 kVp as compared with the antero-posterior projection.

When a localizing cone is used the tube should be angled toward the head and the film displaced accordingly to compensate for the tube angulation.

Fracture Radiographs

Radiograph (893a), antero-posterior and (893b), antero-posterior oblique should be compared. A fracture of the right eighth rib becomes visible in the oblique projection.

8

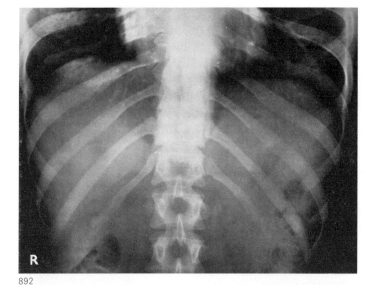
892

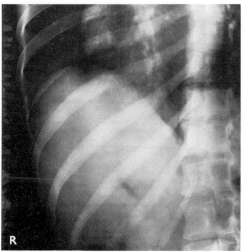
890

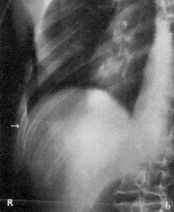

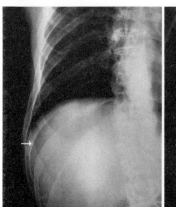
893

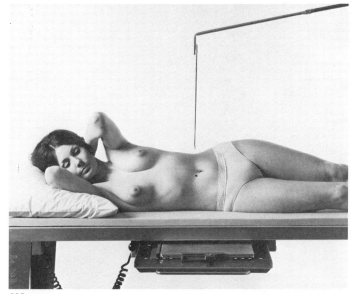

891

8 Bones of the thorax
Ribs

Lateral

Although, in previous editions, there was a description of a lateral projection for the lower ribs, in practice this is never required because there is overlapping of the ribs of the two sides which obscures any bony detail.

The oblique views of the lower ribs are used to obtain further projection for the ribs to be viewed in their full length.

Abnormalities—General

Congenital abnormalities of the ribs are quite common and include splaying of their anterior ends, additional ribs such as cervical ribs or thirteen pairs of ribs. In practice, however, it is only the additional cervical ribs which are of any importance. (Additionally the twelfth rib may be very small or absent.) To be sure of the number of ribs, the antero-posterior film must include the entire dorsal region so that all the ribs can be counted.

Many other conditions also affect the ribs; the lower margin of the ribs may be notched when there is a collateral circulation of arteries or veins (894) or from neurofibromatosis. Metastases from malignant tumours also occur in ribs (895).

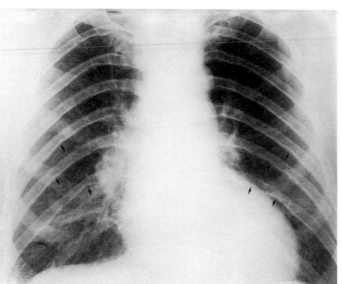

894

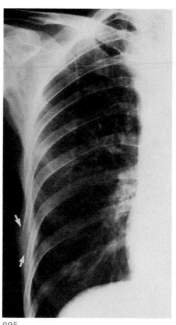

895

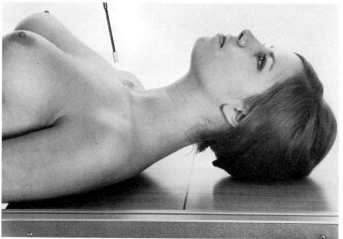

896

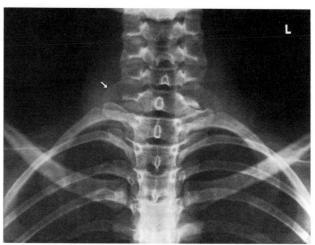

897

Cervical Ribs

When a cervical rib is present it is attached to the seventh cervical vertebra and may be rudimentary (897) or extend over a considerable length with its lower margin at the level of the fifth thoracic vertebra (898); both right and left sides are affected with equal frequency. The erect standing or sitting position is preferred in examinations of this region.

Antero-posterior (basic)

The patient faces the tube with the chin raised and an 18 × 24 cm (8 × 10 ins) cassette is placed transversely to include the fifth cervical to sixth thoracic vertebrae. The patient should be in the true antero-posterior position without any rotation and the whole length of each of the upper ribs must be included.

■ Centre on the sternal notch in the midline with the tube angled 10° toward the head as shown by the oblique line in (896), otherwise small rudimentary cervical ribs as in (897) may be missed (896, 897)

Note—The two radiographs of the same patient showing bilateral cervical ribs are compared (898) without and (899) with a grid. In the film with the grid there is much greater bone detail particularly in the vertebrae and clavicles.

kVp		mAS		Film	Screens	
AP	OBL	AP	OBL			
65	70	10	10	100 cm (40″)	RAPID R	Standard Grid

Antero-posterior oblique

The patient faces the tube and the trunk is rotated through 45° (900).

■ Centre at the level of the sixth cervical vertebra on the side, nearest the film, 3 cm (1¼ ins) from the midline to include from the fifth cervical to fifth thoracic vertebrae. The whole of a cervical rib should be shown on the film (900, 901)

For the oblique projection increase the kilovoltage by 7 kVp as compared with the antero-posterior projection.

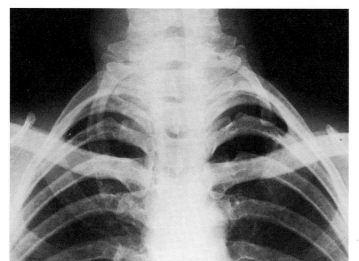

898

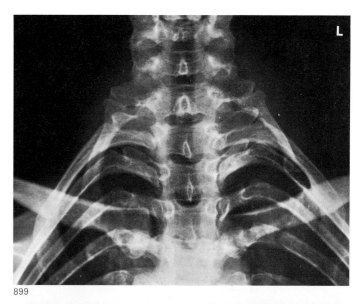

899

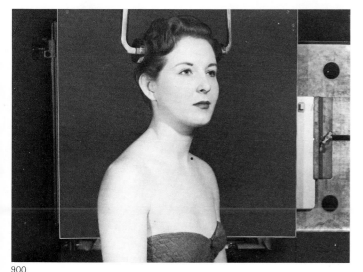

900

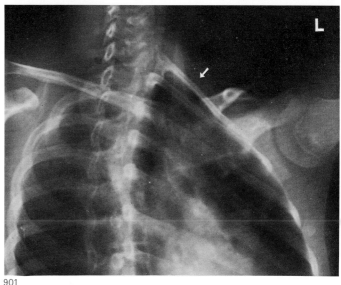

901

Lateral (Cervical ribs)

With the patient in the erect position and the shoulder of the affected side in contact with the vertical Bucky, the shoulders are depressed and the neck stretched upward to allow the seventh cervical region to be seen clear of the trunk. An 18 × 24 cm (8 × 10 ins) cassette is placed transversely to include the fifth cervical to fifth thoracic vertebrae.

■ Centre to the third cervical vertebra (902,903)

The examination for cervical ribs is now seldom required as a separate examination and their demonstration on routine views of the cervical spine or on a chest film is now considered adequate.

Costal Cartilages

There is marked variation in costal cartilage calcification as demonstrated radiographically. In the majority of young subjects, costal cartilage is invisible. There is an obvious difference in the appearance of costal cartilage calcification in men and women; in men the calcification tends to be at the margin whereas in women it is at the centre. In the middle-aged and elderly where costal cartilage calcification is common their overlying shadows must not be mistaken for renal, gallbladder or pancreatic calcifications.

Cervical Ribs

kVp		mAS			Film	Screens	
AP	LAT	AP	LAT	FFD	ILFORD	ILFORD	Grid
65	80	10	10	100 cm (40″)	RAPID R	Standard	Grid

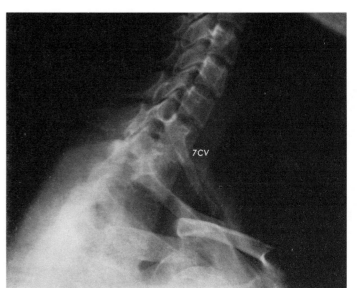
903

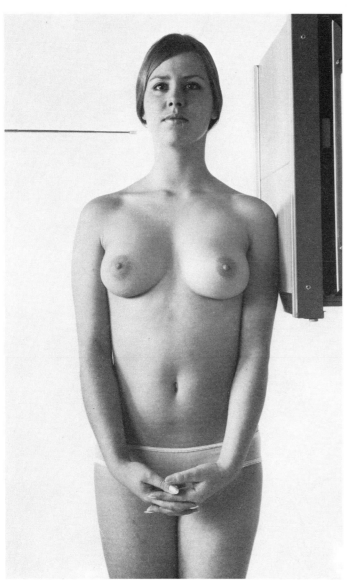
902

250

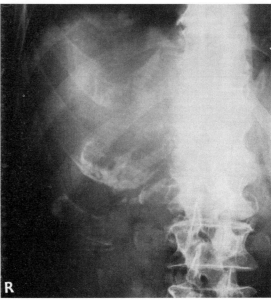
904

9

SKULL

9 SECTION 9

SKULL

General

The radiographic examination of the skull deals with both the cranium and the facial bones which are usually examined separately. The examination of the mandible is dealt with in Section 10.

The bony cranium enclosing the brain is similar to a box with sides, top and bottom. The base is the most complex surface and presents special problems to the radiographer, particularly the demonstration of the temporal bones.

The numerous small facial bones enclose a number of air-filled cavities known as the paranasal sinuses, some of which are large like the antra and others like the ethmoids are numerous and small.

For good radiography a knowledge of the anatomy of the skull is essential and it is often necessary to refer to a dry skull to plan a projection or for trial exposures. Consequently all radiographic departments must have a dry skull readily available.

To aid the student in understanding skull projections, photographs of standard positions each with a complementary series of radiographs of a dry skull are shown in this section and includes different tube angulations on correctly positioned subjects.

For standard radiographic projections of the skull there are recognized planes and lines between fixed visible, palpable or measurable anatomical points acting as a guide for each projection.

Anatomical Terminology
The terminology used is based upon the recommendations of the Commission of Neuroradiology of Milan (1961) and avoids the use of eponyms (proper names) as far as possible but when used are shown in brackets.

There are three lines and four planes of particular importance in positioning the skull for radiographic projections.

Median-sagittal plane
The median-sagittal plane, or line, divides the head vertically, from the front backwards, into two symmetrical halves. When the head is positioned correctly this plane is parallel to the film for the lateral projection (905) and at right angles to the film for the antero-posterior, or postero-anterior (906) projections.

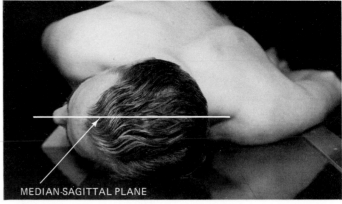

MEDIAN-SAGITTAL PLANE

905

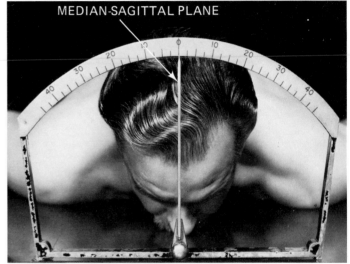

MEDIAN-SAGITTAL PLANE

906

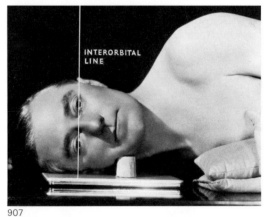

INTERORBITAL LINE

907

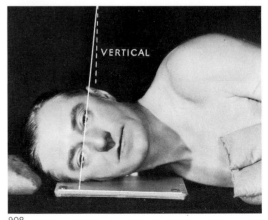

VERTICAL

908

252

Interorbital or Interpupillary line

The interorbital line extends between the centre of the two orbits or the centre of the two pupils and is at right angles to the median-sagittal plane. When the interorbital line is perpendicular to the film the head is correctly placed for the true lateral position from vertex to lower jaw (907). Compensatory tube angulation is required for any deviation from this position. Thus, when the axial ray is projected parallel to the interorbital line and at right angles to the median sagittal plane, a true lateral projection will result (908).

Base lines (A) (B)

The two generally used lines meet at an angle of approximately 10° and are known as the orbito-meatal base line (OMBL) and the anthropomorphic base line (ABL). For any intended projection it must be clearly stated which of these two lines is referred to in the radiographic projection.

(A) Orbito-Meatal base line (OMBL)

The orbito-meatal base line extends from the outer canthus of the eye to the central point of the external auditory meatus (EAM) being referred to as the radiographic base line (909), or "base line" and is the reference from which any angle is measured to adjust the position of the head. The terms "nose-chin" and "nose-forehead" are approximate only, will vary with facial contours and are inadequate for accurate descriptions of radiographic projections. However, in most cases, the "base line" will be at right angles to the film when the patient is in the "nose-forehead" position.

(B) Anthropomorphic base line (ABL)

The anthropomorphic base line extends from the infra-orbital margin to the upper border of the external auditory meatus (EAM), accepted in March, 1877, as the line of Frankfurt or as Reid's base line (911) and referred to as the "anatomical base line".

Note—The positions of the principal planes, lines and points are shown diagrammatically in anterior (910) and lateral (911) projections of the skull.

Tube angulation

The term cranio-caudal is used to indicate the direction of tube angulation towards the feet and the reverse, caudo-cranial toward the head and are often shortened to caudal and cephalad.

When tube angulation is required for a projection, the tube must first be tilted to the required angulation and then centred.

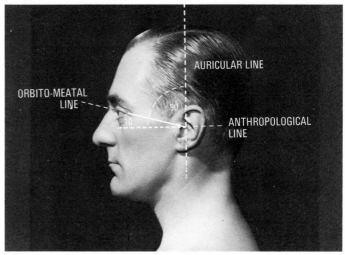

909

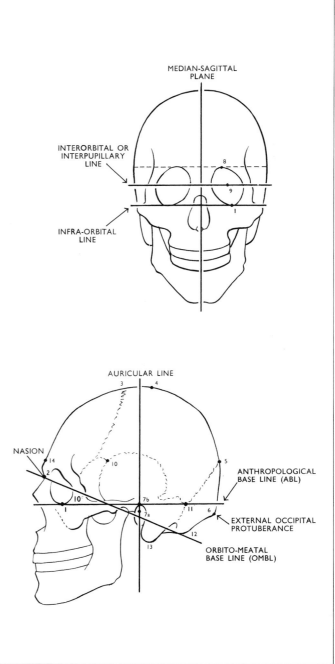

910/911

Preparation
Before the examination all opacities should be removed from the head and neck including hair pins and clips, ear-rings, dentures, necklaces and collar-studs.

Posture
The skull can be examined with the patient either erect or horizontal but most patients are more easily examined in the erect position. The erect views are done in the sitting position and the patient must 'sit up' with the spine as straight as possible. However, in Accident and Emergency cases, where there is injury to other parts of the body and the patient is on a trolley, horizontal supine views are taken.

Exposure conditions
The exposures for the general examination of the skull, as with other areas of the body, have been selected at the most suitable kilovoltage with the milliampere seconds being varied to suit the speed of the film-screen combination and a focus-film distance of 100 cm (40 ins).

Intensifying screens and a radiographic grid are essential for skull radiography while localizing cones or small aperture diaphragms will improve definition.

The head should be immobilized with the help of non-opaque pads of various shapes and sizes and a compression band. Head clamps are also occasionally used. However, in the illustrations to avoid obscuring the position of the patient, the use of immobilization accessories is limited.

Positioning terminology
The positions are named according to the direction of the X-ray beam through the head. In the occipito-frontal projection the X-ray beam enters at the occiput and leaves at the frontal bone, similarly, the occipito-mental and submento-vertical. In these projections the central ray is normally at right angles to the film. The lateral projections are named according to the side nearest the film. In projections where the tube is angled in relation to the film the particular angle prefixes the position of the head e.g. 20° occipito-frontal.

Basic positions
The routine projections are indicated as (basic) to distinguish them from alternative projections included in the text.

Radiation to the lens
Wherever possible skull radiographs must be taken in the postero-anterior position to minimize X-radiation to the lens and applies particularly to high dose examinations such as tomography.

The usual dose to the lens in the occipito-frontal projection is 5 millirads and in the fronto-occipital projection 1000 millirads for a single exposure. The comparative figures for tomography are approximately 4 millirads in the P-A and 700 millirads in the A-P projections per section.

Selected radiographs
A series of radiographs (912) to (920) are taken from the following pages to compare the various projections with each other.

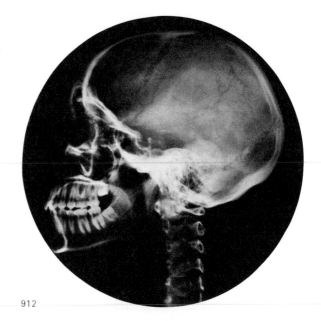

912

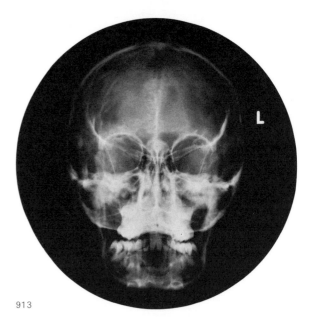

913

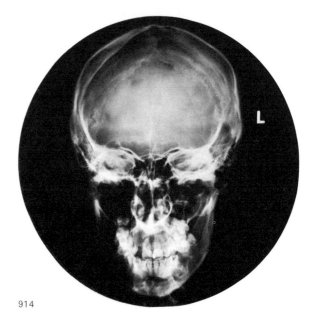

914

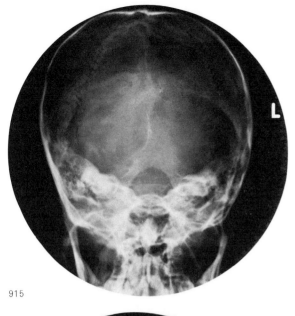

915

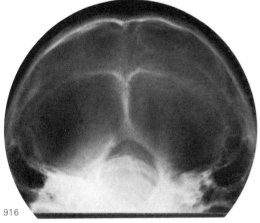

916

(912) Lateral, page 256
(913) 20° occipito-frontal, page 258
(914) Occipito-frontal, page 257.

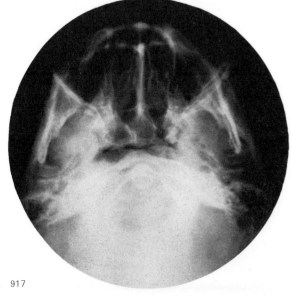

917

(915) 30° fronto-occipital, half-axial, page 259
(916) 30° occipito-vertical page 279
(917) 5° submento-vertical, axial, pages 260–261

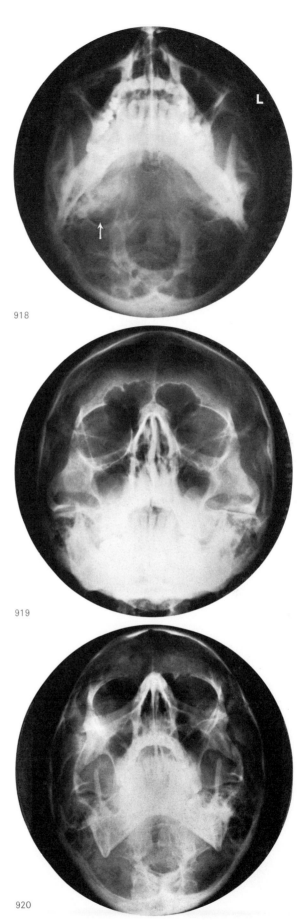

918

919

920

(918) 20° submento-vertical, page 280
(919) Occipito-mental, page 262
(920) 30° Occipito-mental, page 263

Cranium

There are many possible projections to obtain views of the sides, front, top, back and base of the cranium (921) in order to show the lateral, frontal, fronto-parietal, occipital-parietal, occipital and basal regions. However, in practice, only a small number of the possible projections are done depending on the clinical indications.

The commonly used views for the cranium are 20° occipito-frontal (931), 30° fronto-occipital (934) (half axial, Towne's), lateral (924) and 5° submento-vertical (941).

Lateral (basic)

With the patient prone or erect the head is turned with the affected side toward the film. In the prone position the uppermost shoulder is raised and supported on pads. The head is adjusted to the true lateral position with the median plane parallel and the inter-orbital line at right angles to the film. A non-opaque wedge placed under the jaw steadies the head in position (922). Where it is not possible to adjust the head to a true lateral position as in thick-set subjects, the tube must be angled until the central ray is parallel to the inter-orbital line and the cassette adjusted accordingly.

Illustration (923) shows the correct position of the skull in relation to the X-ray tube and film.

■ Centre midway between the glabella and occipital protuberance, the cassette is placed transversely and is displaced towards the vertex (922, 923, 924)

			Cranium Lateral		
kVp	mAS	FFD	Film ILFORD	Screens ILFORD	Grid
65	40	100 cm (40″)	RAPID R	Standard	Grid

Radiograph (924) shows the cranium and facial bones of the two sides superimposed. In the illustration there is perfect superimposition so that the teeth and the mandible overshadow each other.

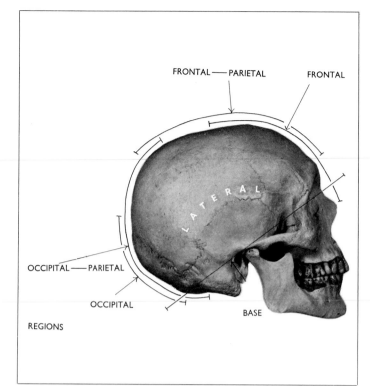
FRONTAL — PARIETAL   FRONTAL

OCCIPITAL — PARIETAL

OCCIPITAL

BASE

REGIONS

921

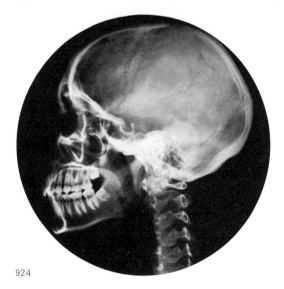
922

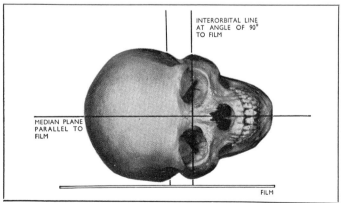
INTERORBITAL LINE AT ANGLE OF 90° TO FILM

MEDIAN PLANE PARALLEL TO FILM

FILM

923

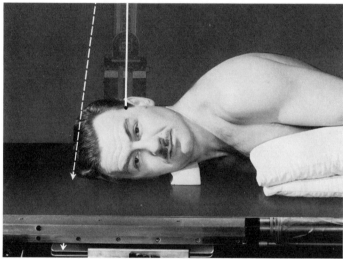
924

Occipito-frontal (basic)

In this commonly used projection of the cranium the occiput and frontal bone are superimposed and the upper margin of the petrous temporal bone coincides with the superior orbital margin so that the internal auditory meatuses are projected through the orbits. It is taken in the nose-forehead position and usually called the occipito-frontal projection particularly as the orbito-meatal line is at right angles to the film.

With the patient erect or prone the head is adjusted so that both the nose and forehead touch the couch and the radiographic baseline is at right angles to the film. When the patient is prone the hands should be clasped under the chest to help immobilization by supporting the patient.

■ Centre in the midline at a point 5 cm (2 ins) below the baseline. The cassette is placed lengthwise and displaced towards the head, the upper border of the cassette being 5 cm (2 ins) beyond the vertex (925, 926, 927)

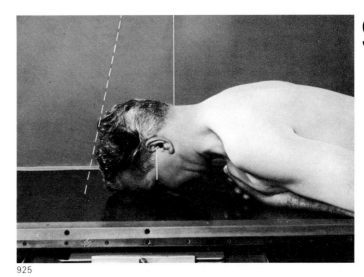

925

O–F

kVp	mAS	FFD	Film ILFORD	Screens ILFORD	Grid
75	40	100 cm (40″)	RAPID R	Standard	Grid

Note—Radiographs of two different patients (927) and (928) were taken at different kilovoltages, the former being at (70 kVp and 30 mAs) and the latter at (120 kVp and 7 mAs). In the higher kilovoltage film there is greater penetration and less contrast.

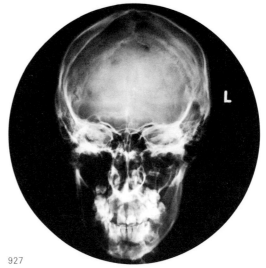

927

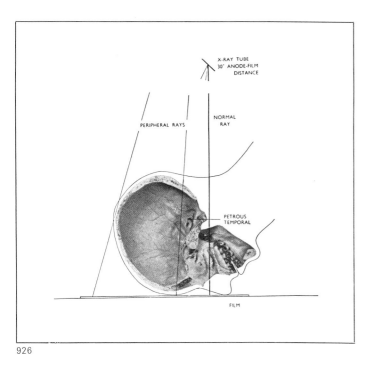

926

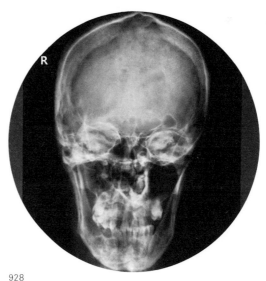

928

Cranium (basic)

20° Occipito-frontal

In this position the petrous temporal bones are projected below the levels of the orbits, the upper margin of the petrous temporals being superimposed upon the inferior orbital margins to give a clear view of the orbits and is therefore a commonly used projection in the routine examination of the skull.

This position (929) should be compared with the previous projection (925) and the corresponding radiographs (931,932) show the difference in appearance of the orbit.

With the patient erect or prone, the head is adjusted so that both the nose and forehead touch the couch and the radiographic baseline is at right angles to the film. When the patient is prone the hands should be clasped under the chest to help immobilization by supporting the patient.

■ Angle the tube 20° toward the feet and centre in the mid line on the nasion (naso-frontal articulation). The cassette is placed lengthwise with its upper border immediately above the vertex (929,930,931).

20° O–F

kVp	mAS	FFD	Film ILFORD	Screens ILFORD	Grid
75	50	100 cm (40″)	Rapid R	Standard	Grid

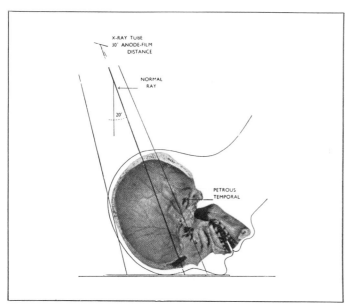

930

The effect of tube angulation in projecting the petrous temporal bones below the orbits is clearly shown. If the radiographs of the dry skull (1022, page 278) and (1027, page 279) are compared with each other, it will be seen that in (1027) with no tube angulation the internal auditory meatuses are seen within the orbit whereas in (1022) a clear unimpeded view of the orbits has been obtained.

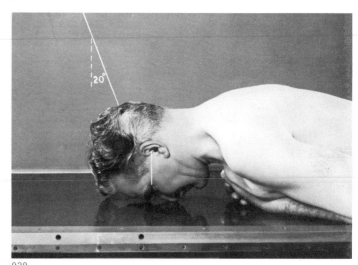

929

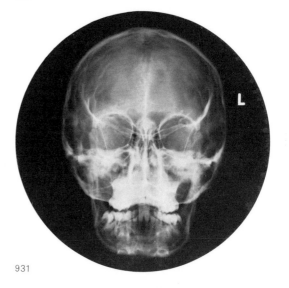

931

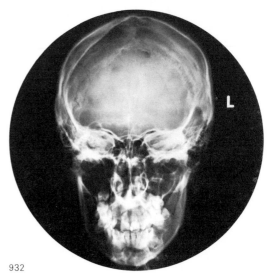

932

Fronto-occipital

This projection is used for a detailed view of the occipital bone and is best obtained with the central ray angled towards the feet. With a 30° tube angulation the petrous temporal bone is seen either side of the foramen magnum projected well above the orbits. The posterior clinoids are seen within the foramen magnum (934). However, with no tube angulation the superior orbital margin coincides with the upper border of the petrous temporal and the internal auditory meatuses are seen through the orbits.

30° Fronto-occipital (basic)
(Half-axial, Townes)

With the patient erect or supine and the chin well down on the chest, the head is adjusted so that the radiographic baseline is at right angles to the film. When the patient is supine a suitable non-opaque pad may be placed under the head to tilt the chin down. Thick-set subjects will need larger pads to obtain an adequate degree of tilt.

■ With the tube angled 30° centre in the midline to the foramen magnum. The cassette is placed lengthwise with its upper margin immediately above the vertex.

Ideally the baseline must be at right angles to the film, however, when this is not possible the tube angulation must be adjusted to compensate for the position of the head.

9

Fronto-occipital

This projection is not commonly used because of increased X-radiation to the eyes. With the patient erect or supine the head is adjusted so that the radiographic baseline is at right angles to the film. When the patient is supine a suitable non-opaque pad may be placed under the head with the chin down.

■ Centre in the midline at the hair line with the central ray at right angles to the couch top or vertical Bucky. The film is placed lengthwise with its upper border 5 cm (2 ins) above the vertex (935,936)

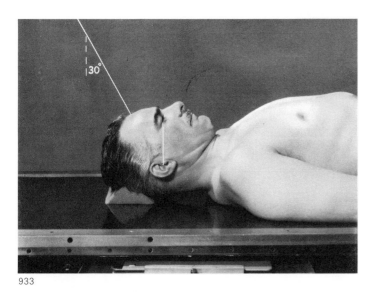

933

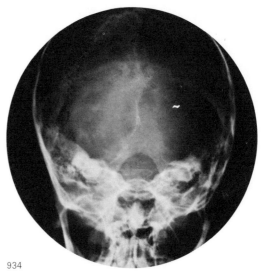

934

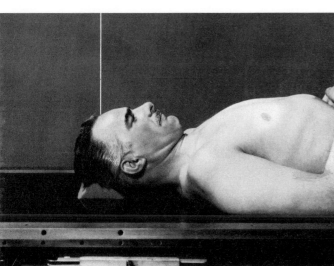

935

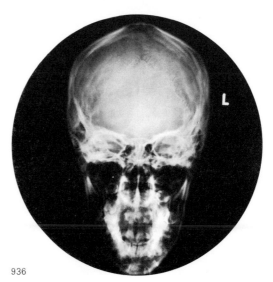

936

259

5° Submento-vertical (basic)
(Axial)

In this position the base of the skull is demonstrated (941) including the basal foramina and petrous temporal bones. The temporo-mandibular joint should be projected in front of the auditory ossicles and the anterior part of the mandible should form an arch across the superimposed maxillary antra and orbits.

With the patient erect or supine the head is hyper-extended until the vertex of the skull is in contact with the couch. In the supine position the shoulders need to be sufficiently raised to bring the radiographic baseline parallel to the film. There is considerable variation between different patients in the ease with which this position can be achieved and tube angulation must be adjusted accordingly.

With an adjustable pedestal Bucky it is easy to position the patient correctly by lowering the Bucky to a suitable level (938).

The Bucky top may also be tilted towards the head to obtain a correct projection.

■ Centre in the midline between the angles of the jaw with the central ray at an angle of 95° to the base-line. The cassette is placed lengthwise with its lower border immediately below the occipital protuberance (937, 938, 939, 940)

SMV

kVp	mAS	FFD	Film ILFORD	Screens ILFORD	Grid
85	50	100 cm (40″)	RAPID R	Standard	Grid

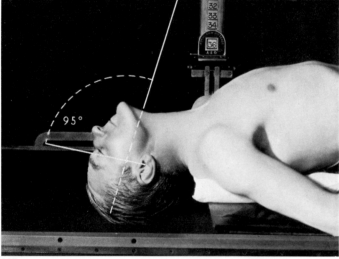

937

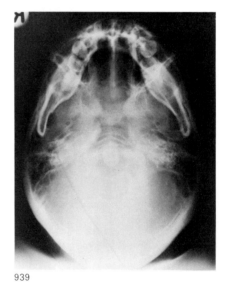

939

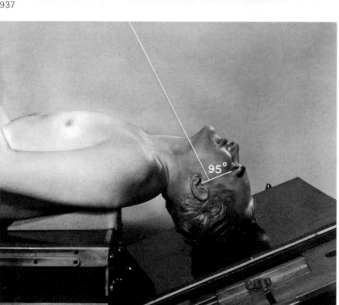

938

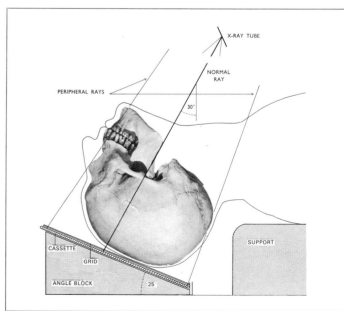

940

260

A radiograph of the skull (941) and an annotated diagram (942) should assist the student in recognizing the radiographic anatomy.

In this view the maxillary antra are superimposed on the orbits and are shown on either side of the nasal cavity and ethmoid sinuses, with the sphenoidal sinuses lying immediately behind the nasal cavities. The pituitary fossa is largely projected over the sphenoidal sinus and the anterior part of the mandible across the maxillary antra and orbits. The zygomatic arch forms the outer margin of the anterior part of the skull with the middle cranial fossa medial to it. The vertical ramus of the mandible is projected over the middle fossa and posteriorly the temporo-mandibular joint abuts against the anterior margin of the petrous temporal. The foramen ovale and foramen spinosum lie medially just behind the pterygoid. The petrous temporal bone is the densest part of the skull and lies on either side of the foramen magnum with the odontoid peg visible in its anterior part. The atlas (C.1) is projected between the petrous temporals, inside the foramen magnum with the posterior fossa lying posteriorly. A careful examination of the film when correctly positioned and exposed should show the auditory ossicles lying within the middle ear just behind the temporo-mandibular joints.

9

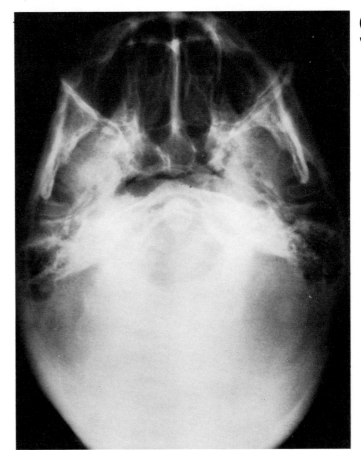

941

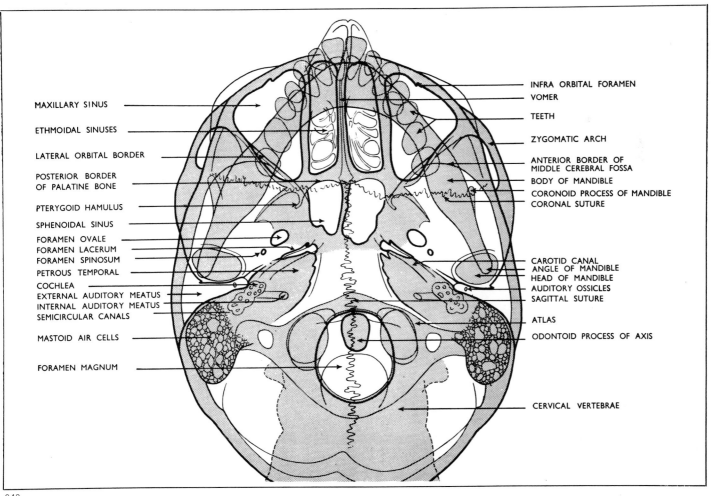

MAXILLARY SINUS

ETHMOIDAL SINUSES

LATERAL ORBITAL BORDER

POSTERIOR BORDER OF PALATINE BONE

PTERYGOID HAMULUS

SPHENOIDAL SINUS

FORAMEN OVALE
FORAMEN LACERUM
FORAMEN SPINOSUM
PETROUS TEMPORAL
COCHLEA
EXTERNAL AUDITORY MEATUS
INTERNAL AUDITORY MEATUS
SEMICIRCULAR CANALS

MASTOID AIR CELLS

FORAMEN MAGNUM

INFRA ORBITAL FORAMEN
VOMER

TEETH

ZYGOMATIC ARCH

ANTERIOR BORDER OF MIDDLE CEREBRAL FOSSA
BODY OF MANDIBLE
CORONOID PROCESS OF MANDIBLE
CORONAL SUTURE

CAROTID CANAL
ANGLE OF MANDIBLE
HEAD OF MANDIBLE
AUDITORY OSSICLES
SAGITTAL SUTURE

ATLAS

ODONTOID PROCESS OF AXIS

CERVICAL VERTEBRAE

942

Facial Bones

Minor fractures of facial bones are not visible on the lateral projection because of the overlying bone and soft tissue shadowing. In the postero-anterior projections superimposition of dense structures is avoided by correct positioning.

Wherever possible views of the face should be done in the erect position otherwise there must be one view taken with a horizontal beam to exclude a fluid level in a paranasal sinus.

Occipito-mental (basic)

This projection shows the orbits, the nasal region, the maxillae and the zygomatic bones.

With the patient erect or prone the head is adjusted to the nose-chin position. The median sagittal plane is at right angles and the radiographic baseline at 45° to the cassette.

■ Centre in the midline through the vertex of the skull and to the nasion (943, 944, 945)

The dry skull is aligned with the radiographic baseline at 45° to the couch top and shows how the denser structures of the skull such as the petrous temporal bones are projected below the antra (946).

Occipito-mental (basic), O-M

kVp	mAS	FFD	Film ILFORD	Screens ILFORD	Grid
75	50	100 cm (40″)	RAPID R	Standard	Grid

Minor fractures may not be visible and the only clue to the presence of a bone injury may be a fluid level in one of the paranasal sinuses. If the film is not done in the erect position or with a horizontal ray this sign will be missed. Gas in the orbit (emphysema) is another sign which may indicate that a fracture is present even though fracture itself is not visible.

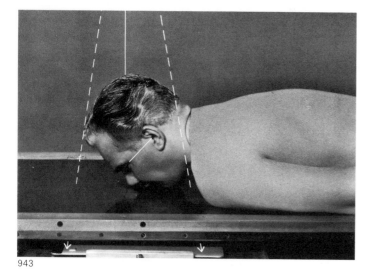
943

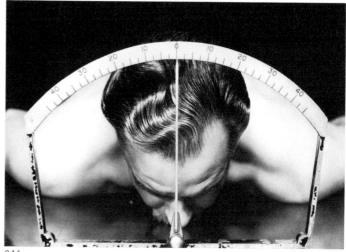
944

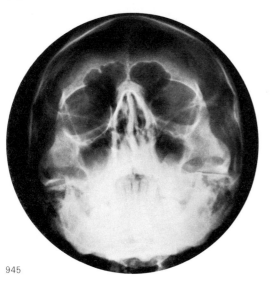
945

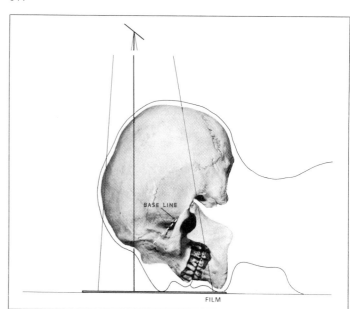
946

30° Occipito-mental (basic)

By tilting the tube 30° in addition to the radiographic baseline being 45°, the lower orbital margins and the zygomatic arches can be demonstrated more clearly (947, 948).

With the patient erect or prone the head is adjusted to the nose-chin position, the median saggital plane being at right angles and the radiographic base-line at 45° to the film.

■ Angle the tube 30° to the feet and centre in the midline to the junction of the nose and upper lip (947, 948)

30° O–M

kVp	mAS	FFD	Film ILFORD	Screems ILFORD	Grid
80	50	100 cm (40")	RAPID R	Standard	Grid

30° Fronto-occipital
(Half-axial, Townes)

This projection has been previously described on page 259 (935) and is now known as the Townes view. For a better view of the zygomatic arches the centring point should be the glabella with appropriate downward displacement of the film. The X-ray beam should be coned to improve image quality (950).

30° O–F

kVp	mAS	FFD	Film ILFORD	Screens ILFORD	Grid
80	50	100 cm (40")	RAPID R	Standard	Grid

Injuries

Two radiographs (949, 30° occipito-mental) (950, half-axial) show a fracture of the right zygomatic arch.

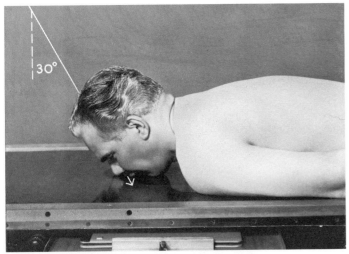

947

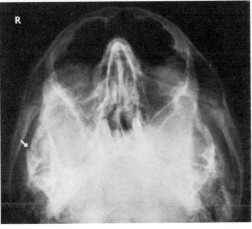

949

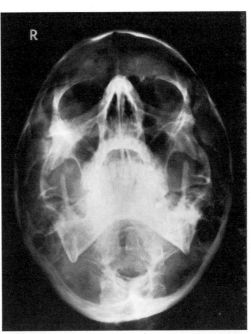

948

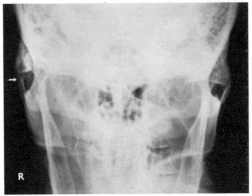

950

Lateral

In this position there is overlapping of the bones of the two sides and minor fractures are not usually visible. A horizontal ray film is therefore particularly important not to overlook a fluid level in the paranasal sinuses, however, the lateral projection can also be done with the patient prone (951).

With the patient erect or horizontal the head is in the true lateral position, with the median-sagittal plane parallel and the interorbital line at right angles to the film, as for the lateral (basic) projection of the skull.

The supine lateral projection is shown on page 272 (978).

■ Centre over the body of the zygoma (951,952)

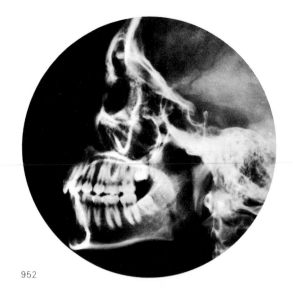

952

Face Lateral

kVp	mAS	FFD	Film ILFORD	Screens ILFORD	Grid
60	20	100 cm (40″)	RAPID R	Standard	Grid

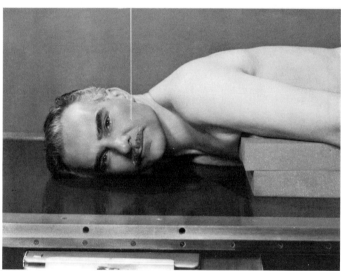

951

In this view the exposure for the bones of the face will not show the nasal bones or soft tissues. Either a separate radiograph with a reduced exposure must be done or a suitable non-screen film can be placed on the cassette and exposed simultaneously. The screen film will show the facial bones (953) while the non-screen film shows the soft tissues and nasal bones (954).

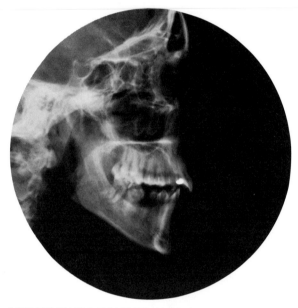

NEGATIVE FOR BONE STRUCTURE
953

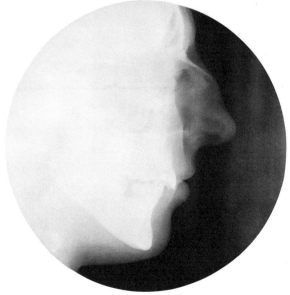

NEGATIVE FOR SOFT TISSUE STRUCTURE
954

Oblique

Films taken from the oblique position are recognized additional projections which can be used to demonstrate minor fractures to facial bones.

With the patient erect or prone and in the nose/forehead position, the head is adjusted so the median sagittal plane and the readiographic base line are both at right angles to the film. The head is then turned through 40° to the affected side making sure that the nose and chin are in contact with the couch. This brings the supra orbital margin, the tip of the nose, the zygoma and the chin into the same plane (955).

When the patient is prone the appropriate shoulder is raised on a pad for support to bring the opposite side of the face towards the film; the head should be immobilized.

■ With the tube angled 10° toward the head centre through the mastoid process remote from the film (956, 957).

			Film	Screens	
kVp	mAS	FFD	ILFORD	ILFORD	Grid
65	20	100 cm (40″)	RAPID R	Standard	Grid

Oblique

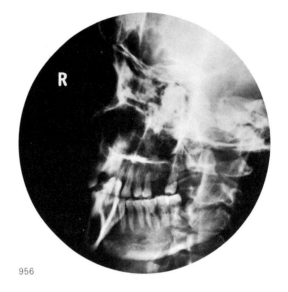

956

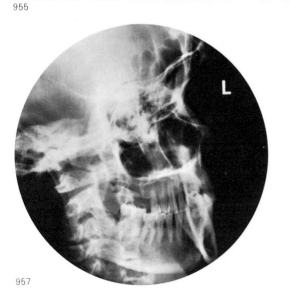

955

957

Nasal

Nose Lateral

kVp	mAS	FFD	Film ILFORD	Screens ILFORD	Grid
60	10	100 cm (40")	ILFEX 90 (NS)	—	—

Lateral (basic)

(1) With the head in the true lateral position an appropriate sized non-screen film is placed immediately below the nose on the couch (958,960,961).

(2) An occlusal or dental film in contact with the bone is supported on a sandbag or non opaque pad. The success of this position depends largely on being able to use the flexibility of double wrap film (959). This view is not commonly used particularly in modern departments with only automatic processing because the small sized film will not go through the processor.

Fracture radiograph

Radiograph (961) shows a depressed fracture of the nose but the examination is incomplete without the supero-inferior projection (962, 965).

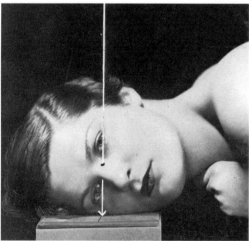

958

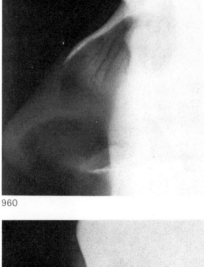

960

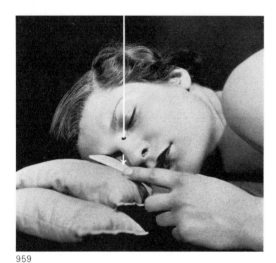

959

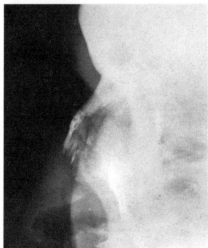

961

Supero-inferior

This view is by far the most important to show fractures of the nose. However, in some patients, particularly children, the small nasal bone cannot be projected beyond the maxilla and upper teeth. A suitable non-screen film is held between the teeth so that it will be at approximately 110° to the x-ray beam.

With the patient erect or supine the central ray is adjusted to be at a tangent to the forehead in the midline, passing through the angle between the nose and the upper lip.

■ Centre through the root of the nose with a focus-film distance of 100 cm (40 ins).

The dry skull is aligned to show how the nasal bones are projected anteriorly to the maxilla and the upper teeth (964).

Fracture radiographs

Two radiographs (966) show a fracture of the nose in two planes at right angles to each other.

9

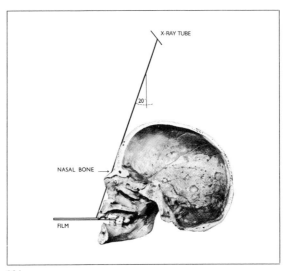
964

Nose Sup—Inf

kVp	mAS	FFD	Film ILFORD	Screens ILFORD	Grid
65 —	30	100 cm (40″)	ILFEX (NS)	—	—

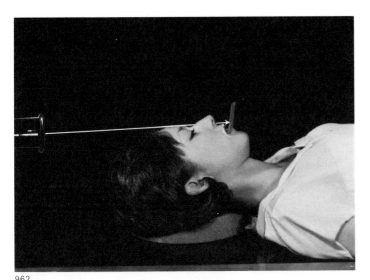
962

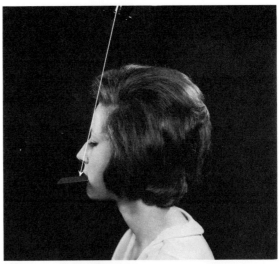
963

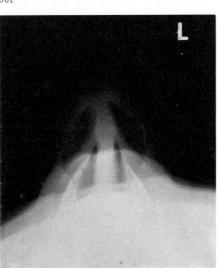
965

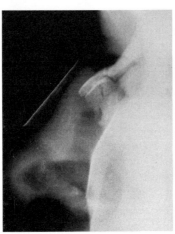
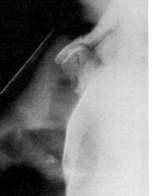
966

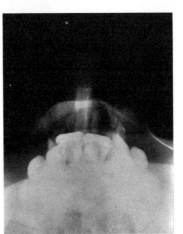

Maxillae

kVp	mAS	FFD	Film ILFORD	Screens ILFORD	Grid
65	30	17 cm (6·5 ins)	Occlusal	—	—

Intra-oral
Greater detail of the hard palate and roots of the upper teeth may be shown by using intra-oral occlusal films.

(1) Central
The patient is seated with a head support behind the occiput and the occlusal plane lying horizontally.

With the central ray in the midline at 75° to the occlusal plane the film is placed transversely between the jaw, as far back as possible and held lightly between the teeth.

■ Centre in the midline through the tip of the nose, with the central ray at 75° to the film (967,968).

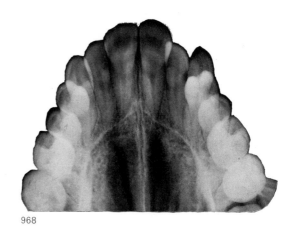
968

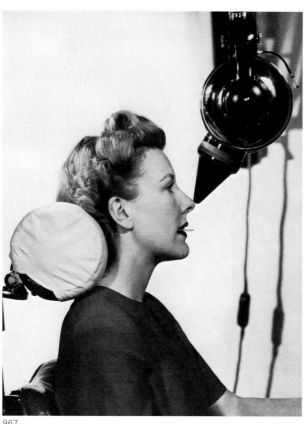
967

(2) Right and left

With the patient in the same position as previously described the occlusal film is held transversely between the teeth but more over to the right or left as required.

■ Centre over the outer canthus of the eye with the tube angled 65° to the centre of the film.

Although these projections are not confined to dental equipment and can be done in the department with larger units, positioning of the tube is much easier with a dental unit.

In the department a larger focus-film distance has to be used because the tube head has an associated light beam diaphragm.

Maxillae Oblique

kVp	mAS	FFD	Film ILFORD	Screens ILFORD	Grid
65	25	17 cm (6·5 ins)	Occlusal	—	—

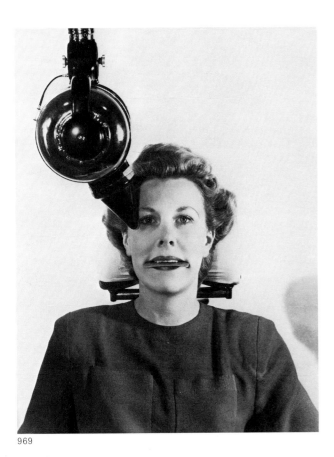

969

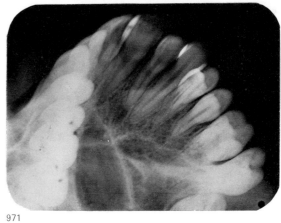

970

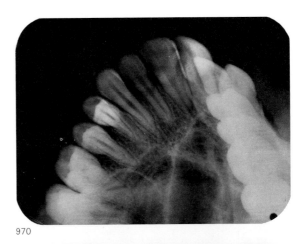

971

In the investigation of malocclusion and facial disproportion caused by developmental defects (972) a wide radiographic field is required. Radiography is essential in the initial diagnosis, in monitoring progress of the condition and the effects of treatment.

For monitoring the results of treatment it is essential to take serial radiographs under standardized conditions for true comparative pictures. Variations in technique will make any measurements on serial radiographs valueless because both the measurements and the relationship can be altered by slight changes of projection or of the position of the patient.

A true lateral facial view is the most useful projection. The occipito-frontal view is the most commonly used additional film particularly in assessing the mandible.

The Craniostat and its uses

To produce truly comparable follow-up films a special head holding device is used in orthodontic hospitals. The apparatus shown in (973) is relatively simple and is made up of two parallel arms to which are attached ear plugs so that the head is supported in the same position on each occasion the patient is radiographed, with a constant relationship to the film and the tube.

For the Lateral View

Reid's base line should be horizontal so that the posterior margin of the mandible clears the cervical spine. An adjustable horizontal line on the front of the film support helps to adjust the head so that the lower orbital margin and the superior border of the external auditory meatuses (Reid's base line) are in the same horizontal plane.

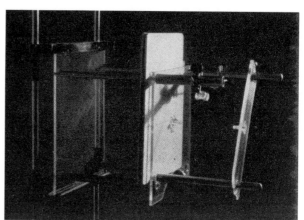
973

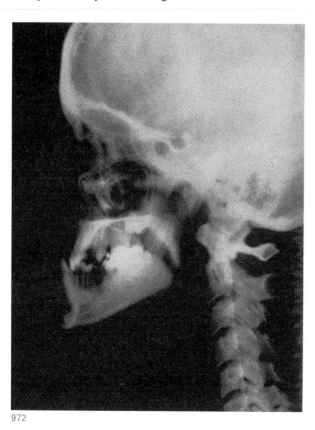
972

In (974) a child is correctly positioned in a Craniostat but the supports for the nasion and occipital bone are not shown on the photograph. The horizontal line on the marked Perspex sheet is in front of the cassette at the level of Reid's base line.

In radiograph (975) a lateral radiograph of the face is shown taken with the aid of a craniostat and the nasion support in position.

More elaborate craniostats are used in special centres and are incorporated in the x-ray equipment together with Potter-Bucky diaphragms. Radiograph (976) was taken on such an apparatus and there is a line diagram of the film (977) plotting the angulation of the incisors and other bony points.

9

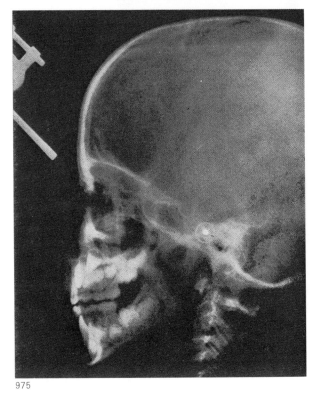

974

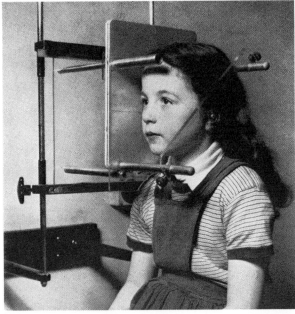

975

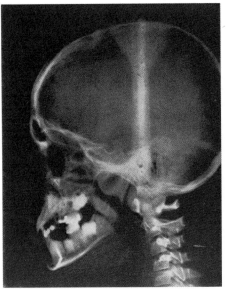

976

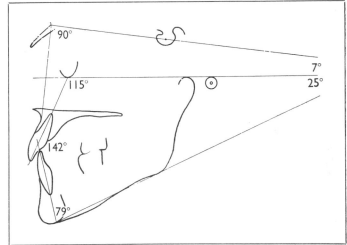

977

271

Lateral

In all cases of trauma to the skull when the patient is supine and cannot be moved, a film is placed vertically against the lateral aspect of the head. A horizontal beam at right angles to the film is used.

■ Centre midway between the glabella and the occipital protuberance (978,979)

Note—A horizontal ray lateral is essential in all cases of head trauma to exclude an air/fluid level in one of the paranasal sinuses or in the ventricles of the brain.

Occipito-frontal

When an occipito-frontal view is required on a patient on a casualty stretcher the head can be raised on a non-opaque pad and turned to face the film which is placed vertically. The orbito-meatal line should be at right angles to the film. Raise the shoulder furthest from the couch top on a pad to maintain the head comfortably in position.

■ Centre from the horizontal position 5 cm (2 ins) below the base line and at right angles to the film (980,981)

Note—Satisfactory radiographs can be obtained when using a stationary grid as in (980) or when using the vertical Bucky. It is essential to raise the head on a non-opaque pad to allow the cassette to be placed low enough to include the side of the head nearest the couch.

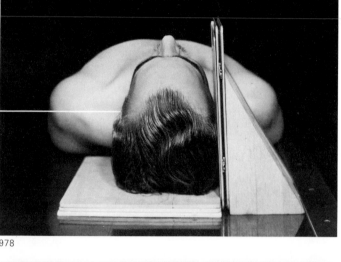

978

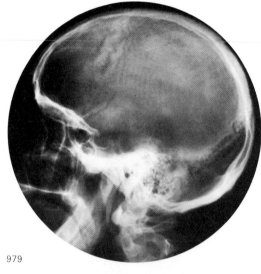

979

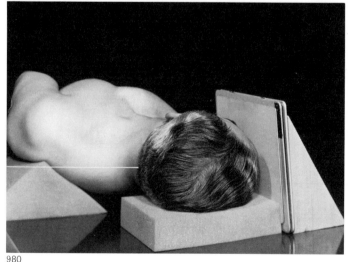

980

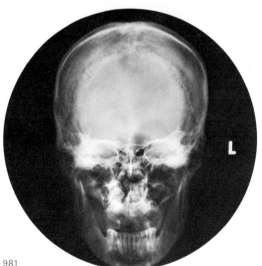

981

Fronto-occipital

With seriously injured patients, where the head must not be turned to the side, a reverse occipito-frontal position is used. With the patient supine, the head is raised on a small non-opaque pad to slightly flex the neck bringing the chin toward the chest and the radiographic baseline at right angles to the table top. This allows the head to be flexed slightly forward with the chin towards the chest, thus preventing undue strain on the neck in establishing the baseline/film relationship while greatly assisting immobilization. Sandbags on either side, separated from the head by non-opaque pads will assist immobilization.

■ Centre in the midline with the tube vertical over the vertex of the skull (983, 984)

20° Mento-occipital

9

In patients who cannot be moved, a 20° mento-occipital view is required to show the facial bones. Ideally the chin should be raised until the radiographic baseline is at 45° to the film, but if the patient's head cannot be sufficiently extended additional tube angulation will be needed to compensate.

■ Centre in the midline over the mouth with the central ray 20° to the head (985, 986)

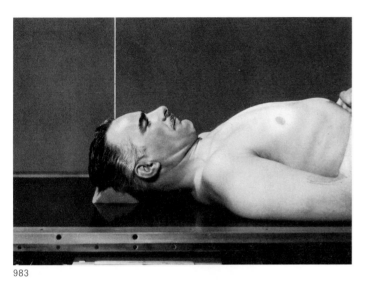

983

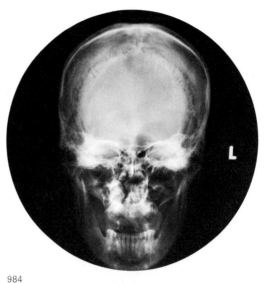

984

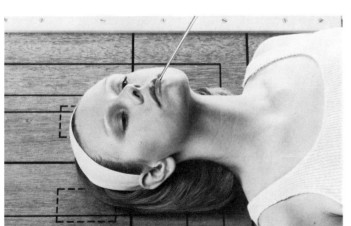

985

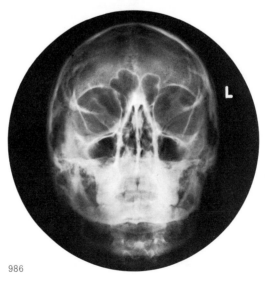

986

Additional views

Zygomatic arches

Where the arches cannot be shown free from overlying structures in either the 30° fronto-occipital projection or in the submento-vertical view, each arch will need to be radiographed separately.

Submento vertical

With the patient seated and the head extended the vertex is in contact with the vertical Bucky. The radiographic baseline is parallel with the film and the head rotated 15° away from the affected side.

■ Centre to the angle of the jaw of the affected side and radiograph each side in turn.

Reduce the kilovoltage by 15 kVp as compared with the submento-vertical (basic) view (987).

Vertico-mental

With the patient prone the head is extended, the chin touching the table top. Rotate the head 15° away from the side being examined.

■ Centre at right angles to the radiographic baseline through each arch in turn (988,989)

Reduce the kilovoltage by 15 kVp compared with the submento vertical (basic) projection.

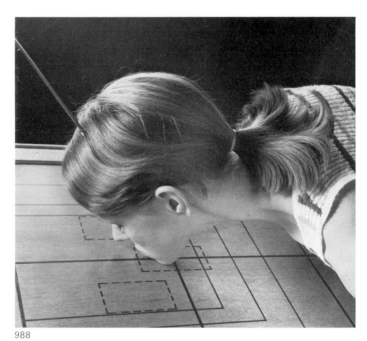

987

988

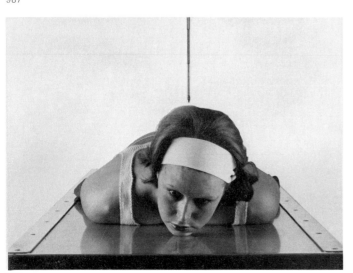

989

Pineal Body

When calcified, the pineal is visible on the lateral view and may then also be seen on frontal projections for estimation of displacement from the midline. Pineal shift is used as an indication of cerebral space occupying lesions. For the estimation of pineal shift it is important to have a true frontal projection without rotation.

Space occupying lesions can be due to tumours or as a result of a trauma. However, if the pineal is not visible on the lateral view it will not be seen on the frontal view. In radiographs (991–994) the pineal is shifted due to a subdural haematoma caused by a head injury. The subdural haematoma acts as a space occupying lesion which shifts the pineal away from the lesion. Surgical clips are visible in the post-operative radigraphs but the pineal shift is still present and after air encephalography (994) the displaced cerebral ventricles are demonstrated.

With the introduction of computed tomography the demonstration of space occupying lesion with deviation and distortion of the ventricular system and the pineal has been greatly simplified (995b).

9

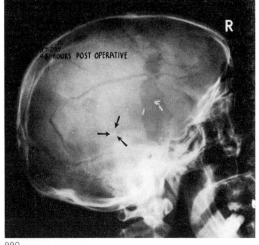

990

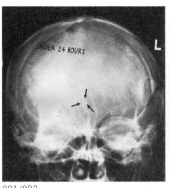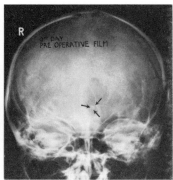

991/992

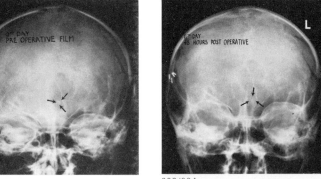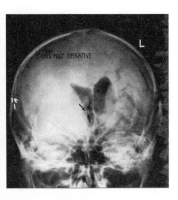

993/994

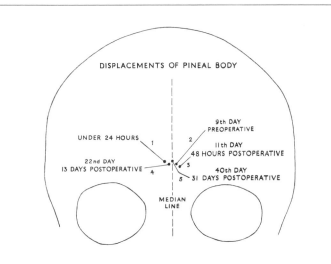

995a

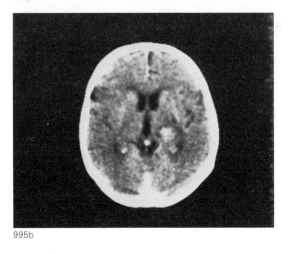

995b

275

Sella Turcica

(Pituitary fossa)

A view of the dry skull (997) shows the sella turcica lying in the centre of the inner aspect of the base of the skull. It is a shallow depression called the pituitary fossa and contains the pituitary gland. The anterior clinoids are on either side of the tuberculum sellae which forms the anterior and upper part of the pituitary fossa. The dorsum sellae with the posterior clinoids forms its posterior boundary. The floor of the pituitary fossa appears as a white line called the lamina dura lying above the sphenoidal sinus.

Lateral (basic)

The sella turcica is shown through the squamous part of the temporal bone and a coned view should be taken to show the

bony detail. The head must be maintained in the true lateral position, with the median sagittal plane parallel and the interorbital line at right angles to the film. With the patient erect the head can be kept in position by use of the head clamp (996), and in the horizontal position by placing a non-opaque pad under the jaw and a sandbag against the vertex of the skull.

■ Centre 2·5 cm (1 in) in front of and above the external auditory meatus, using a small localizing cone (996, 997, 998, 999)

Sella Turcica Lateral

kVp	mAS	FFD	Film ILFORD	Screens ILFORD	Grid
65	40	100 cm (40″)	RAPID R	Standard	Grid

68   100 mA   2/5 SEC   40″   IUP Room

Radiograph (999) was taken with a small localizing cone to show the bony detail and radiograph (998) with a larger cone to show bony landmarks.

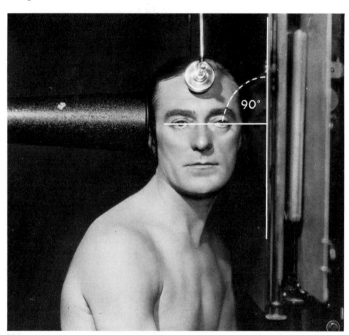

996

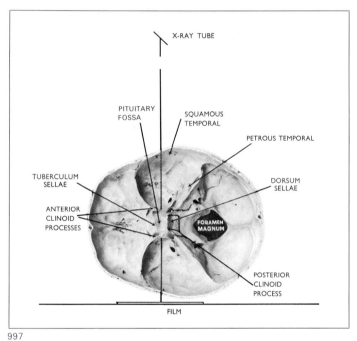

997

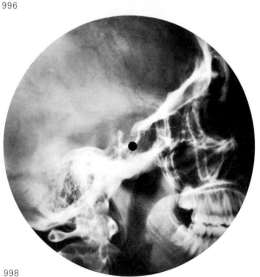

998

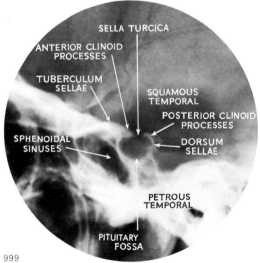

999

The variations in size and appearance of the sella turcica are shown in radiograph (1000).

Frontal Views

The pituitary fossa is easily seen on the lateral radiograph but on the frontal view is hidden by the dense bone at the base of the skull. In frontal projections the pituitary fossa can be seen either through the frontal and sphenoidal sinuses or through the foramen magnum.

The floor of the pituitary fossa is usually best seen through the sphenoidal sinus whereas the dorsum sellae is shown through the foramen magnum.

The sphenoidal air cells lie in front of and below the pituitary fossa and are trans-radiant by comparison appearing as darker areas (1002) which act as the landmark to locate the sella turcica.

10° Occipito-frontal

With the patient erect or prone the head is placed in the nose-forehead position; the median sagittal plane and the radiographic baseline are at right angles to the film.

■ With the tube angled 10° towards the head, centre in the midline 5 cms (2 ins) below the occipital protuberance to allow the axial ray to pass through the glabella (1001, 1002, 1003)

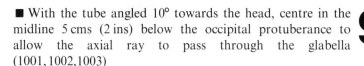

10° O–F

kVp	mAS	FFD	Film ILFORD	Screens ILFORD	Grid
75	40	100 cm (40″)	RAPID R	Standard	Grid

84 100 mA @ 2/5 sec IUP Room

A diagram superimposed on the midline section of a dry skull (1003) has been positioned to show the sella turcica and the central ray projected through the frontal bone above the nasion.

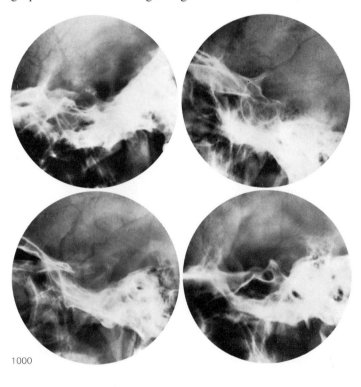

1000

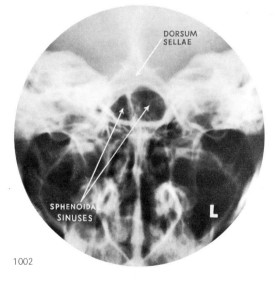

1001

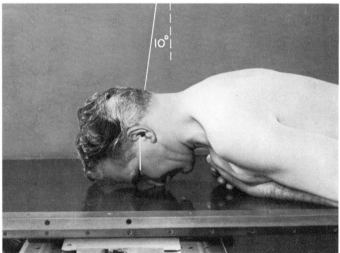

DORSUM SELLAE

SPHENOIDAL SINUSES

L

1002

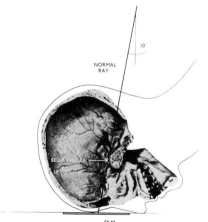

NORMAL RAY

10°

SELLA TURCICA

FILM

1003

30° Fronto-occipital
(Half-axial)

With the patient erect or supine and the chin well down toward the chest, the median sagittal plane and radiographic baseline are both positioned at right angles to the film. A full description of this view is given on page 259.

■ With the tube angled 30° to the radiographic baseline, centre in the midline through the glabella, pituitary fossa and the foramen magnum. Use a small localizing cone (1004, 1005, 1006, 1007)

30° F—O					
kVp	mAS	FFD	Film ILFORD	Screens ILFORD	Grid
80	40	100 cm (40")	RAPID R	Standard	Grid

Radiograph (1007) was taken with a small localizing cone to show the bone detail and radiograph (1005) with a larger cone to show bony landmarks.

A diagram superimposed on the midline section of a dry skull (1006) has been positioned to show how the sella turcica is projected through the foramen magnum.

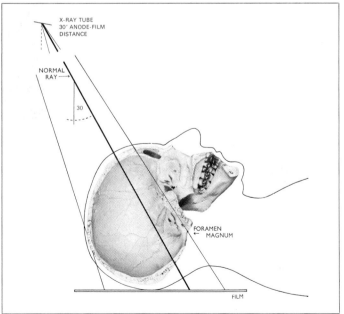

1004

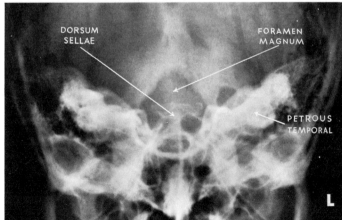

1005

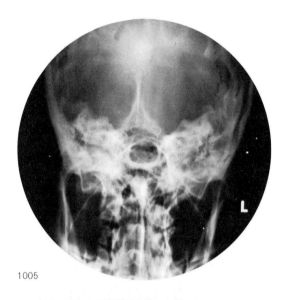

1007

1006

Occipital Bone
Occipito-vertical

An infrequently used position to show the occipital bone is shown in (1008,1010).

With the patient in the prone position and the trunk raised on pillows, the neck is flexed to bring the vertex of the skull into contact with the X-ray couch and the base line to film angle at approximately 50°.

This view is more easily done with the patient erect using head clamps for fixation. With the head in contact with the bucky the chin is tucked well in; the median sagittal plane is at right angles and the radiographic base line at 50° to the film.

■ Centre in the midline 2 cm (1 in) below the occipital protuberance (1008, 1009, 1010)

Radiograph (1009) shows the mastoid air cells on either side at the level of the foramen magnum.

Illustration (1010a) shows the relationship between occipital bone, X-ray tube and film.

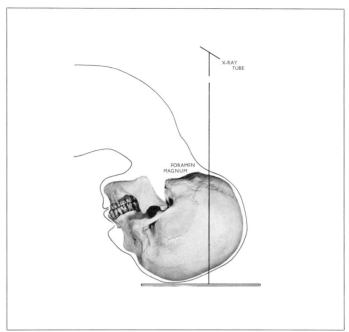

1010a

Occipito Vertical

kVp	mAS	FFD	Film ILFORD	Screens ILFORD	Grid
75	30	100 cm (40″)	RAPID R	Standard	Grid

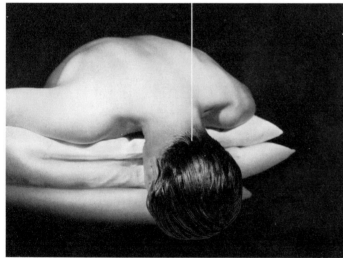

1008

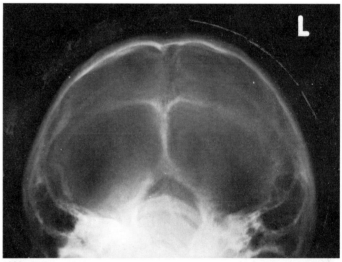

1009

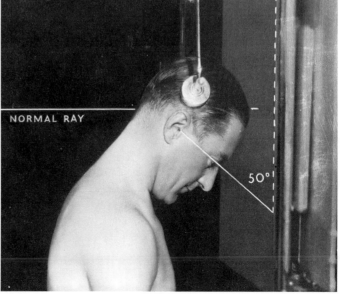

1010

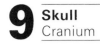

Jugular Foramina

20° Submento-vertical
The jugular foramina may be seen with a modified basic projection appearing on a radiograph as dark areas on each side of the anterior part of the foramen magnum but on the routine basic projections are obscured by the petrous temporal bones. In this modified projection with the tube tilted caudally the foramina lie between the petrous bones anteriorly and the transverse process of the atlas posteriorly.

With the patient erect or supine the neck is extended to bring the vertex of the skull into contact with the Bucky and with the radiographic baseline parallel to the film.

Jugular Foramina 20° SMV

kVp	mAS	FFD	Film ILFORD	Screens ILFORD	Grid
80	40	100 cm (40″)	RAPID R	Standard	Grid

■ With the tube angled 20° caudally (70° to the radiographic base line) centre in the midline at the level of the external auditory meatuses. Use a narrow slit diaphragm or a small localizing cone

The same projection is produced by reducing the extension of the neck so that the radiographic baseline is at 20° to the film. The central ray must then be perpendicular to the cassette midway between the external auditory meatuses. This position is preferable in patients with a short neck.

Lateral
With the head in the true lateral position, rotate the face 15° toward the film and tilt the tube 15° toward the feet.

■ Centre 2 cm (1 in) above and behind the external auditory meatus remote from the film, taking the right and left sides in turn. The foramina will be shown just below the external auditory meatus and anterior to the mastoid process (1014, 1015)

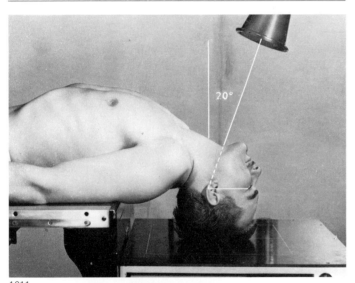

1011

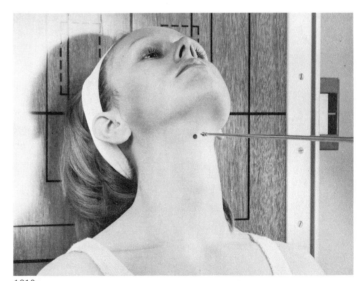

1012

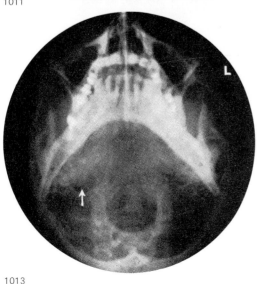

280
1013

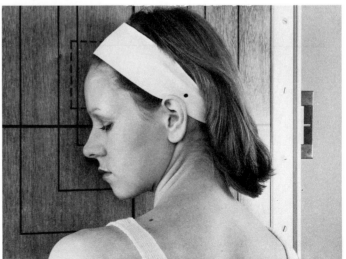

1014

Localized Tangential Projections

For most patients the routine lateral and frontal projections will be taken even when there is an obvious protruding lesion (1016a, b). However, to demonstrate any underlying bone involvement localized tangential views are required to show the inner and outer tables of the skull.

■ Centre over the lesion using a small localizing cone (1017, 1018); this projection can be used for any part of the cranial vault

Radiograph (1018) shows the soft tissue mass and the underlying associated bone destruction. An opaque marker has been used on the skin over the mass.

Note—The exposure should be reduced by approximately 10 kVp. To show both the soft tissue and the bone detail a non-screen film is placed in front of the cassette and both exposed simultaneously.

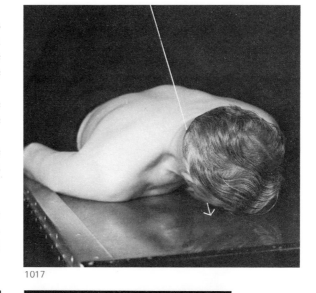

1017

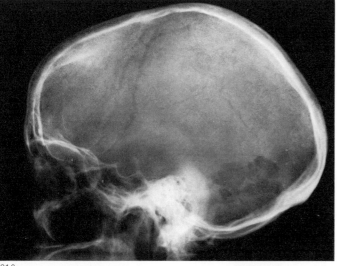

1016a

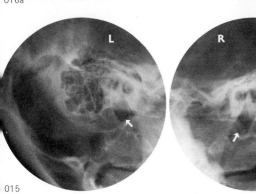

1015

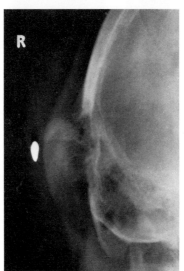

1018

Dry bone projections

A series of radiographs of the dry skull (1019 to 1024) shows the varying relationship of the structures of the cranium as the tube angle is changed from 0° to 30°, as shown in photograph (1019). Notice the varying appearance of the frontal sinuses, the orbital rim, the lesser wings of the sphenoids within the orbital cavities, and the changing position of the petrous temporals. At the commonly used angle of 20°, the upper petrous borders should be at the level of the lower border of the orbits (1022).

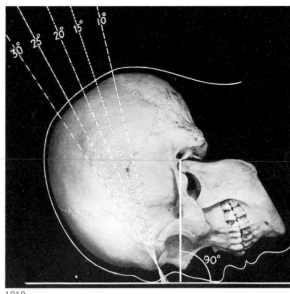

1019

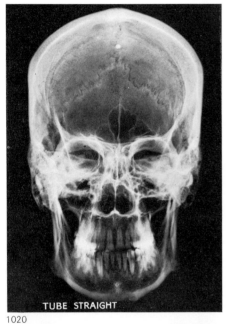

TUBE STRAIGHT

1020

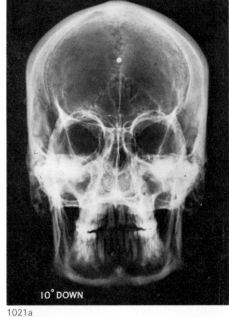

10° DOWN

1021a

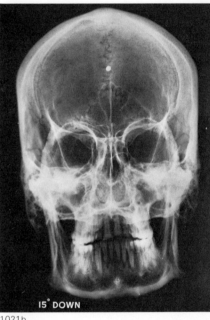

15° DOWN

1021b

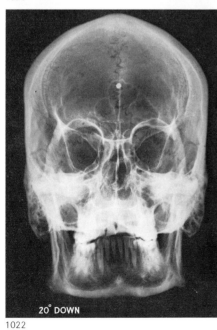

20° DOWN

1022

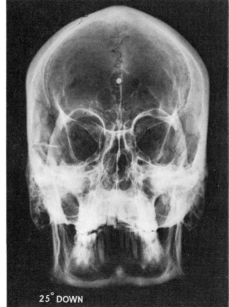

25° DOWN

1023

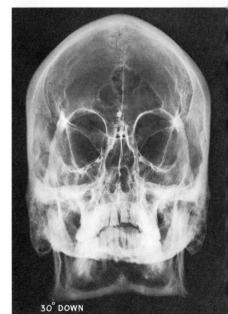

30° DOWN

1024

Dry bone projections

In the occipito-frontal (basic) view the normal centring point is 5 cm (2 ins) below the radiographic baseline with the central ray parallel to it. Provided the central ray remains parallel to the baseline there is only a small change in the appearance of the radiograph as the centring point is changed. However, as can be seen from the previous illustrations (1020–1024), even a slight change in tube tilt can produce a marked change in the appearance of the radiograph. When the orbits are to be shown the dense petrous bone is projected below the inferior orbital margin but when the internal auditory meatuses are to be visualized they must be projected within the orbits.

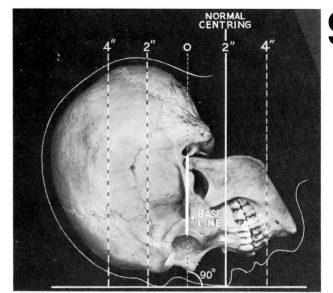

1025

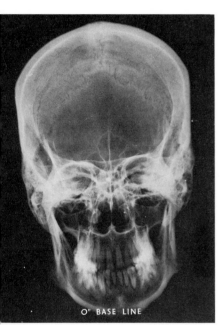

O" BASE LINE

1026

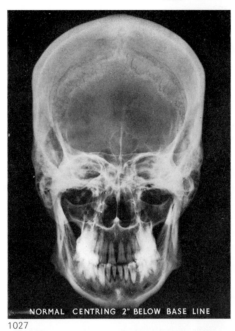

NORMAL CENTRING 2" BELOW BASE LINE

1027

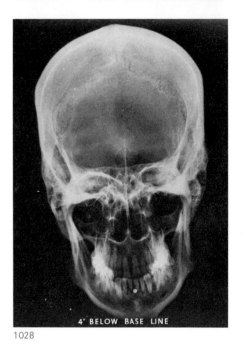

4" BELOW BASE LINE

1028

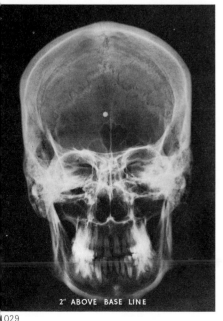

2" ABOVE BASE LINE

1029

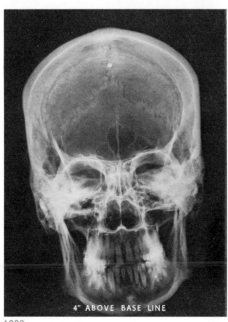

4" ABOVE BASE LINE

1030

Dry bone projections

The photograph (1035) of a dry skull shows a series of tube angles in the fronto-occipital position from which four projections (1031–1034) have been selected to show the varying radiographic appearances. Photograph (1036) shows a series of angles for the reverse position (occipito-frontal) and the equivalent four projections (1037–1040) for comparison.

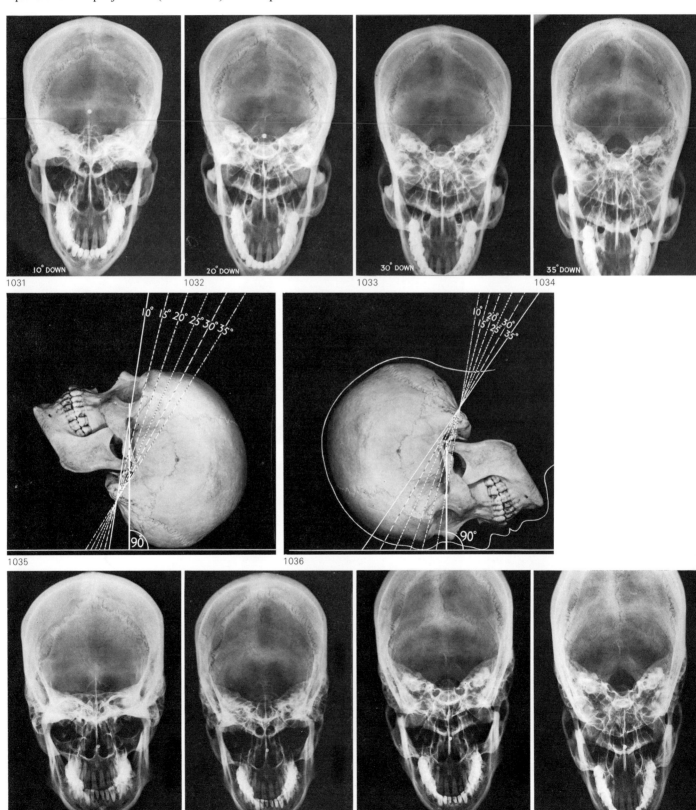

1031 1032 1033 1034

1035 1036

1037 1038 1039 1040

Dry bone projections

The photograph (1041) is of a dry skull in the occipito-mental position with varying tube angles and is followed by the comparable radiographs (1042,1045). With a 10° angle the petrous temporals are projected well below the antra (1043) and with greater angulation the zygomatic arches and inferior orbital margins are more clearly shown.

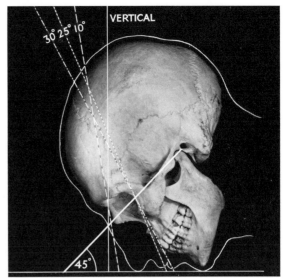

VERTICAL

30° 25° 10°

45°

1041

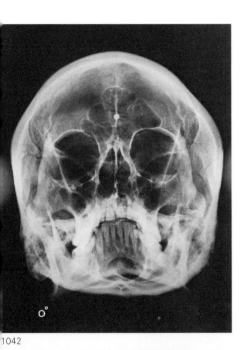

0°

1042

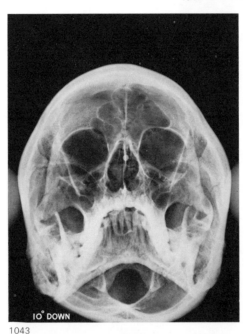

10° DOWN

1043

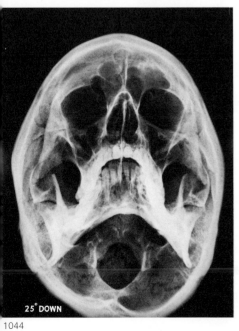

25° DOWN

1044

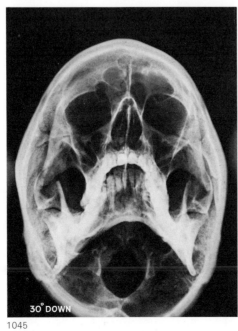

30° DOWN

1045

Photograph (1050) is a range of tube angulations for the demonstration of the jugular foramina (1051–1053).

Dry bone projections
Submento-vertical

The photograph (1049) is of a dry skull in the submento-vertical position with varying tube angles to show the base of the skull. The corresponding radiographs are (1046–1048).

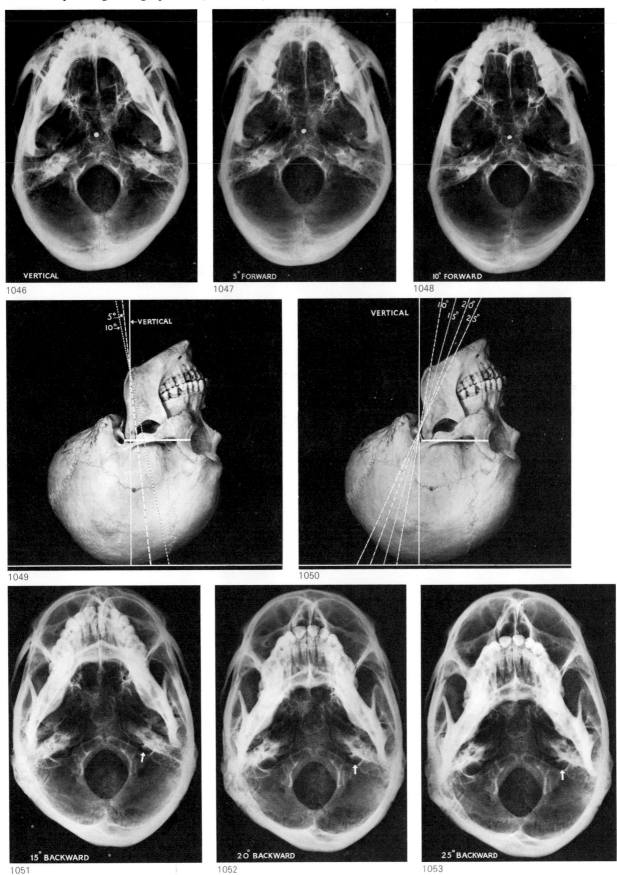

1046 VERTICAL
1047 5° FORWARD
1048 10° FORWARD

1049
1050

1051 15° BACKWARD
1052 20° BACKWARD
1053 25° BACKWARD

286

10

PARANASAL SINUSES

PARANASAL SINUSES

Anatomy

The maxillary antra, ethmoids, frontal and sphenoidal sinuses together form the paranasal or accessory nasal sinuses which are air filled cavities within the facial bones lined with mucous membrane and communicating with the upper respiratory tract. Being air-filled they appear on the radiographs as radiolucent shadows or dark areas. The paranasal sinuses are irregular in shape and vary in appearance from subject to subject, the maxillary antra are by far the most constant in appearance.

The positions of the paranasal sinuses are indicated on the dry skull in the frontal, lateral and supero-inferior views (1054, 1055, 1056)

Maxillary Antra

The maxillary sinuses or antra are two large cavities inside the maxillary bone one on either side of the nose. They extend from below the orbits to above the roof of the mouth and, posteriorly, to the pterygoid plate (1054, 1055)

The occipito-mental, occipito-frontal and lateral projections are used to show the maxillary antra.

Frontal Sinuses

The two frontal sinuses are in the frontal bone adjacent to the fronto-nasal articulation. They are divided by a thin asymmetrical septum so that the sinus on one side is larger than the other. However, in some subjects, the frontal sinuses are extremely small while in others they are very large spreading extensively above the roof of the orbit (1054, 1055) occasionally one or both may be absent.

The 15° occipito-frontal, occipito-mental, 20° submento-vertical and lateral projections may be used to show the frontal sinuses.

Ethmoidal Sinuses

The ethmoidal air cells are divided into three groups anterior, middle and posterior. The numerous ethmoidal air cells are situated deeply at the root of the nose and form the lateral walls of the superior nasal cavities. They vary in size, shape and number from as few as four to as many as 15 on each side (1054, 1055). On the lateral view (1055) the posterior margin can be seen to extend towards the sphenoidal sinus.

The 15° occipito-frontal, oblique right and left, submento-vertical, vertico-submental and lateral projections may be used to show the ethmoid sinuses.

Sphenoidal Sinuses

The sphenoidal sinuses lie immediately below the sella turcica which is in the centre of the floor of the cranium as shown in the saggital section of the dry skull (1055). They show considerable variation in size and shape and the intervening septum is asymetrical being deflected to one side.

On the lateral view the sphenoidal sinuses are superimposed and show as a dark, kidney-shaped image lying below the pituitary fossa. The submento-vertical view of the skull shows the sinuses lying side by side and projected over the pituitary fossa.

The lateral, submento-vertical, vertico-submental and 10° occipito-frontal projections can be used to show the sphenoidal sinuses.

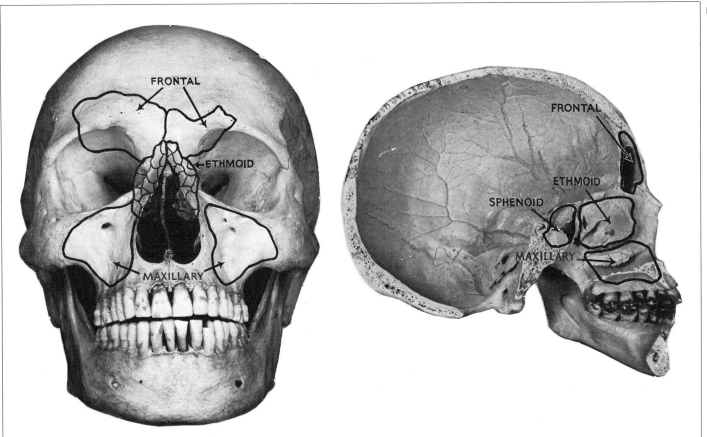

1054

1055

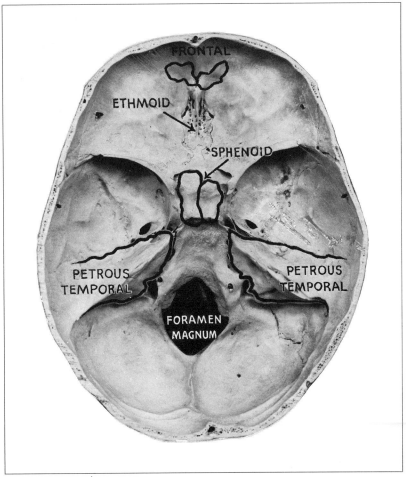

1056

Planes, lines and landmarks

A number of different projections are required to show all the paranasal sinuses. To obtain comparable views there must be accuracy in positioning the patient and aligning the X-ray beam. It is, therefore, essential to use fixed points and planes which are common to all subjects (1057, 1058, 1059).

These were previously described in Section 9 but the following planes are particularly important for paranasal sinuses.

Median-sagittal plane

The median-sagittal plane divides the head vertically into two halves and in the antero-posterior and postero-anterior projections must be at right angles to the film while in the lateral views it lies exactly parallel (1057).

Interorbital line

The interorbital or interpupillary line extends between the centre of the two orbits or pupils (1057) at right angles to the median-sagittal plane. In the lateral view this line must, wherever possible, be at right angles to the film. However if the head cannot be adjusted to bring the interorbital line perpendicular to the film then the tube should be angled so that the central ray is parallel to the interorbital line.

In this book the orbito-meatal line (OMBL) is used as the radiographic base line (1058) and not the anthropomorphic base line.

Orbito-meatal base line (OMBL)

The orbito-meatal base line extends from the outer canthus (OC) of the eye to the central point of the external auditory meatus (EAM) (1058). It is used as a base line to indicate the angle at which the head should be adjusted in relation to the film. The terms 'nose-chin' and 'nose-forehead' are approximate only since facial contours vary especially with length of nose and the prominence of forehead and chin. Without a check on the base line angle, projections will be inaccurate.

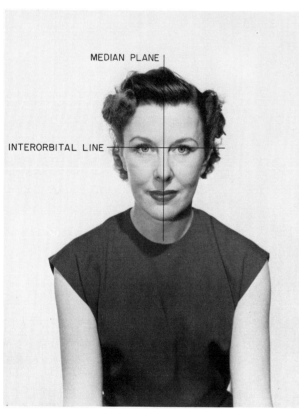

1057

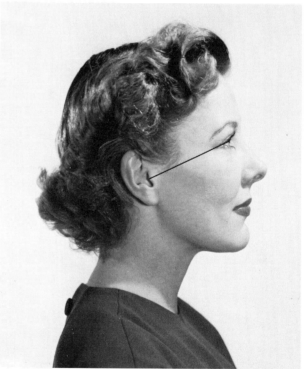

1058

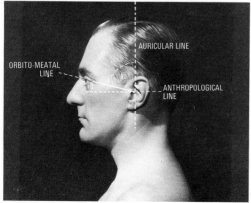

1059

Facial types

The three drawings of the head in the lateral view show the position of the orbito-meatal line or radiographic base line (RBL) which extends from the outer canthus of the eye to the centre of the external auditory meatus. Variations of the 'nose-forehead' line and the 'nose-chin' line are shown on each drawing. There is a great difference not only in the angle of intersection of these lines but also in their relationship to the radiographic base line.

In (1060) when the nose-forehead line is parallel to the film the radiographic base line is at a right angle and when the nose-chin line is parallel to the film then the radiographic base line is at 45°.

However in (1061) with a flat type of face there is an almost straight line from the forehead to the chin and to bring the radiographic base line to a right angle to the film the chin must be tucked in, thus bringing the nose away from the cassette.

On the other hand in (1062). In a subject with a prominent nose both the forehead and the chin will be away from the cassette when the radiographic base line is at right angles to the cassette.

10

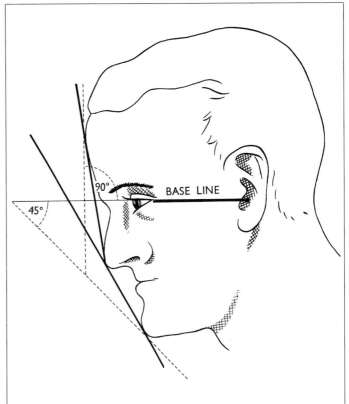

1061

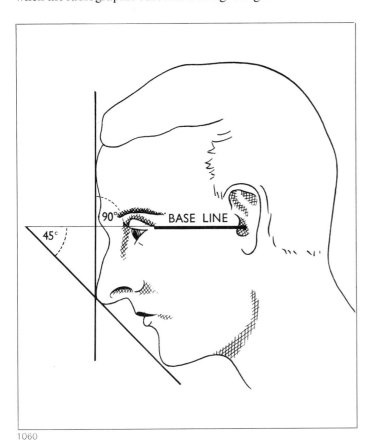

1060

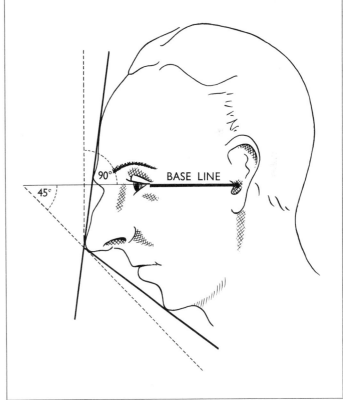

1062

Positioning terminology

It will be appreciated from the previous pages that the terms 'nose-chin' and 'nose-forehead' are imprecise being only a guide to the position of the head in relation to the film. For a correct description of the projection the base line to film angle must be specified.

(1) Occipito-Mental (O.M.)

or 'nose-chin' is the accepted term which indicates that the base line is at an angle of 45° to the film. The occipital region overshadows the mandible in this view.

(2) Occipito-Frontal (O.F.)

or 'nose-forehead' is the accepted term which indicates that the angle between base line and film is 90°. The occipital region overshadows the frontal bone in this view.

(3) Lateral

The median-sagittal plane is parallel and the inter-orbital line at right angles to the film.

(4) Submento-Vertical (S.M.V.)

is the accepted term which indicates that the vertex of the skull is toward the cassette and that the base line is as nearly parallel to the film as possible in the particular subject. The mandible overshadows the frontal bone in this view.

(5) Vertico-Submental

is the accepted term which indicates that the inferior margin of the symphysis menti is towards the cassette and overshadows the frontal bone. The base line-film angle is as nearly parallel to the film as possible in the particular subject.

(6) Oblique

is the accepted term which indicates that the head is rotated so that the median sagittal plane is 40° to the film and the radiographic base line is raised 30° by extending the head. In this position the superior orbital margin, zygomatic bone, mandible and the tip of the nose tend to lie in a plane parallel to the cassette. The central ray passes through the temporal region towards the orbit of each side in turn.

Technique
Erect or Horizontal

In the vast majority of cases the patient will be radiographed in the erect position which is by far the most convenient method for routine examinations. The illustrations are therefore shown in this way, but, clearly, whether the projections are taken with the patient erect or horizontal the tube/patient/film alignment will be similar and the radiographs need only be turned through 90°. When fluid levels are to be demonstrated a horizontal beam must be used and in the erect views the central ray must be kept horizontal. If the central ray is angled then a fluid level will become invisible. However with the patient horizontal the projections must be modified to include a horizontal ray view which is usually used for the lateral radiograph.

Number of Exposures

In the majority of subjects the sinuses can be shown in two or three views which usually includes the occipito-mental and lateral. However in special circumstances further projections will be needed particularly for the eithmoid sinuses.

Right and Left

Important—A right or left marker must be included on every film; 0·5 cm ($\frac{1}{4}$ in) letters are recommended.

Size of Film

Small films especially 13×18 cm ($6\frac{1}{2} \times 8\frac{1}{2}$ ins) are preferred, larger films being wasteful.

Arrangement in text

In the text each position is described and illustrated with photographs, radiographs and line drawings, the position of the sinuses being indicated on the radiographs. The six positions of the head together with the 12 variations of tube position are tabulated and the 12 resulting radiographs are shown on pages 308–310. The more frequently used projections are indicated as (Basic).

Sinus Protractor

The sinus protractor is designed for use on a flat surface and is large enough for the indicating arm to correspond with the base line of the subject. The range of the arc is restricted, for convenience, to the range of angles required for sinus technique.

Equipment

With a modern skull unit paranasal sinus examinations are greatly simplified as they provide for comfortable positioning and immobilization of the patient as well as accurate centring and positioning of the tube. With this equipment the tube although freely movable in several directions always remains centred to the centre of the Potter-Bucky diaphragm and is ideal for positioning the patient in the erect position.

However, even with a universal or erect Bucky, it is still possible to obtain accurate projections by careful attention to detail. In the majority of accident and emergency departments examinations will be done on a vertical Bucky when the patient is erect or on an ordinary Bucky table when the patient is horizontal.

Automatic selection of exposure is available on some modern equipment.

Grid

Sinus radiography is usually carried out using a Potter-Bucky diaphragm.

Localizing cone

It is essential to use a localizing cone with a small aperture, excluding all structures except those immediately adjacent to the sinuses being radiographed, thereby reducing scatter to a minimum. The use of a long cone touching the head simplifies tube centring.

The Head-clamp

The head can be immobilized by an adjustable head clamp and is an asset in some patients but may be difficult to manipulate.

The head is placed in position with the head-clamp central and projecting far enough to grasp the head at the correct angle. The patient should be warned that the clamp is being tightened sufficiently to only steady the head and there should be no discomfort from extreme pressure. The clamp should be tightened with the right hand, while the left hand on one side of the head-piece checks the pressure applied to the head. When rotation of the head is required with the clamp applied, the central thumbscrew is loosened sufficiently to allow the clamp to be moved under pressure. With a hand on each side of the head-piece the head is firmly rotated to the required angle, as indicated by the protractor, and the thumb-screw then tightened to prevent further movement.

The moving parts should be kept well lubricated, and the head-clamp should be mounted on a fixed part of the stand to enable the Potter-Bucky diaphragm and cassette tray to be moved independently of the positioned and immobilized patient.

Patient

Before the examination all extraneous opacities must be removed including artificial dentures, spectacles, hearing aid, ear-rings, hair clips and hair pins, neck ornaments and collar studs.

Important—The set must be in the correct position, accessory equipment near at hand, and the exposure factors selected before positioning the patient for sinus views. Sinus view positions are often difficult to maintain and the patient must be kept in the required position for the minimum amount of time.

Exposure factors

The exposure factors quoted in this section apply to an adult subject having average head measurements.

10

293

Occipito-Mental (basic)
Maxillary and Frontal sinuses

With the patient erect, facing the film and the median sagittal plane at right angles to the cassette, the chin is raised to bring the radiographic base line to 45° to the film.

Using a skull unit the Bucky platform is centred to the lower orbital margin and, with the patient immobilized, the exposure can be made.

However, with a vertical Bucky, before fully positioning the patient, the cassette must be central in the Bucky tray, locked in position, and centred to the lower orbital margin. Then the X-ray tube is centred to the cassette. The patient's head should be immobilized by using a head clamp (1063) or a Bucky band.

Although this is often called the nose chin projection it should be noted that it is uncommon for both the nose and chin to make contact with the table-top when the radiographic base-line is at 45° to it.

Ideally this projection should be done with the mouth open to show the sphenoidal sinus.

■ Centre above the occipital protuberance, at the level of the lower and anterior margin of the orbits (1063, 1064, 1065)

The mid-line section of the dry skull (1065) shows how the petrous temporals are projected below the maxillae to demonstrate the maxillary and frontal sinuses (1064). The radiograph is not acceptable when parts of the maxillary sinuses are obscured by the petrous temporals (1066). To produce an acceptable radiograph either there must be further extension of the head to raise the chin or caudal angulation of the tube to project the petrous temporals below the antra as was shown in the series of dry skull projections in Section 9 p. 285.

O–M

kVp	mAS	FFD	Film ILFORD	Screens ILFORD	Grid
75	50	100 cm (40″)	RAPID R	Standard	Grid

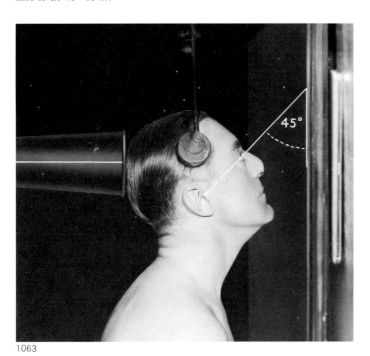

1063

1065

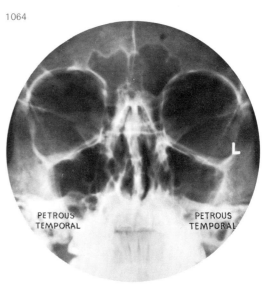

1064

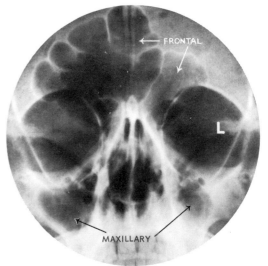

1066

Occipito-Frontal
Maxillary, Ethmoidal and Sphenoidal sinuses

With the patient erect and the median sagittal plane at right angles to the cassette the head is flexed to bring the radiographic base-line perpendicular to the film.

Using a skull unit the Bucky platform is centred to the nasion and, with the patient immobilized the exposure can be made.

However, with a vertical Bucky, before fully positioning the patient, the cassette must be central in the Bucky, locked in position and centred to the Nasion and the X-ray tube must be centred to the cassette. The patient's head should be immobilized either by using a head clamp (1067) or a Bucky band.

Slight downward inclination of the forehead raises the posterior parts of the base of the skull so that the petrous temporals are projected through the orbits. The maxillary and ethmoid sinuses are seen below the base of the skull.

■ Centre 4 cm (1½ ins) below the occipital protuberance through the nape of the neck at the level of the nasion (1067, 1068, 1069)

kVp	mAS	FFD	Film ILFORD	Screens ILFORD	Grid
75	40	100 cm (40")	RAPID R	Standard	Grid

The dry skull (1068) shows how the maxillary antra are projected below the base of the skull with the frontal sinuses close to the film.

In the resulting radiograph (1069) the maxillary antra are shown beneath the dense skull base with the anterior ethmoidal cells above them and the sphenoidal sinuses adjacent to the mid-line. The lower parts of the frontal sinuses are obscured in this projection and the petrous temporal bones are projected through the orbits. The dorsum sellae and the clinoid processes are seen above the sphenoidal sinus.

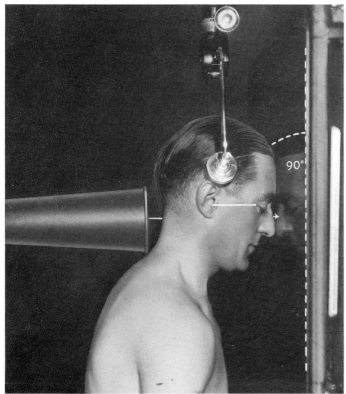

1067

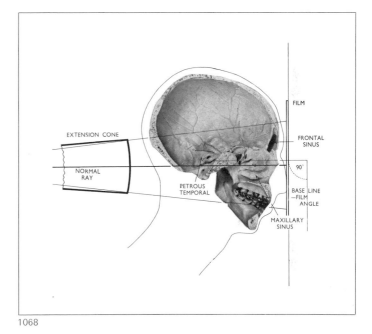

1068

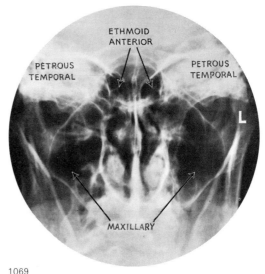

1069

15° Occipito-Frontal (basic)
Frontal and Ethmoidal sinuses

Using a vertical Bucky the patient is in the same position as for the previous projection with the radiographic base-line at right angles to the film. There is only a variation in tube centring and angulation for this projection. With a 15° caudal angulation, the tube is centred above the external occipital protuberance and to the nasion. The petrous temporal bones are now projected over the lower third of the orbits but overshadow the upper parts of the maxillary antra, giving a clear view of the frontal and ethmoidal air cells without undue distortion because the frontal region is close to the film and parallel with it.

To obtain the same projection with a skull unit the radiographic base-line is raised 15° to the horizontal by slight extension of the neck, and the Bucky platform is tilted to bring it perpendicular to the base line, the tube remains horizontal. Because a horizontal ray is used this manoeuvre is advantageous as it would clearly demonstrate a fluid level.

■ Centre 2 cm (1 in) above the external occipital protuberance and to the naison

With the vertical Bucky the tube is angled 15° towards the feet; with the skull unit the tube remains horizontal and the Bucky platform is angled 15°.

When using a vertical Bucky the film is displaced toward the feet to bring the central ray to the centre of the cassette.

The dry skull (1072) shows how the petrous temporals are projected through the lower thirds of the orbits. The frontal and anterior ethmoidal sinuses are undistorted and projected above the base of the skull. This is also shown in a series of dry skull projections in Section 9 Page 282 and should be compared with the resulting radiograph (1071) and the radiograph of the previous projection (1067) and (1071, 1073)

15° OF

kVp	mAS	FFD	Film ILFORD	Screens ILFORD	Grid
75	40	100 cm (40″)	RAPID R	Standard	Grid

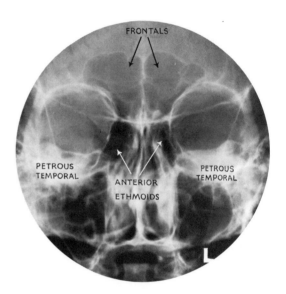

1071

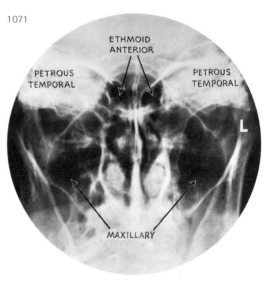

1073

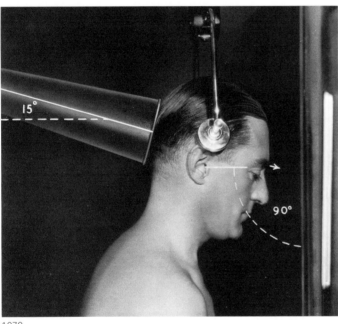

1070

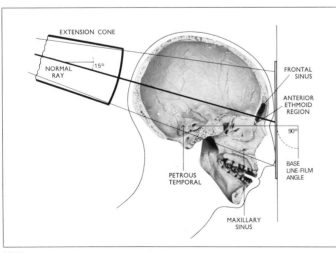

1072

Lateral (basic)—all sinuses

With the patient erect the head is turned from the occipitomental into the lateral position with the side of the head in contact with the Bucky platform. The median sagittal plane must be parallel and the interorbital line at right angles to the film. When the head clamp is used it is applied to the central occipital region posteriorly and above the level of the frontal sinuses anteriorly.

■ Centre 2 cm (1 in) posterior to the outer canthus of the eye along the radiographic base-line (1074, 1075, 1076)

<table>
<tr><th colspan="7">Lateral</th></tr>
<tr><th>kVp</th><th>mAS</th><th>FFD</th><th>Film
ILFORD</th><th>Screens
ILFORD</th><th>Grid</th></tr>
<tr><td>65</td><td>20</td><td>100 cm
(40″)</td><td>RAPID
R</td><td>Standard</td><td>Grid</td></tr>
</table>

In subjects where the correct adjustment of the interorbital line cannot be made the tube is angled to project the central ray parallel to the interorbital line.

In the lateral (basic) projection the right and left sinuses are superimposed.

For a localized projection of the *sphenoidal sinuses* the centring point is adjusted accordingly.

■ Centre 2 cm (1 in) in front of and 2 cm (1 in) above the external auditory meatus, through the squamous portion of the temporal bone, using a small localizing cone (1076(b), 1077)

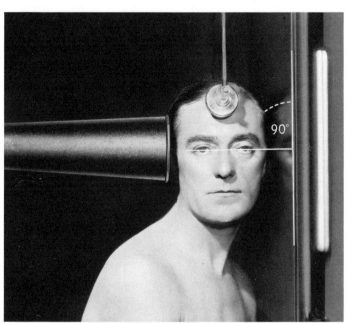

1074

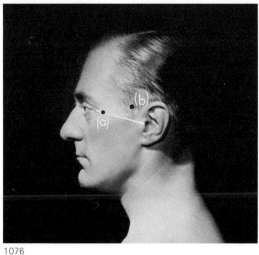

1076

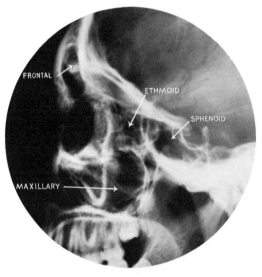

1075

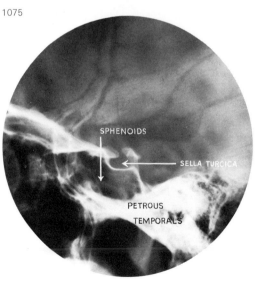

1077

Oblique—Right and left (basic)
Posterior ethmoidal sinuses and Optic foramina

With the patient erect in the nose forehead position and the median sagittal plane at right angles to the film, the chin is raised to bring the radiographic baseline to 30° above the horizontal. The head is then rotated so that the median sagittal plane is 40° to the film. The right and left sides are examined in turn. In this position the side of the face being examined has the nose, eyebrow, zygomatic bone and chin in contact with the Bucky platform.

■ Centre 6 cm (2½ ins) above and behind the tube side external auditory meatus. The central ray passes directly through the orbit nearest to the film (1078, 1079, 1080, 1081)

Oblique					
kVp	mAS	FFD	Film ILFORD	Screens ILFORD	Grid
70	20	100 cm (40")	RAPID R	Standard	Grid

Note—the radiographs show the posterior ethmoidal cells overshadowing the lower part of the orbit and adjacent structures. The position of the optic foramina in relation to the lateral wall of the orbit is used to compare the projections on the two sides (1080, 1081)

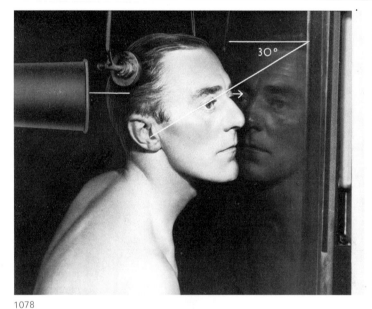

1078

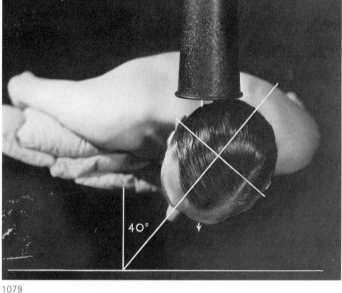

1079

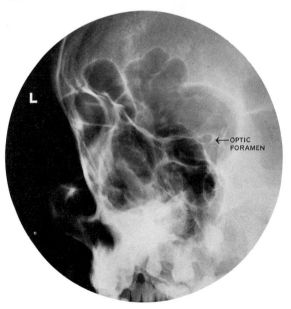

1080

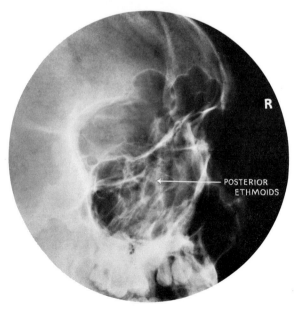

1081

Submento-Vertical (basic)
Sphenoidal and Posterior Ethmoidal sinuses

With the patient erect, facing the tube and the sinus stool approximately 30 cm (12 ins) from the Bucky platform the neck is extended and the back arched to bring the vertex of the skull in contact with the Bucky platform. In the ideal position the baseline and film are parallel (1082). However, tube angulation should be used, if the subject is unable to extend the neck (1083). The stool must be locked in position and the patient's feet must be firmly on the floor to prevent any movement of the stool.

■ With the tube angled 5° and the central ray 95° to the radiographic baseline, centre in the mid-line between the angles of the mandible (1082).

When considerable tube angulation is used the film is displaced towards the head accordingly.

Note—Of the three positions (1082, 1110, 1113) for the sphenoidal sinuses, (1082) is the most commonly employed.

The mid-line section of the dry skull (1083) shows how the sphenoidal and posterior and ethmoidal cells are projected clear of the mandible to overshadow the vertex of the skull. Reference should also be made to the series of dry skull projections Section 9. Page 286.

Radiograph (1084) shows the sphenoidal sinuses either side of the mid-line, (posteriorly) being separated from the foramen magnum by the shadow of the basi-occiput. The posterior ethmoidal cells lie anteriorly within the curve of the mandible which obscures the anterior ethmoid cells.

SMV

kVp	mAS	FFD	Film ILFORD	Screens ILFORD	Grid
85	50	100 cm (40″)	RAPID R	Standard	Grid

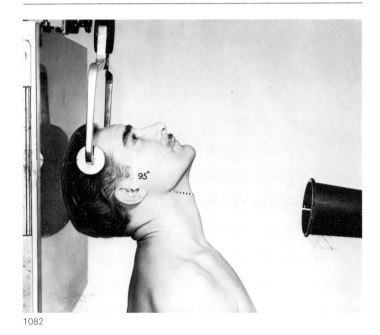

1082

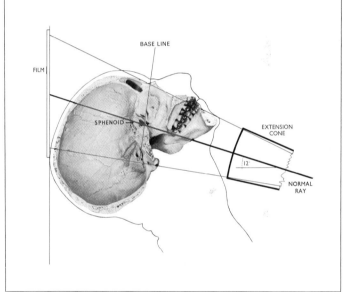

1083

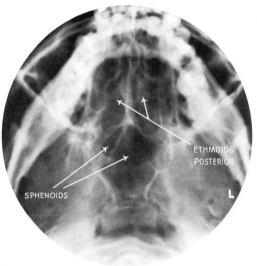

1084

Occipito-Mental
Fluid levels—erect

To confirm the presence of fluid in the maxillary and frontal sinuses an additional projection is required. From the occipito-mental position the median sagittal plane is tilted 30° to the vertical; the head clamps are adjusted to maintain the correct position (1085). The median sagittal plane should remain at right angles to the film keeping the radiographic baseline raised 45° to the horizontal.

■ Centre in the mid-line mid way between the levels of the two lower orbital margins.

When the head is tilted the sinuses must be kept within the limits of the X-ray beam using a small cone (1086).

Two radiographs of the same subject show the erect occipito-mental position (1087) and the laterally flexed occipito-mental position (1088) with fluid in both maxillary antra. Both right and left laterally flexed projections of the sinuses may be taken.

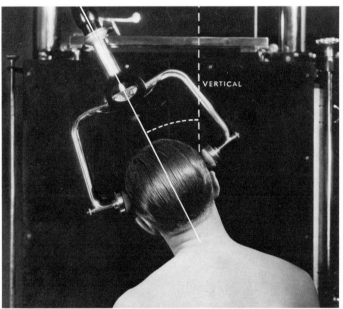

1085

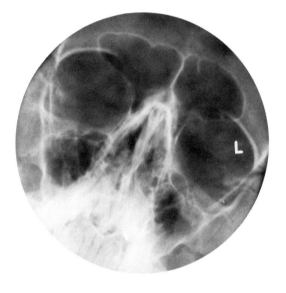

1086

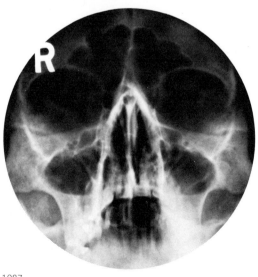

1087

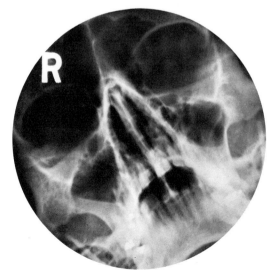

1088

Fluid levels—Horizontal ray

With the patient horizontal fluid levels can also be shown in the frontal projection. The patient must be half prone with the head in the lateral position using a horizontal ray (1089) and a projection equivalent to the occipito-mental position (1063) The film is supported vertically against the face and at right angles to the median sagittal plane. Fluid levels in the frontal sinuses are indicated by arrows on the radiographs (1090) and (1092) taken with a horizontal ray and the patient horizontal, whereas (1091) is taken with a horizontal ray and the patient erect, (1091) and (1092) being radiographs of the same patient.

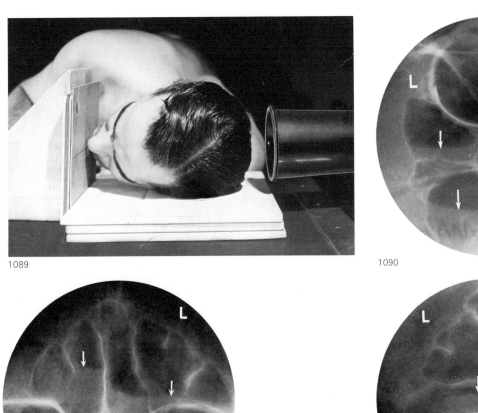

1089

1090

1091

1092

20° Submento-Vertical Anterior ethmoidal sinuses

With the patient in position as for the submento-vertical (basic) view (1082) tube angulation is increased by 15–25° to show the anterior ethmoidal sinuses (1094)

■ Centre within the anterior curve of the mandible and toward the frontal sinuses with the tube angled 20°–30° cephalad (1093, 1094)

Radiograph (1095) shows a frontal view and (1096) a plan projection of the anterior ethmoidal sinuses and part of the frontal sinus.

Dry Skull projections

A photograph of a dry skull (1097) indicates the three tube angles used for the three radiographs (1098, 1099, 1100).

The sphenoidal and ethmoidal sinuses are shown on all three radiographs. 30° angulation (1100) gives the best view of the anterior parts of the sphenoidal sinus and part of the frontal sinus.

All show the ethmoidal sinuses but to the greatest extent, perhaps, with the 30° angulation (1160) which depicts the sinus area within the maximum width between the two sides of the mandible.

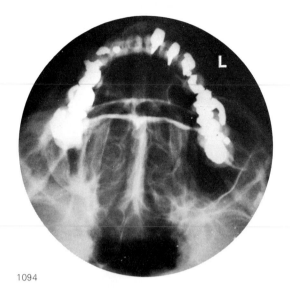

1094

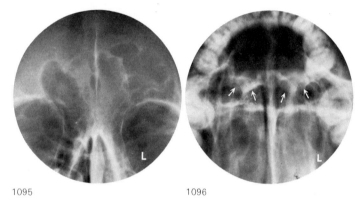

1095   1096

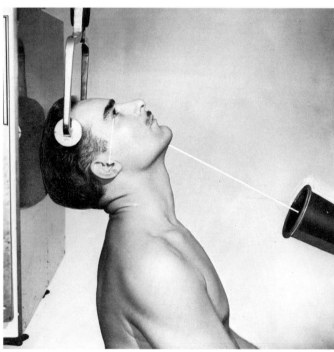

1093

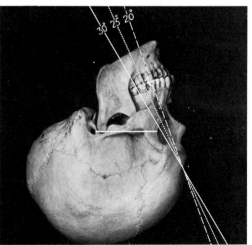

1097

Abnormalities

Six radiographs of one subject show the varying appearances in the different positions and projections.

(1101) in the prone position, occipito-mental; the left antrum is opaque.

(1102) in the erect position, occipito-mental; the frontal sinus has a fluid level (basic).

(1103) in the horizontal position, occipito-mental (1089), the frontal sinus again shows the fluid level.

(1104) in the prone position, 30° occipito-frontal.

(1105) 20° submento-vertical (1093), and

(1106) erect lateral (basic).

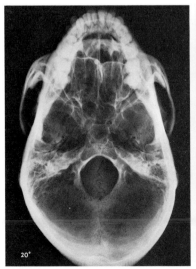

PRONE
1101

ERECT
1102

HORIZONTAL
1103

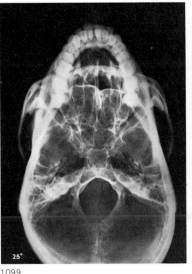

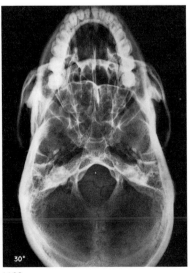

PRONE
1104

ERECT
1105

ERECT
1106

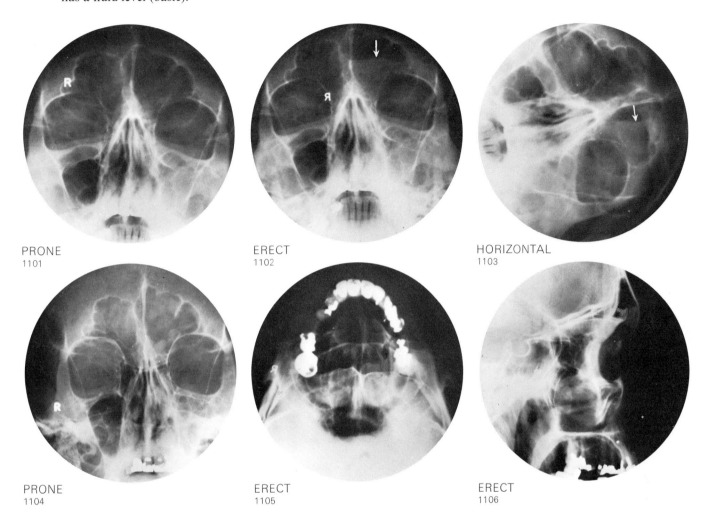

20°
1098

25°
1099

30°
1100

303

Additional Views

10° Occipito-Frontal
Maxillary, Ethmoidal and Sphenoidal sinuses

With the patient erect in a position similar to the 15° occipito-frontal (basic) projection (1067) there is only a variation in tube centring.

■ Centre in the midline 5 cm (2 ins) below the occipital protuberance with the tube angled 10° cephalad. The central ray is directed through the sella turcica and sphenoidal sinuses to the nasion. The position of the pituitary fossa is deduced from the lateral aspect of the head. Centre to the centre of the film (1107, 1008, 1109)

The illustration of the dry skull in sagittal section (1108) shows how the sphenoidal sinuses are projected to overshadow the frontal bone and should be compared with (1109).

If the radiograph taken with this projection (1109) is compared with the film taken with the occipito-frontal projection (1069) the sphenoidal sinuses are shown to better advantage using the 10° upward tube angulation.

				10° O–F		
kVp	mAS	FFD	Film ILFORD	Screens ILFORD	Grid
70	40	100 cm (40″)	RAPID R	Standard	Grid

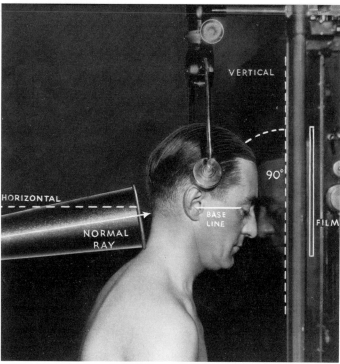

1107

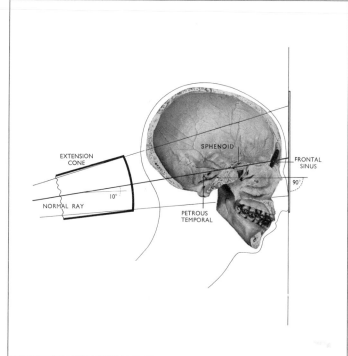

1108

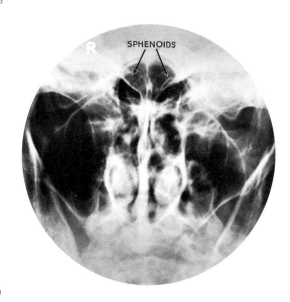

1109

Vertico-Mental—Open mouth
Sphenoidal sinuses

With the patient erect and in a position similar to the occipito-mental (basic) projection (1063) there is only a variation in tube centring and the radiograph is taken with the mouth open. As with the occipito-mental (basic) position the radiographic base line is raised 45° to the horizontal.

■ Centre in the midline with the tube angled approximately 70° to the radiographic base line or 25° caudad. The central ray passes through the vertex of the skull toward the open mouth through a point 2 cm (1 in) above and in front of the external auditory meatus and also 2 cm (1 in) anterior to the external auditory meatus along the radiographic base line to emerge at the centre of the open mouth. The film must be displaced downward to coincide with the direction of the axial ray (1110, 1111, 1112)

The illustration of the dry skull in sagittal section diagram (1111) shows how the shadow of the sphenoidal sinuses are projected through the open mouth.

The sphenoidal sinuses can also be shown in the submento-vertical (basic) (1082) or vertico-submental projection (1113).

Vertico-Mental

kVp	mAS	FFD	Film ILFORD	Screens ILFORD	Grid
70	30	100 cm (40")	RAPID R	Standard	Grid

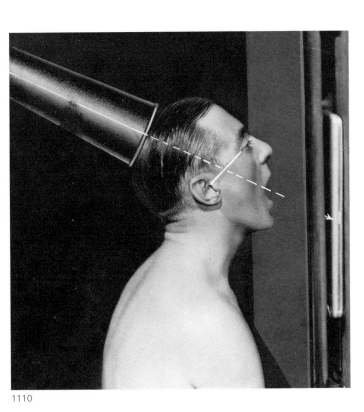

1110

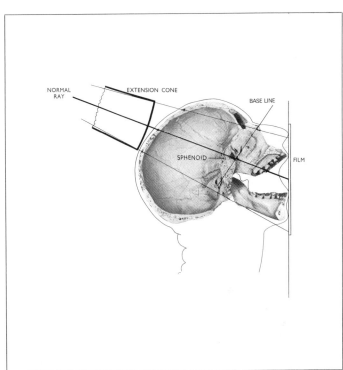

1111

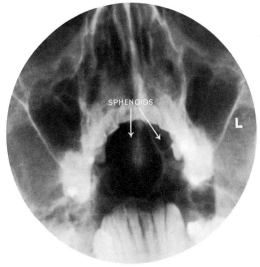

1112

Vertico-Submental
Sphenoidal and Posterior Ethmoidal sinuses

This position is particularly suitable for patients with a long and mobile neck but difficult for the short necked, high shouldered subject.

With the patient erect and facing the film, the neck is extended to bring the inferior border of the symphysis menti into contact with the film support. The angle made by the radiographic baseline with the film should be more than 40° to avoid elongation of the image and undue downward displacement of the cassette.

■ Centre in the midline through the vertex of the skull with the tube angled 95° to the radiographic base line with which it intersects approximately 2 cm (1 in) in front of the external auditory meatus. The tube angle is approximately 30°–40° to the horizontal depending upon how far the head is extended.

The film is displaced toward the feet to allow for the tube angulation (1113, 1114, 1115).

Vertico-Submental					
kVp	mAS	FFD	Film ILFORD	Screens ILFORD	Grid
80	50	100 cm (40″)	RAPID R	Standard	Grid

The dry skull diagram (1114) shows how the sphenoidal and posterior ethmoidal sinuses are projected between the mandibular rami; this being the reverse of the sub-mento vertical projection (1082).

The resulting film (1115) is similar to (1084). Because the mandible is closer to the film its margins are well defined but the gap between the rami is smaller which may obscure the ethmoidal cells particularly if there is insufficient extension of the head or angulation of the tube.

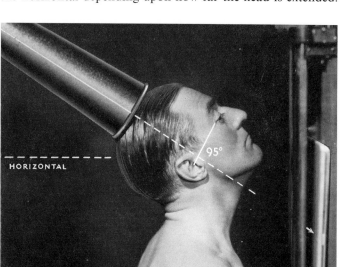

1113

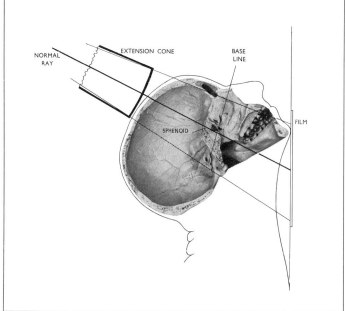

1114

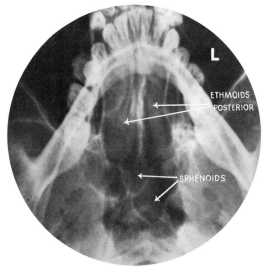

1115

Contrast Studies
Opaque Injections

In the past contrast studies of the paranasal sinuses were performed. Direct injection into the sinuses or the indirect replacement method were used especially to show the floor of the antra.

Direct method

Direct injection of a contrast medium into the sinuses was used mainly for the maxillary antra. Lateral projections were performed with separate injections to avoid superimposition of the opposite side (1116). A frontal view of both antra filled with a contrast medium is shown in (1117).

Indirect (replacement) method

A contrast medium can also be made to enter the paranasal sinuses by indirect or replacement method and is mainly of historical interest (1118).

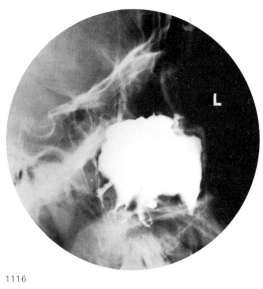

1116

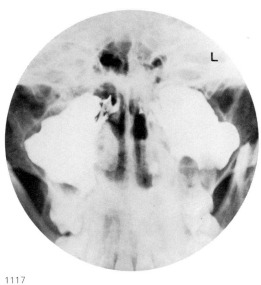

1117

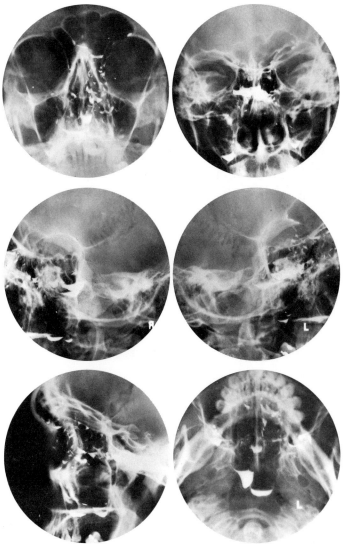

1118

Opaque injections

Detailed views of the sinuses are obtained using modern tomographic equipment and together with computed tomography has completely displaced contrast studies of the paranasal sinuses (1119).

Computed tomography of paranasal sinuses (1119). Black arrow indicate ethmoidal sinuses, S—Sphenoidal sinuses, A—Maxillary antra, P—Polyps and white arrows indicate mucosal thickening in antrum.

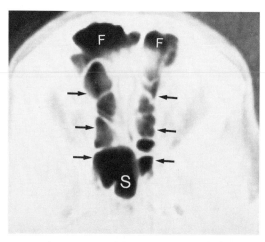

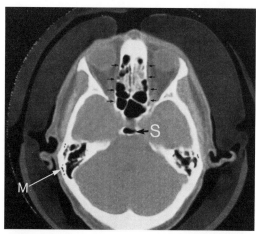

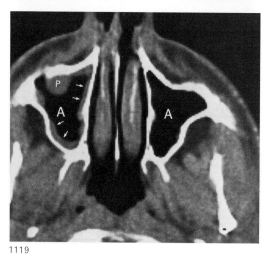

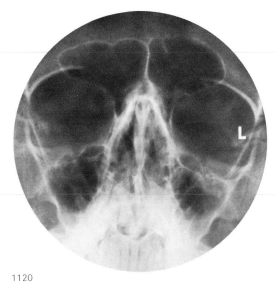

1120

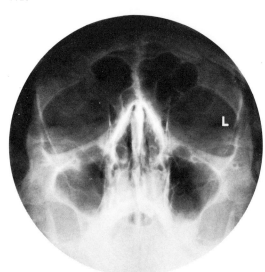

1121

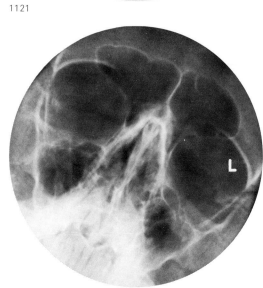

1119

1122

Number	Position	Angle to Film	Centring	Tube Angle	Sinuses Shown
1120	Occipito-Mental (basic)	Base Line 45°	Above occipital protuberance to lower margin orbits	Nil	Frontal Maxillary
1121	10° Occipito-Mental	Base Line 45°	Above occipital protuberance to lower margin orbits	10° down	Maxillary Frontal
1122	Occipito-Mental (fluid levels-erect)	Base Line 45°	Above occipital protuberance to lower margin orbits	Nil or 10° down	Maxillary Frontal for fluid levels
1123	Occipito-Frontal	Base Line 90°	4 cm (1½") below occipital protuberance to antra	Nil	Maxillary Anterior Ethmoidal
1124	10° Occipito-Frontal	Base Line 90°	5 cm (2") below occipital protuberance to nasion	10° up	Maxillary Sphenoidal
1125	15° Occipito-Frontal (basic)	Base Line 90°	Above occipital protuberance to nasion	15° down	Frontal Anterior Ethmoidal
1126	Lateral (basic)	Interorbital Line 90°	2 cm (1") from eye along radiographic Base Line	Nil	All Sinuses
1127	Lateral (localized)	Interorbital Line 90°	2 cm (1") in front of and above EAM	Nil	Sphenoidal
1128	Submento-Vertical (basic)	Base Line parallel to film	In midline between angles of jaw	5° forward 95° to Base Line	Sphenoidal Posterior Ethmoidal
1129	20° Submento-vertical	Base Line parallel to film	Within anterior curve of mandible	20° to 30° forward	Anterior ethmoidal Posterior frontal
1130	Vertico-Submental	Base Line 30° to 40°	Vertex	95° to Base Line	Sphenoidal Posterior Ethmoidal
1131	Vertico-Mental	Base Line 45°	Vertex to open mouth	70° approximate	Sphenoidal
1132	Oblique 40° (R and L)	Base Line 30°	6 cm (2½) above and behind EAM on tube side	Nil	Posterior Ethmoidal
1133	(Basic)	Base Line 30°	6 cm (2½") above and behind EAM on tube side	Optic Foramina	

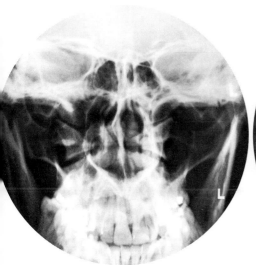

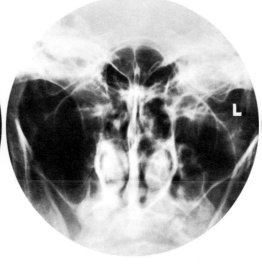

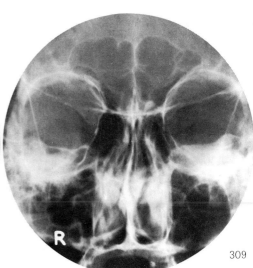

1123

1125

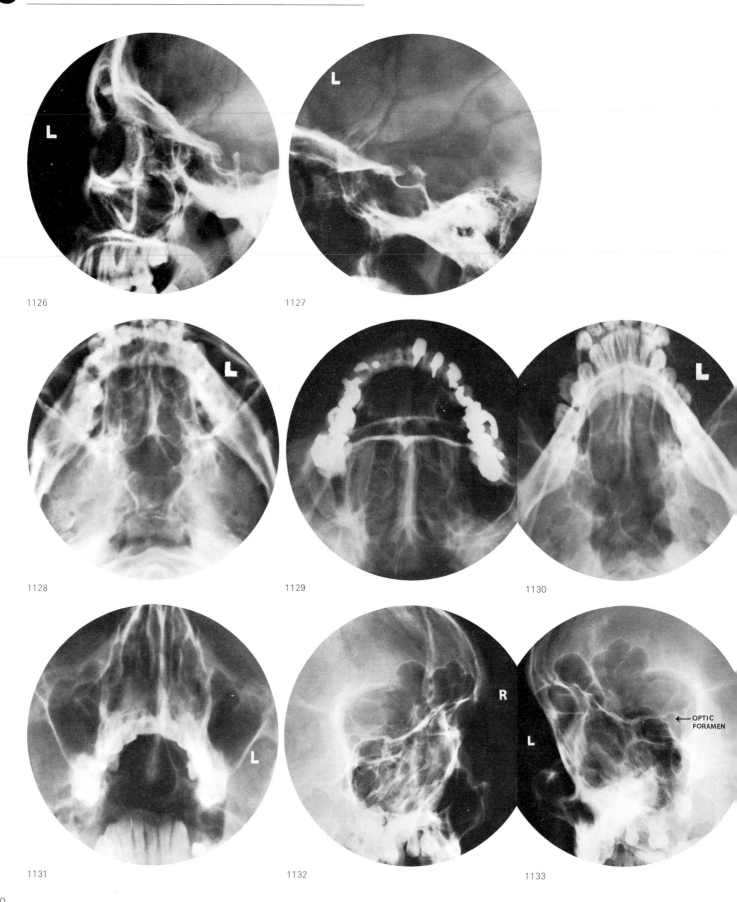

1126

1127

1128

1129

1130

1131

1132

1133

OPTIC FORAMEN

11 SECTION 11

MANDIBLE

The photograph of the dry bone (1134) shows the important radiographic features in the examination of the mandible, namely the symphysis menti uniting the two halves in the anterior midline of the lower jaw, the body extending horizontally backward on each side from the symphysis menti to the ramus, supporting the lower teeth along its upper alveolar margin and the angle formed by the junction between the horizontal and the almost vertical portion of the ramus. The ramus extends upward from the angle having two separate processes superiorly, the condylar process posteriorly, with its smooth superior surface articulating with the temporal bone to form the temporo-mandibular joint, and the coronoid process anteriorly which moves under the zygomatic arch. The two processes are separated by the mandibular notch (1134).

On the true lateral radiograph the two halves of the mandible are superimposed on one another, and on the frontal view the upper cervical vertebrae overshadow the symphysis menti and the adjacent body of the mandible. To show each part of the body various oblique projections are needed, either the X-ray tube may be angled toward the mandible (1135) or the head may be angled in relation to the tube (1136).

The projection required will also depend upon the type of injury and the build of the patient. Patients with a short neck or a relatively immobile cervical spine are difficult to position.

Wherever possible, projections for the mandible should be taken with the patient sitting rather than horizontal, and a moving Bucky should be used for the postero-anterior views although no grid is required for the oblique projections. Where a patient can only be radiographed in the horizontal position the projections for the mandible must be done supine and the frontal view will be an antero-posterior projection, because in the prone position there will be pressure on the painful mandible.

For detailed views of the teeth intra-oral projections are required but to overcome the anatomical curve of the mandible either a series of projections will be needed or ortho-pantomography (see Section 19).

To take the series of radiographs to show the whole of the mandible the head must be rotated to follow the curve of the jaw so that each part of the bone in turn is parallel to the film (1138,1139), the tube being centred to avoid overshadowing by the cervical vertebrae or the opposite side of the mandible. For a complete examination several of the following projections may be needed:

(1140) The ramus, angle and adjacent body.
(1143) The body to the canine socket.
(1154) Postero-anterior general.
(1158) Postero-anterior oblique, to show the symphysis menti and adjacent body.
(1162) Infero-superior general.
(1167) Infero-superior localized occlusal projections.
(1165) Super-inferior, described as Collar Radiography.

The intra-oral and occlusal projections are done on non-screen film; for all other views intensifying screens are required. It is advisable to use a grid or Potter-Bucky for the frontal and submento-vertical projections.

The general extra-oral projections of the mandible are taken to show both displacement fractures and pathological conditions. When, for various reasons it is impossible to place a small film inside the mouth, when the scope of intra-oral film is insufficient to investigate the condition or when confirmation of the relative position of the lesion or displacement is required, the lateral projection of the mandible can be taken with the jaw on a cassette as in (1135) or by using an angle board with the jaw tilted as in (1136). In both positions the right and left sides are examined separately.

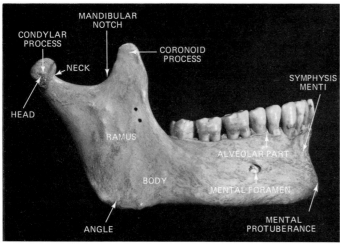

1134

The adjustable angle board (1137) helps in examining the mandible but a sandbag or a triangular non-opaque block can also be used to support the head and cassette in the oblique position.

The adjustable angle board (1137) is hinged and has an adjustable slide which allows a variation in angle up to 25°. When a greater angle is necessary a small block or sandbag is placed under the open end of the angle-board. It also has an adjustable right angle support which allows a small cassette to be placed in the correct position in relation to the mandible which rests on it, taking films of the right and left sides in turn. Because of the slope of the cassette the film marker must be firmly attached.

To show the body and ramus of the mandible from the symphysis menti to the angle and its adjacent ramus, several projections are required. With the median plane of the skull parallel to the film the angle of the mandible and the ramus are shown but the symphysis menti and adjacent border of the body

of the mandible are foreshortened (1139). However, when the face is rotated to bring the body of the mandible against the cassette the symphysis menti and adjacent body is shown to greater advantage (1138). Similar projections can of course be obtained by using the angle board with a perpendicular central ray (1136).

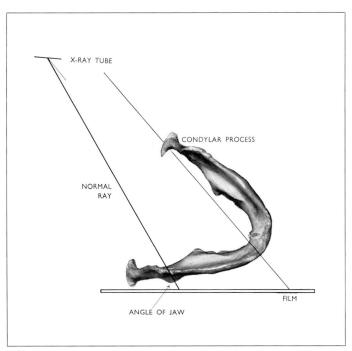

1137

1135

1136

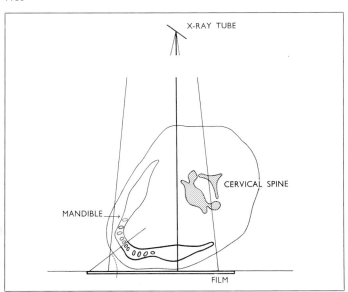

1138

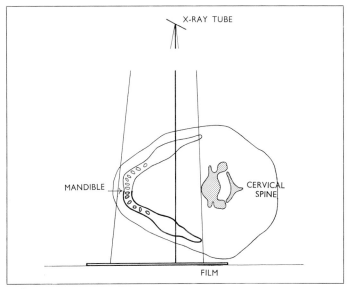

1139

11 Mandible

Ramus, Angle and Adjacent body

1 Variable Angle-board
With the variable angle board at 25° the perpendicular cassette support is adjusted for right and left sides as appropriate. The patient lies half prone (1140) and the head is positioned over the open end of the angle board to bring the median plane of the head parallel and the inter-orbital line perpendicular to the cassette as for a lateral (basic) projection of the skull. The lower border of the mandible should be parallel to and 2 cm (1 in) above the edge of the cassette. A small forward tilt of the chin avoids superimposition of the cervical vertebrae on the ramus.
■ Centre with the tube straight, 5 cm (2 ins) below the angle of the jaw remote from the film (1140, 1141).

2 Head horizontal and Tube angled
With patient half prone and the raised shoulder supported on sandbags, the head is placed in the lateral position on the cassette. For convenience the cassette is raised on a shallow block (1142). Alternatively this projection can be done with the patient seated.
■ With the tube angled 25° toward the head, centre 5 cm (2 ins) below the angle of the jaw remote from the film (1142).

This position gives a satisfactory view of one side of the mandible, the opposite side being projected to a higher level (1141), for an adequate view of the opposite side the patient must be repositioned to obtain a similar radiograph.

To avoid the shadow of the hyoid bone being over the angle of the mandible, the angle of the variable angle board should be reduced to 15°; the tube being angled 10° toward the jaw and centred over the angle of the jaw.

Mandible Head from Tube Angled

kVp	mAS	FFD	Film ILFORD	Screens ILFORD	Grid
60	10	100 cm (40″)	RAPID R	Standard	—

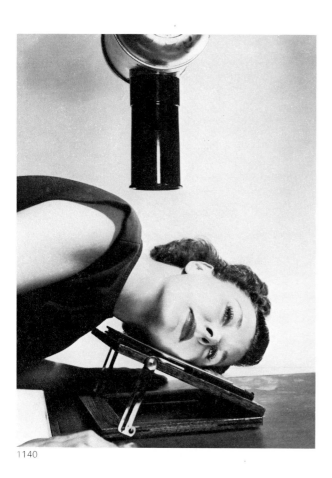

1140

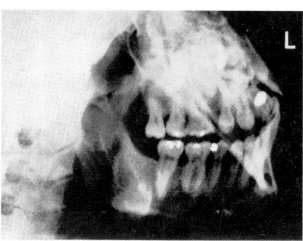

1141

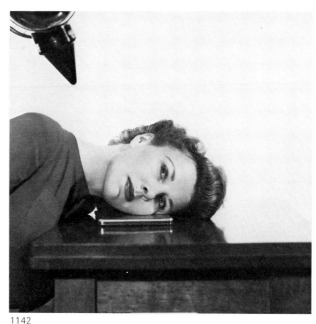

1142

314

Body to Canine socket
1 Variable Angle-board

With the patient in the same general position either standing (1143), or sitting (1144), the face is turned toward the angle board with the body of the mandible in contact with the cassette; the angle board should be steadied with sandbags at both ends.

■ With the tube angled 10° toward the symphysis menti, centre 5 cm (2 ins) below the angle of the jaw remote from the film (1143, 1145a, b.)

Body to Canine

kVp	mAS	FFD	Film ILFORD	Screens ILFORD	Grid
60	10	100 cm (40″)	RAPID R	Standard	—

Note—Short-necked, high-shouldered patients will more easily be positioned on the angle board when allowed to kneel on a stool or to stand being bent forward at the trunk and the hands resting on the couch for support.

2 Head horizontal and Tube angled

With the patient in the same general position either standing (1143), or sitting (1144) the face is turned toward the film, with the body of the mandible being in contact with the cassette. To help in positioning the patient the cassette is raised on a small pad or block of wood.

■ With the tube angled 20° toward the head and 10° toward the face, centre 5 cm (2 ins) below the angle of the jaw remote from the film (1144).

Radiograph (1145b) shows the body of the mandible but the ramus is overshadowed by the cervical vertebrae. The molar region of the maxilla of the same side is also clearly shown. This projection should be compared with (1141).

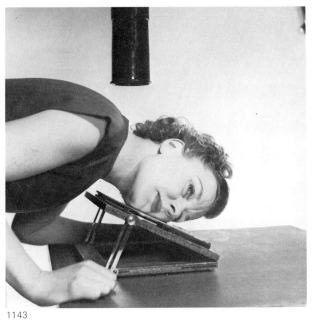

1143

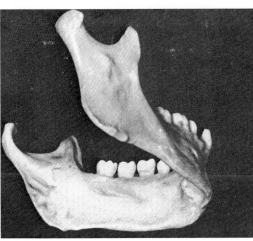

1145(a)

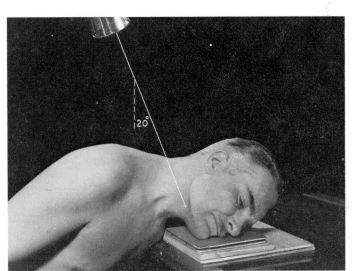

1144

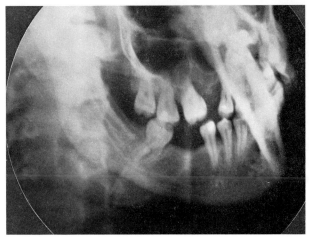

1145(b)

Patient supine, Head horizontal

With the patient supine the head is turned toward the side being examined, the median plane is parallel to the cassette which is raised and angled to support the head in comfort; the opposite shoulder is supported on sandbags.

This position is particularly suitable for short-necked patients, is easily maintained, and there is less strain than in the positions previously described. The shoulders are well removed from the X-ray field, centring being simplified.

■ With the central ray angled 60° to the film and toward the head, centre 5 cm (2 ins) below the angle of the jaw remote from the film (1146, 1147).

Patient Supine, Head Vertical

When a lateral view of the mandible is required with the patient supine the cassette is supported vertically beside the jaw parallel with the median plane of the head for the projection of the ramus and adjacent body (1148, 1149)

For the more anterior part of the body of the mandible the head is turned toward the film to allow the body of the mandible to make contact with the cassette.

■ With a horizontal ray and the tube angled 30° toward the head, centre 5 cm (2 ins) below the angle of the jaw remote from the film, (1148, 1149)

When the patient cannot be moved into the lateral or prone positions, the frontal projection must be taken antero-posterior and not postero-anterior and with perhaps a modified slightly oblique projection.

			Film	Screens	
kVp	mAS	FFD	ILFORD	ILFORD	Grid
60	10	100 cm (40″)	RAPID R	Standard	—

Pt Supine

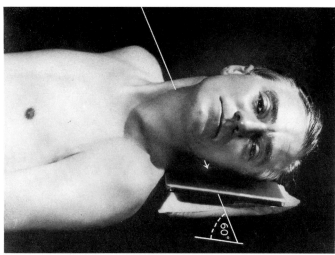

1146

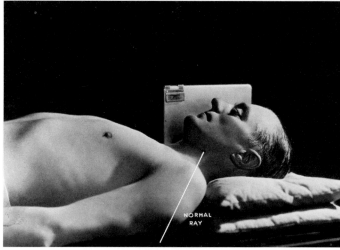

1148

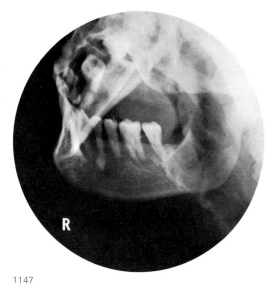

1147

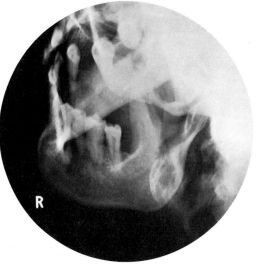

1149

Injuries

As in other regions of the body, radiographic examination of the mandible should include two projections, whenever possible, at right angles to each other (1151, 1153). When X-raying the mandible, however, for suspected fracture the opposite side also requires examination (1150, 1151).

The lateral radiograph (1150) is taken for the anterior part of the body of the mandible (compare 1145b) and shows a fracture just anterior to the root of the right canine whereas in (1151) taken for the ramus of the mandible another fracture is seen at the angle of the left mandible (compare 1141). The true lateral projection (1152) with the two sides of the mandible super-imposed, shows the fractures but it is not possible to lateralize these although it does give a good view of their alignment. On the postero-anterior view (1153) the position of the fractures are demonstrated with slight lateral displacement of the ramus of the mandible on the left side.

Dental Unit

Dental units have small focus tubes which allow examinations at a short focus film distance without much loss of detail. Because of the mobility of dental unit tube heads examinations can be done with the patient seated in a dental chair. In the vast majority of cases these units are used for examination of the teeth with intra-oral films but large films of the mandible can also be taken. The same general principles then apply in the various projections of the mandible with regard to the relative positions of the patient, the film, and the tube.

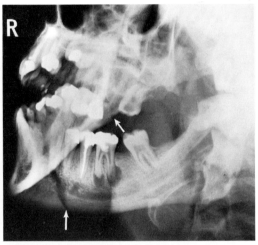

1150

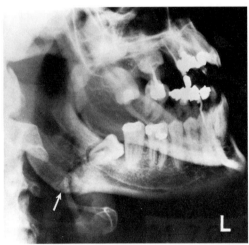

1151

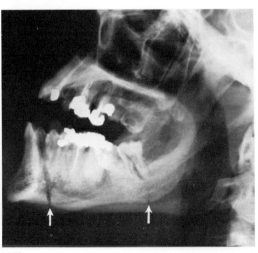

1152

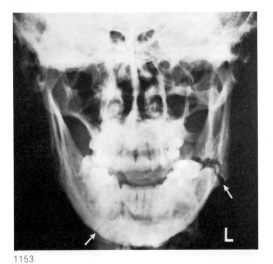

1153

317

Postero-anterior

When the patient has a fracture of the mandible a postero-anterior projection can be done in the erect position (1154) but is not usually possible when the patient is prone. However, a projection with the film horizontal can be done where detail of the anterior part of the mandible is required but no erect Bucky is available (1155).

With the patient in the nose-forehead position both the median sagittal plane and the radiographic baseline are at right angles to the film.

■ Centre in the midline between the angles of the mandible approximately 7·5 cm (3 ins) below the external occipital protuberance. The baseline of the skull is then projected above the condyles of the mandible.

					P-A	
kVp	mAS	FFD	Film ILFORD	Screens ILFORD	Grid
70	30	100 cm (40″)	RAPID R	Standard	Grid

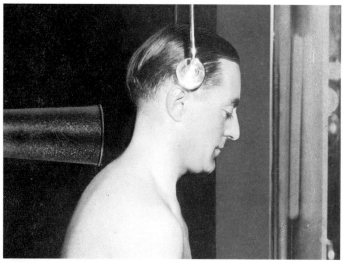

1154

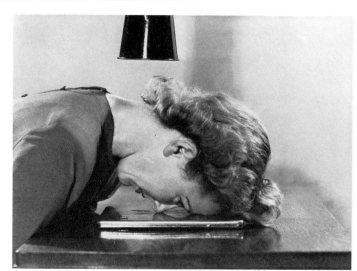

1155

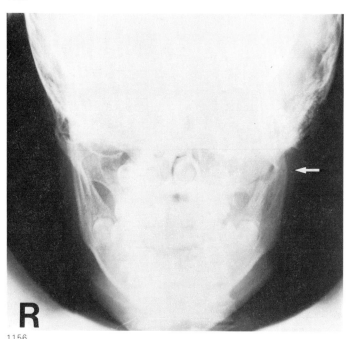

1156

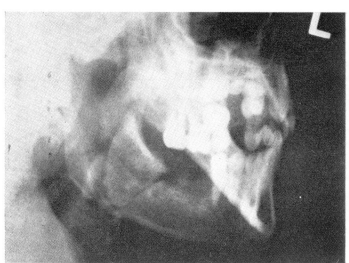

1157

Postero-anterior oblique

The symphysis menti may be projected clear of the cervical vertebrae by turning the head 20° toward right or left side, as indicated in the cross-sectional diagram (1159) to produce radiograph (1160)

■ Centre 5 cm (2 ins) from the midline and directly through the mandibular symphysis for right and left sides in turn (1158, 1159, 1160, 1161)

For this projection the kilovoltage should be reduced by 5 kVp compared with the postero-anterior projection. The use of grid is optional. Radiographs (1160 and 1161) were taken with a grid.

The diagram (1159) shows how rotation of the head and centring the tube separates the shadow of the symphysis menti from that of the cervical vertebrae.

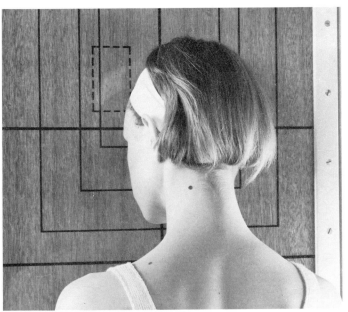

1158

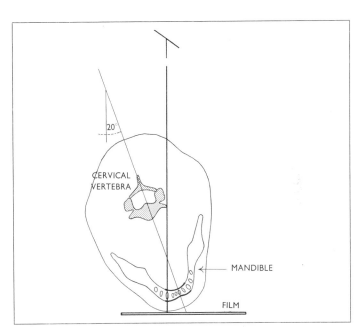

1159

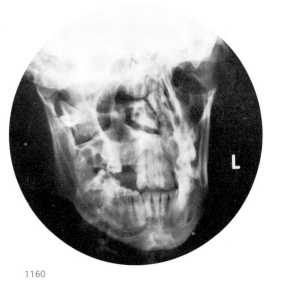

1160

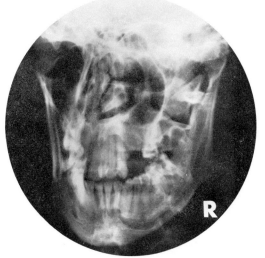

1161

Infero-superior—General

This is the projection to show the body of the mandible particularly the relationship of the two sides to each other and to the symphysis menti. Displacements in the antero-posterior plane can be assessed on this view which can be done with the patient in either the erect or horizontal position.

With the patient erect or supine the neck is extended to bring the vertex of the skull into contact with the film support, the radiographic base-line parallel and the median sagittal plane at right angles to the film. In the supine position it may not be possible to bring the radiographic baseline parallel to the film, the tube should then be angled to compensate, producing a modified projection (1164)

■ Centre in the midline between the angles of the jaw with the central ray approximately 95° to the baseline (1162).

Supero-inferior, Collar radiography

A specially shaped notched cassette can be used in an alternative technique to show the mandible in the vertico-submental projection (1165).

The special cassette is shaped to enclose the neck below the mandible and is placed on an adjustable table top at a height suitable for the patient to rest the lower jaw on the cassette which protrudes to enclose the neck of the patient (1166).

Note—It is necessary to trim the film to the cassette shape as required.

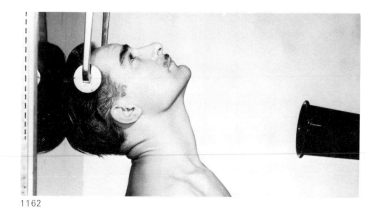

1162

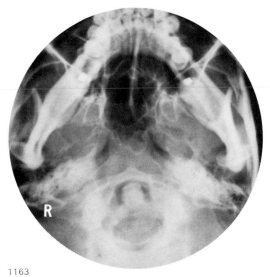

1163

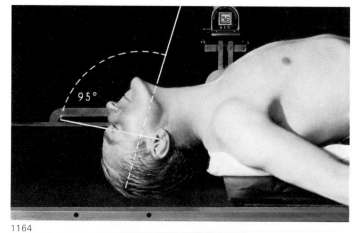

1164

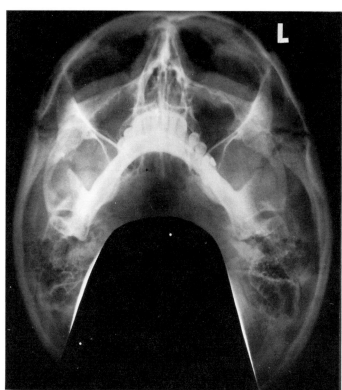

1166

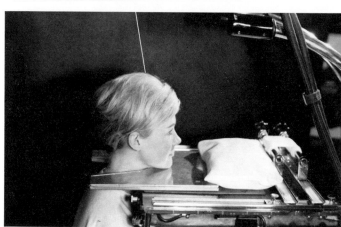

1165

Inferosuperior—Intra-oral (1)

A localized projection of the anterior part of the body of the mandible and the symphysis menti is obtained with an occlusal film between the upper and lower jaws and is usually done with a dental unit. Any ventral or dorsal displacement in relation to the general line of the mandible will be shown.

Using a dental unit and chair the patient's neck is extended over the head-rest and the tube head is placed well down over the chest. The X-ray beam is directed at right angles to the occlusal film.

This projection can also be done with large X-ray units and without a dental chair, but the patient must nevertheless be placed in the position shown in (1167), or with the patient horizontal and the neck extended over a pillow or sandbags. The occlusal film is placed transversely and well back in the jaw, being held in position between the lightly closed teeth.

■ Centre at right angles to the occlusal film, from the submental aspect (1167, 1168)

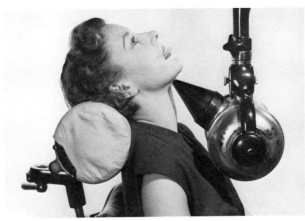

1167

Inf-Sup.

kVp	mAS	FFD	Film ILFORD	Screens ILFORD	Grid
65	10	85 cm (30″)	Occlusal	—	—

Note—It is only possible to do this projection when an occlusal film can be introduced into the mouth and held between the jaws otherwise, the infero-superior (general) position (1162) or the alternative technique (1165) will be required.

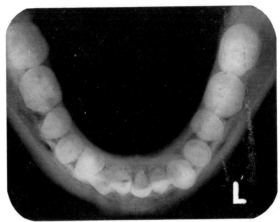

1168

Infero-superior—Intra-oral (2)

For a detailed view of the bone adjacent to the symphysis menti an occlusal film is held in the same position as previously described (1167) but the tube is centred obliquely through the jaw at an angle of 45° to the film (1169, 1170)

Note—Because of the difficulty of including R or L markers on an occlusal radiograph, the occlusal film must always be placed with the embossed "." facing the tube on the right side of the patient so that the dot on the film always occurs on the same side.

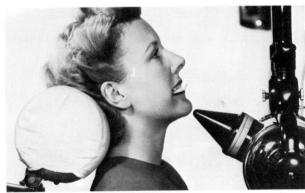

1169

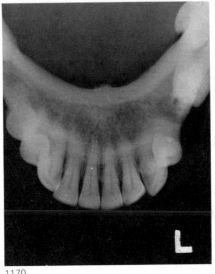

1170

Temporo-Mandibular joints

The condylar processes of the mandible articulate with the temporal bones to form the temporo-mandibular joints lying anterior to the right and left external auditory meatuses (1174). These joints, on the true lateral view, are obscured by the dense petrous temporal bones and each joint must therefore be projected separately free from overlying densities but avoiding undue distortion.

Head straight—Tube angled (basic)

With the patient half-prone the shoulder nearest the tube is raised and the chest supported on sandbags, the head is placed in the true lateral position with the median sagittal plane parallel and the radiographic baseline at right angles to the direction of the beam from the angled tubed (1171).

■ With the tube angled 25° towards the feet, centre 5 cm (2 ins) above the joint remote from the film so the central ray passes directly through the joint in contact with the film. Use a small localizing cone (1171, 1172, 1173)

			T-M Jt.		
kVp	mAS	FFD	Film ILFORD	Screens ILFORD	Grid
70	40	100 cm (40″)	RAPID R	Standard	Grid

Using the position described the following radiographs may be taken:
(a) With the jaws clenched (teeth in contact—RC, LC)
(b) The jaws relaxed (teeth in contact R, L)
(c) At rest with teeth apart (R, L)
(d) With the jaws open (RO, LO)
(e) With the jaws open (wedge between teeth RO, LO)

The views of the temporo-mandibular joint with the jaws open may be taken with a bite block between the jaws (1172) or more commonly without, but in a similar position.

The films should be labelled to show how the radiographs were taken corresponding to the positions (a) to (e) and also for side as indicated by the letters shown above.

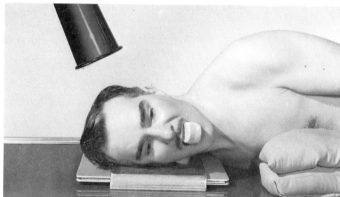

1171

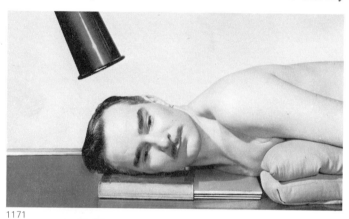

1173

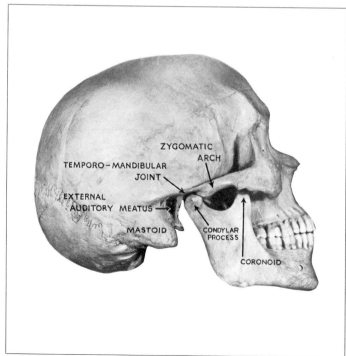

1174

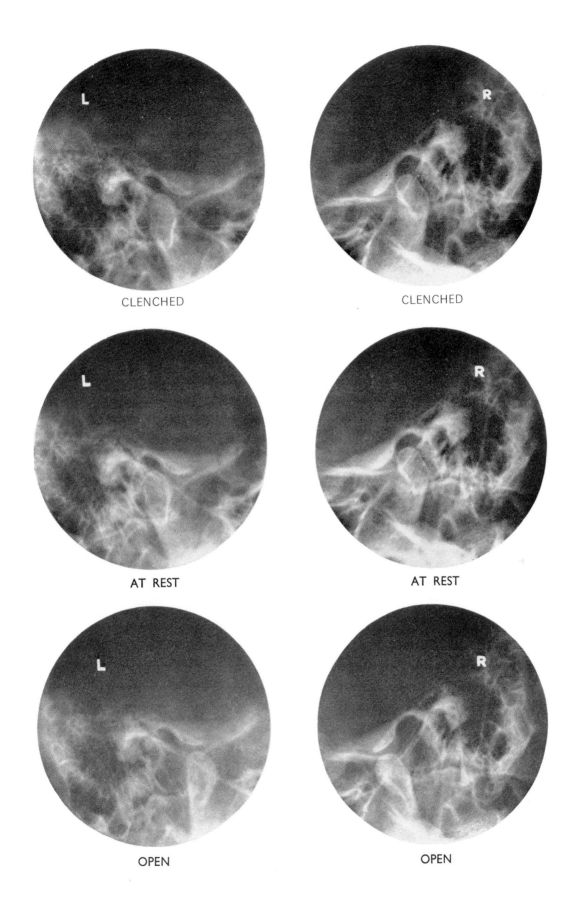

CLENCHED   CLENCHED

AT REST   AT REST

OPEN   OPEN

323

(2) Short distance technique

If the focus-film distance is reduced to 30 cm (12 ins) the image of the joint nearest the tube is diffused while the joint adjacent to the film is clearly defined.

A modified extension cone on the X-ray tube is attached to a specially designed craniostat and fitted to a cassette tunnel by two right-angled arms. The head is then immobilized in the correct position to produce a standard series of six projections for the temporo-mandibular joints. Three exposures are taken of each (1178, 1179).

The surface of the cassette tunnel is covered with lead, apart from the exposure aperture measuring 5 × 7 cm (2 × 3 ins) in its lower part.

An adjustable plastic ear plug decentralized by 1 cm (½ in) maintains the position of the head in relation to the film. The median sagittal plane and anthropomorphic base line are parallel, and the inter-orbital line perpendicular to the film (1176).

A modified diaphragm with a 2 mm aluminium filter and a circular aperture 2·5 cm (1 in) in diameter with surrounding lead fits into the craniostat at a caudal angle of 15° for centring 5 cm (2 ins) above the external auditory meatus on the side nearest the tube. After positioning the patient with the ear plug in the external auditory meatus three exposures of the lower half of the film are made (1177) with the jaw clenched, at rest and open. The cassette is moved 5 cm (2 ins) for each exposure (1178). The patient is then repositioned to face in the opposite direction and the position of the cassette is reversed so three similar exposures can be made of the opposite joint. The single 13 × 18 cm (6½ × 8½ ins) film then shows the six exposures. The radiograph is then divided transversely and rejoined to make viewing easier (1179).

With a focus-film distance of 30 cm (12 ins) a filter is most important because it greatly reduces the radiation dose. For each sequence of three exposures comparing the use of a 1 mm aluminium filter at 60 kVp with a 3 mm aluminium filter at 70 kVp the dosage is reduced from 15 mr to 6 mr.

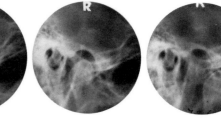

1177

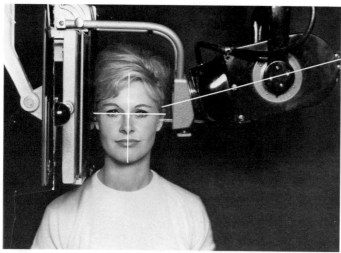

1176

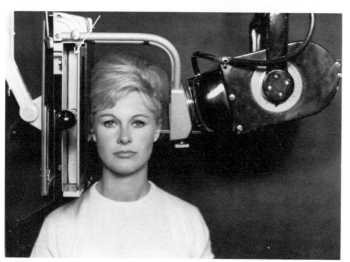

1178

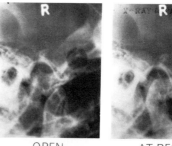
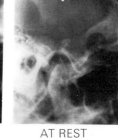
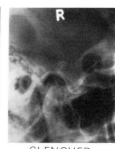
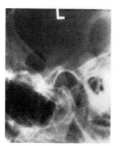
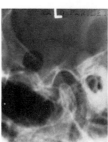
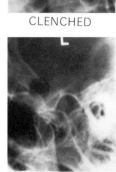

OPEN   AT REST   CLENCHED

CLENCHED   AT REST   OPEN

1179

In (1176) the cassette is in the first position with the mouth "clenched"; the cassette is then withdrawn by 5 cm (2 ins) for the second exposure "at rest" and on withdrawing the cassette by a further 5 cm (2 ins) a third exposure is taken with the mouth "open".

Patient prone—Tube angled

From the true lateral position the face is directed 20° toward the table top. By feeling the temporo-mandibular joint nearest the cassette, it is positioned to the centre of the table top.

■ Angle the tube 20° cephalad and centre to the temporo-mandibular joint in contact with the table top (1180, 1181)

Patient supine—Tube angled

With the patient supine and the raised shoulder supported on sandbags, from the lateral position tilt the head so that the parietal region is in contact with the cassette.

■ With the tube angled 30° toward the head centre to the temporo-mandibular joint nearest to the film. As previously each side is exposed separately with the jaw both open and closed (1182, 1183)

TM Jt. Pt. Supine

kVp	mAS	FFD	Film ILFORD	Screems ILFORD	Grid
60	10	100 cm (40")	RAPID R	Standard	—

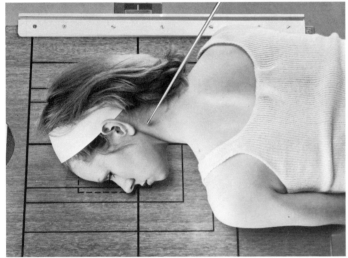

1180

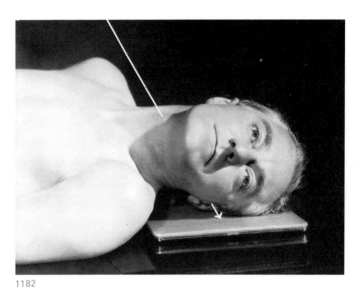

1182

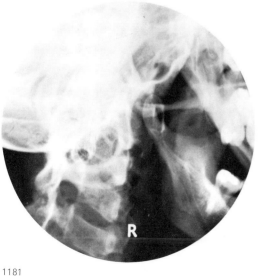

1181

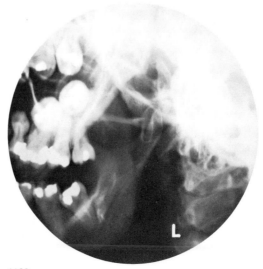

1183

Frontal Views

Although both sides are shown together on the frontal views the joints are not well visualized because of the overlying mastoid processes.

Postero-anterior

With the patient horizontal or erect and in the nose-forehead position the median sagittal plane and radiographic baseline are positioned at right angles to the film.

■ Centre in the midline 7·5 cm (3 ins) below the baseline with the tube angled 10° cephalad for the central ray to pass midway between the tempro-mandibular joints (1184, 1185, 1186)

The radiograph (1185) is taken with the mouth open and (1186) with the mouth closed.

Antero-posterior

A frontal view of the temporo-mandibular joints can also be done using a modification of the 30° fronto-occipital (Towne's) projection.

With the patient horizontal or erect the median sagittal plane and the radiographic baseline are positioned at right angles to the film.

■ With the tube angled 30° caudad, centre in the midline above the glabella to a point midway between the temporo-mandibular joints (1187, 1188, 1189)

Note—In the frontal views little is gained by doing both open and closed projections though these have been illustrated (1185, 1186, 1188 1189).

P-A; AP

kVp		mAS			Film	Screens	
AP	PA	AP	PA	FFD	ILFORD	ILFORD	Grid
80	80	50	40	100 cm (40")	RAPID R	Standard	Grid

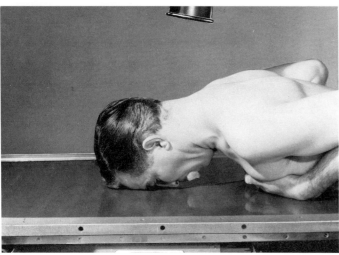

1184

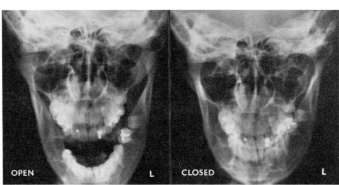

1185   1186

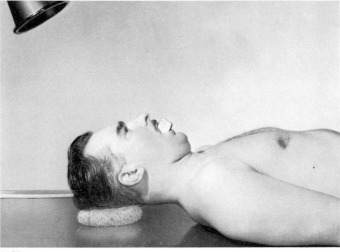

1187

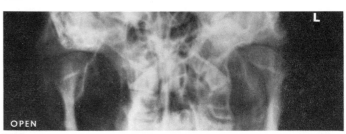

1188

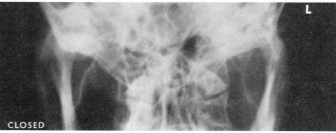

1189

Injuries

In the frontal view (1190) bilateral fractures of the condylar processes are shown (arrows). In (1191a) a film of the left side has been taken using the projection (1171) with the patient prone, head straight and tube angled; (1191b) shows a similar projection of the right side, however the fracture is only clearly seen in radiograph (1191c) taken with the patient supine, the head tilted laterally and the tube angled (see 1182).

Tomography

The temporo-mandibular joints are much more clearly seen on tomograms and the series of radiographs (1193) are of tomographic cuts of both sides with the mouth closed and mouth open. The examination was performed with the head in the true lateral position.

Figure (1192) shows a cassette tunnel which can be used to take four routine exposures of the temporo-mandibular joints on a single 25 × 20 cm (10 × 8 ins) film.

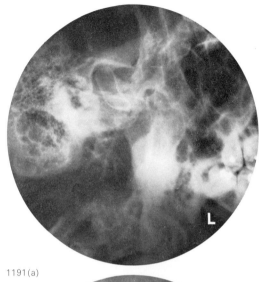

1191(a)

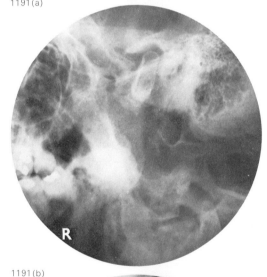

1191(b)

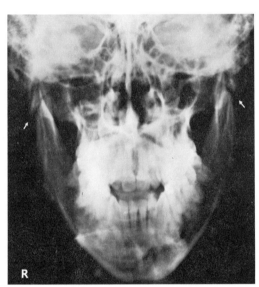

1190

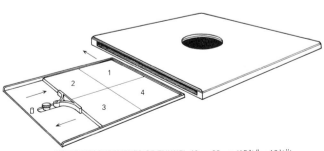

INSIDE MEASUREMENTS OF TUNNEL 40 × 33 cm (15⁷/₈″× 12⁷/₈″)
DIAMETER OF APERATURE 9.5 cm (3³/₄″)
INSIDE MEASUREMENTS OF CASSETTE TRAY 28 × 32 cm (11″× 12³/₄″)
ADJUSTABLE CLIP TO HOLD CASSETTE FOR 25 × 20 cm (10″× 8″) FILM

1192

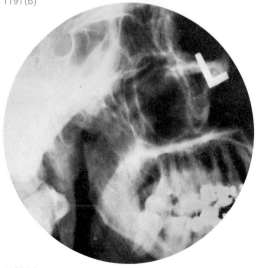

1191(c)

11

327

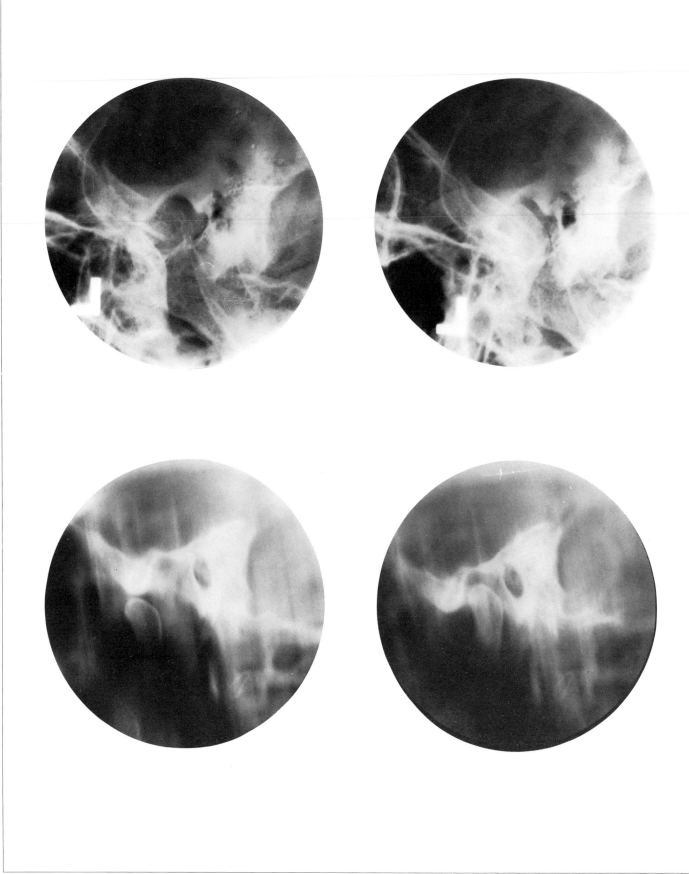

12
SUBJECT TYPES

SUBJECT TYPES

The position of the internal organs, especially the stomach, colon, gall-bladder, and kidneys is greatly influenced by the physique and the age of the patient.

In the short stockily built individual the stomach tends to be high in the abdomen and horizontal, the transverse colon is in a similar position so that there is not much overlapping of its ascending and descending parts and the left colic flexure is high under the left hemi-diaphragm. Similarly the gall-bladder tends to lie transversely and is often seen end on appearing spherical and laterally placed and is also high in the abdomen. The thorax is short and broad otherwise there is less variation in the position of the internal structures than in the abdomen (1202, 1203).

In the long thin subject the stomach is J-shaped and often in the erect position, the lower part of the body of the stomach lies over the sacrum. To show the stomach in the erect position a large film will be required to cover the area from the diaphragm to the anterior superior iliac spine. The colon is also low in position with marked sagging of the transverse colon into the bony pelvis. The gall-bladder is elongated and appears to lie parallel to the spine, is also low in position often being at the level of the fourth and fifth lumbar vertebrae. The thorax is long and narrow (1200, 1201) and there is often a depressed sternum.

Between these two extremes there is a spectrum of intermediate types. It is important to appreciate the variations in the position of the internal abdominal organs for accurate radiography especially when examining the gall bladder, which is done without fluoroscopy to locate its position.

Mill has described 4 types of bodily habitus, Hypersthenic, Sthenic, Asthenic, and Hyposthenic. In each of these types the internal organs tend to follow a particular pattern.

Two radiographs of a stomach, after drinking barium, (1194, 1195) show the difference between the Hypersthenic or stockily built individual and the Hyposthenic or long thin individual. In the Hypersthenic type (1194) the stomach is more horizontal and the duodenal loop lies below the greater curve whereas in the Hyposthenic type (1195) the stomach is J-shaped overlying the duodenal loop and reaching below the level of the iliac crest. Quite clearly a different size film will be required to show the stomach in the Hypersthenic compared with the Hyposthenic individual.

1 Hypersthenic

This type of subject is massively built; the thorax is broad from side to side, relatively shallow from above downward but deep from back to front. The lungs are correspondingly broad at the bases and the apices barely show above the clavicles. The heart is broad and squat with its long axis lying transversely.

The dome of the diaphragm is high and the lower costal margin is at a high level with a wide angle. The stomach and transverse colon are usually in the upper part of the abdomen and the colon shows without overshadowing of the flexures. The gall-

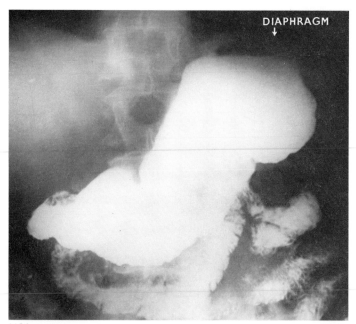

1194

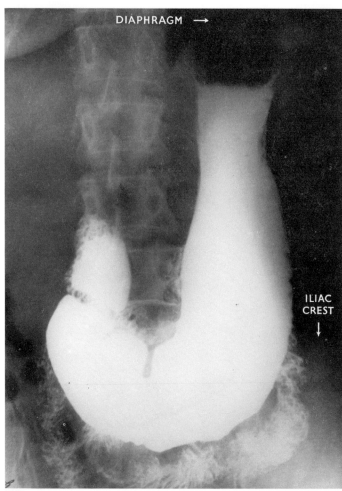

1195

bladder is horizontal, high in the abdomen and well away from the midline. This is the least common type not exceeding 5% of the population (1196).

2 Sthenic

This type is similar to the hypersthenic type but not as broad in proportion to the height (1197). This is the most common type, about 48% of the population being in this group.

3 Asthenic

The asthenic type has a markedly elongated and narrow thorax with elongated lungs and the apices well above the clavicles. The heart is vertical and appears long and slender. The costal angle is narrow being usually less than a right angle with a low

dome of diaphragm and the lower costal margin is close to the level of the iliac crests. The abdominal cavity is shallow, with the greatest capacity in the pelvis. In the erect position the stomach is well down and reaches well below the iliac crest often down into the pelvic cavity. The colon is low and chiefly in the pelvis with marked overlapping of its different parts. The gall-bladder is vertical in position, low down and close to the midline. 12% of the population are in this group (1198).

4 Hyposthenic

These subjects are similar to the asthenic but with less marked features. Approximately 30% of the population fall into this group (1199).

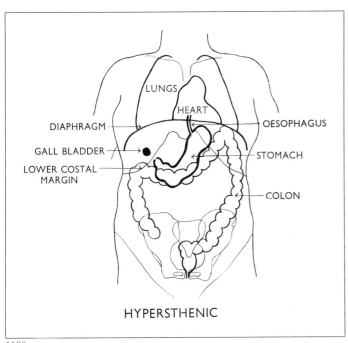

HYPERSTHENIC

1196

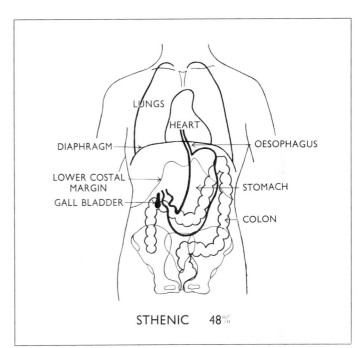

STHENIC   48%

1197

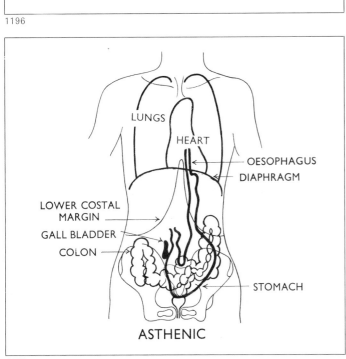

ASTHENIC

1198

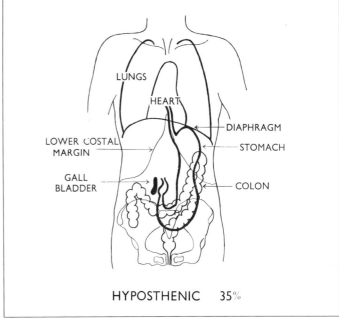

HYPOSTHENIC   35%

1199

A postero-anterior and lateral radiograph of two subjects, both eighteen years of age, show the differences between asthenic (1200, 1201) and hyposthenic (1202, 1203) individuals.

In the asthenic subject the lung fields appear larger than in the hyposthenic type in the frontal view but the chest is considerably narrower from back to front in the asthenic subject.

The asthenic type (1200) required a full length 35 × 43 cm (14 × 17 ins) film whereas for the hyposthenic type (1202) only a 35 × 35 cm (14 × 14 ins) film was needed.

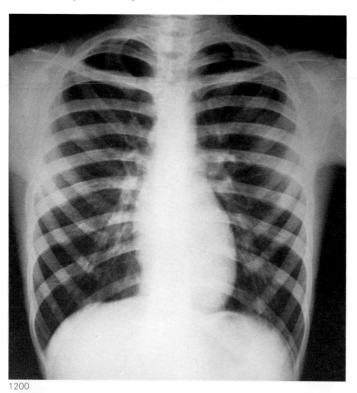

1200

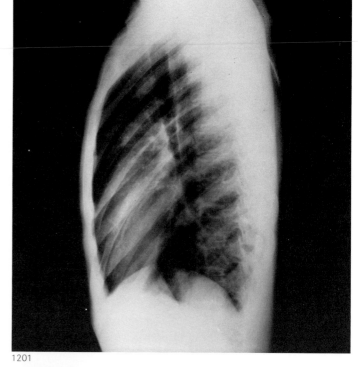

1201

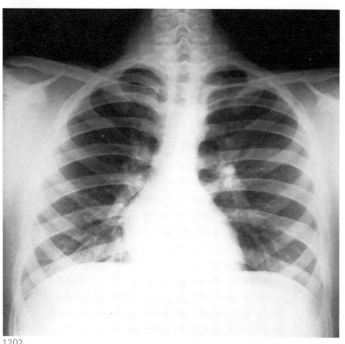

1202

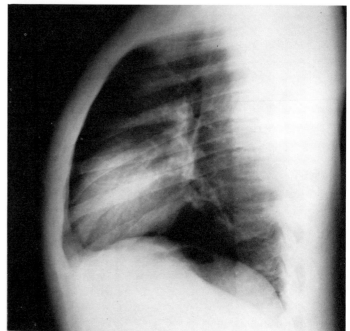

1203

13

HEART AND AORTA

HEART AND AORTA

The heart is a hollow, muscular organ which with the roots of the aorta and pulmonary artery is enclosed in a fibroserous sac, the pericardium and is situated a little to the left of the midline in the middle mediastinum resting on the anterior aspect of the dome of the diaphragm.

The heart acts as a pump and with rythmic contractions propels the blood throughout the circulatory system of blood vessels. There are approximately 60 to 80 heart beats per minute. Thus for the average individual the heart cycle is 0·8 second and the exposure time of a chest radiograph must therefore be well below the time of a cardiac cycle to avoid movement blurring.

The heart has four chambers, the right and left atria above and the right and left ventricles below. The atria are separated by the interatrial septum and the ventricles by the inter-ventricular septum. Blood flows from the right atrium into the right ventricle through the tricuspid valve and from the left atrium to the left ventricle through the mitral valve. In the normal subject there is no communication between the right and left atria or the right and left ventricles (1204).

The left ventricle pumps the blood into the aorta which gives off the major arteries and as these divide the vessels become smaller being then called arterioles. From the arterioles the blood flows into capillaries; which join up again to form venules which in turn become veins, joining together to form the inferior vena cava in the lower part and the superior vena cava in the upper part of the body. Superior and inferior venae cavae drain into the right atrium. From the right atrium the blood is propelled into the right ventricle and thence to the pulmonary artery, pulmonary arterioles and capillaries, where they join up to form the pulmonary venules and then the pulmonary veins which drain into the left atrium. The blood flows from the left atrium into the left ventricle thus completing the circulation of the blood which was first described by William Harvey in 1628.

The thoracic aorta is the largest of the great vessels and is divided into three parts, the ascending aorta, the arch and the descending aorta. The descending aorta starts at the level of the fourth thoracic vertebra and is divided into the thoracic portion lying above the diaphragm and the abdominal portion below.

On the chest radiograph the heart is seen as a pear shaped structure of soft tissue density with its broad base adjacent to the diaphragm and its narrower upper part overlying the spine. In the hyposthenic type the heart is long and thin whereas in asthenic individual it tends to be broad and horizontal (see page 332). The size and shape of the heart also varies with respiration and the position of the patient. In inspiration the heart appears smaller and more vertical (1205) and changing from the erect to the horizontal position the heart appears larger and more horizontal (1206). Comparing a postero-anterior radiograph with an antero-posterior radiograph the heart appears smaller in the postero-anterior radiograph because there is less magnification as it lies nearer the anterior chest wall.

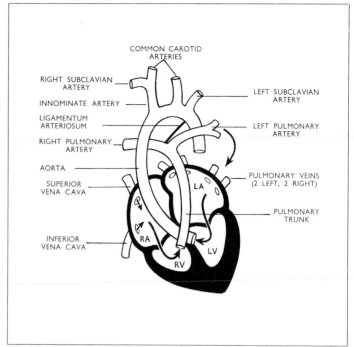

1204

The thoracic aorta is shown in its full length in the left postero-anterior oblique position with the ascending aorta lying anteriorly, the arch reaching to below the level of the clavicles and the descending aorta being partially superimposed on the dorsal vertebrae. In the postero-anterior projection the arch of the aorta is seen end on as a circular shadow just to the left of the dorsal vertebrae at the level of D6. The anterior margin of the barium filled oesophagus acts as a marker for the posterior margin of the heart in the right anterior oblique position and can be shown both on fluoroscopy and on radiographic examination.

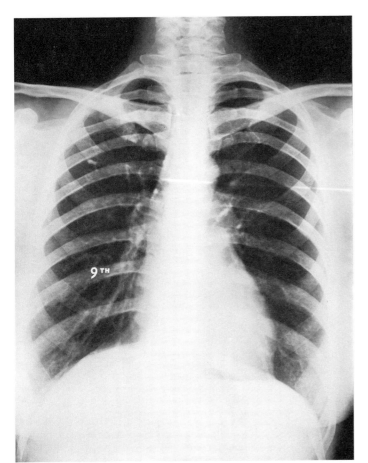

ERECT
1205

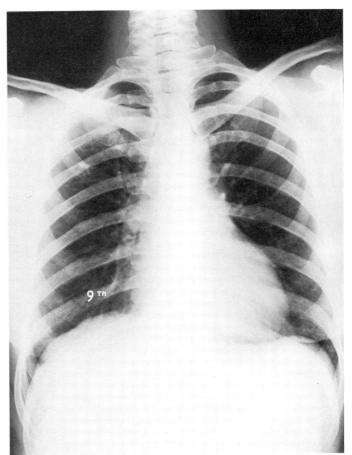

PRONE
1206

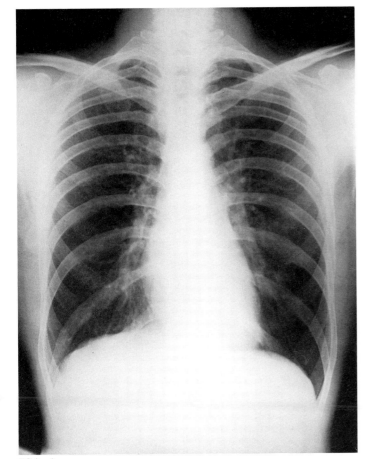

72 inches
1207

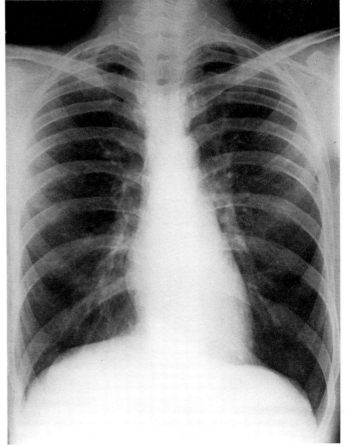

30 inches
1208

13 Heart and aorta

Technique

Radiographs of the chest to show the heart should be more penetrated than for the lungs. The exposure factors are adjusted for either a slightly increased kilo-voltage or an increased mAs to give a darker film.

Chest radiographs are normally taken in deep inspiration using exposure time of a fraction of a second (·04–·01). The focus-film distance is 180 cm (72 ins) to avoid heart magnification in the postero-anterior projection and is referred to as teleradiography (1207). Two films of the same patient exposed at a 180 cm (72 ins) and 75 cm (30 ins) show the difference in radiographic size of the heart with different focus film distances.

Oblique projections of the thorax for heart examinations are normally done at a focus film distance of 150 cm (60 ins).

For the penetrated views of the heart examinations are normally also done at a focus film distance of 150 cm (60 ins).

For penetrated views of the heart a grid is used and greater definition can be obtained with adequate coning.

The exposure factors quoted in this section refer to an adult subject of average physique.

Postero-anterior

This projection is usually done with the patient standing but may be done with the patient seated.

With the patient facing the film and the arms encircling it the chin is placed over the top edge of the cassette to ensure close proximity of the heart to the film. Alternatively the position of the patient may be similar to that for a postero-anterior lung radiograph (Section 14).

■ Centre, in the midline, at the level of the sixth thoracic vertebra (1209, 1210)

			PA		
kVp	mAS	FFD	Film ILFORD	Screens ILFORD	Grid
70	15	180 cm (72″)	RAPID R	Fast	—

The exposure is made in inspiration and it is most important that the thorax is perfectly symmetrical in this view. Rotation of the trunk to right or left, which can be seen on the radiograph by the asymetrical position of the sterno-clavicular joint, will cause distortion to the position of the heart on the radiograph.

Lateral

The patient is turned to bring the left side toward the film, with the arms folded over the head, or raised above the head, to rest on a horizontal bar.

The median plane of the trunk should be parallel to the film. The patient is viewed both from the back and from the side to ensure that the median plane of the trunk is parallel to the film.

■ Centre midway between the front and back, to the axilla at the level of the sixth thoracic vertebra (1211, 1212)

Note—A moving or stationary grid is required to overcome the excessive secondary radiation from photon scatter in large subjects for both the postero-anterior and lateral projections.

Attention must be paid to adequate coning and the correct size film must be used depending on the size and bodily habitus of the patient.

			Lateral		
kVp	mAS	FFD	Film ILFORD	Screens ILFORD	Grid
80	60	150 cm (50″)	RAPID R	Fast	Grid

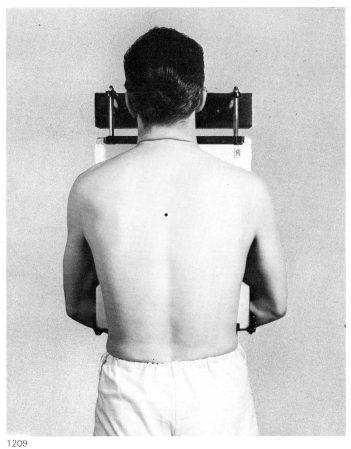

1209

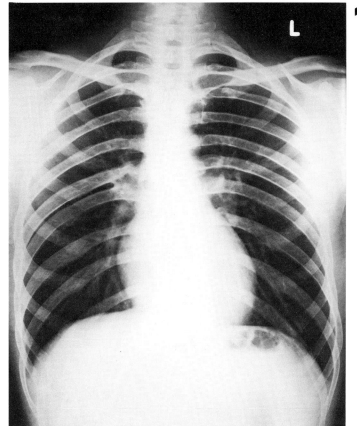

1210

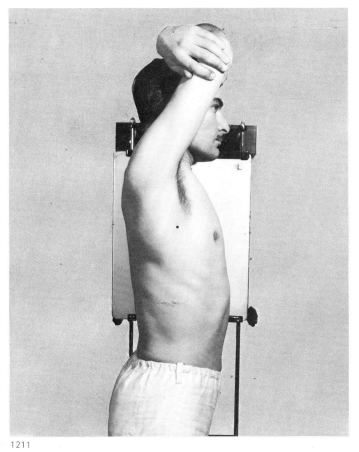

1211

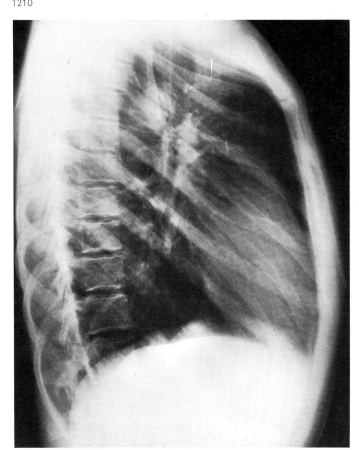

1212

Postero-anterior oblique

There is considerable variation in the relationship of the descending aorta, the heart and ascending aorta in this projection. However the average angle of rotation in relation to the postero-anterior position is 60° for the right postero-anterior oblique and 70° for the left postero-anterior oblique (1289, 1293).

The focus-film distance for the oblique projections should be 150 cm (60 ins). The oblique positions are used to separate the heart, aorta, and vertebral column without overshadowing. In the right postero-anterior oblique position the anterior margin of barium filled oesophagus is intimately related to the posterior margin of the aortic knuckle and heart border.

Right postero-anterior (first) oblique (R.A.O.)

With the patient facing the film, the right side of the patient is kept in contact with the cassette and the trunk rotated to bring the left side away from the film to form an angle of 60°.

■ Centre midway between the vertebral column and the left axilla to the level of the sixth thoracic vertebra (1213, 1215)

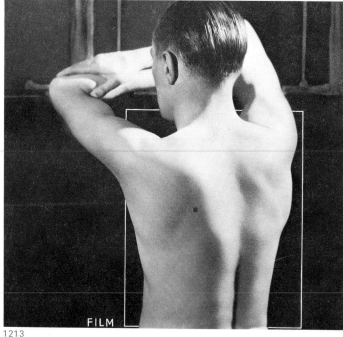
FILM
1213

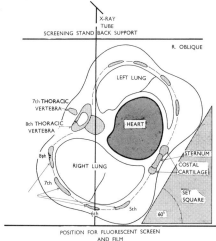
1214

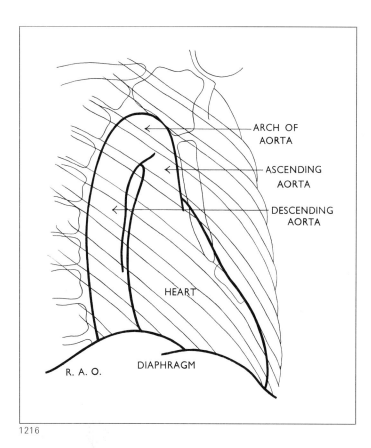
ARCH OF AORTA

ASCENDING AORTA

DESCENDING AORTA

HEART

R. A. O. DIAPHRAGM

1216

The labelled line diagrams (1216, 1220) show the positions of the aorta and heart in the 2 oblique projections.

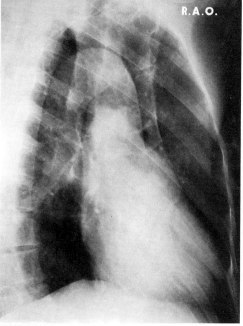
RIGHT OBLIQUE
1215

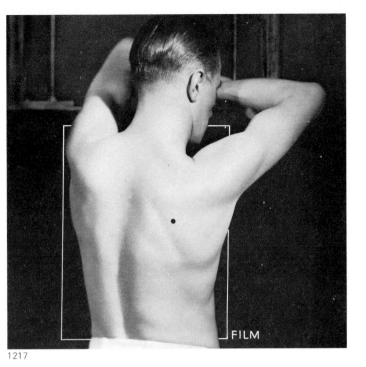

1217

Left postero-anterior (second) oblique (L.A.O.) 13

With the patient facing the film, the left side is kept in contact with the cassette and the trunk rotated to bring the right side away from the film to form an angle of 70°.

In this position the aortic arch is opened out to show the transradiant aortic window lying immediately below and the aortic triangle above the aortic arch.

■ Centre midway between the vertebral column and the right axilla at the level of the sixth thoracic vertebra (1217, 1218, 1219, 1220)

Diagrams of axial sections at the level of the heart (1214, 1218) show the relationship between the X-ray tube, patient and film. A set square is shown in position which can be used to assess the angle the trunk makes with the cassette.

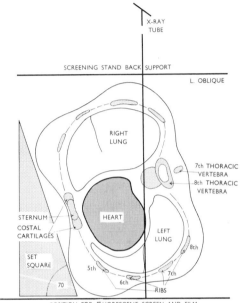

1218

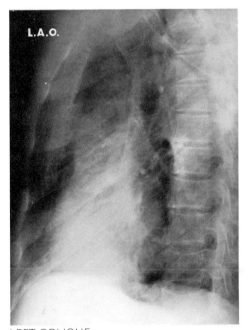

LEFT OBLIQUE
1219

1220

AORTIC TRIANGLE

ARCH OF AORTA

AORTIC WINDOW

ASCENDING AORTA

DESCENDING AORTA

HEART

L. A. O.

DIAPHRAGM

Oblique

kVp		mAS			Film	Screens	
RAO	LAO	RAO	LAO	FFD	ILFORD	ILFORD	Grid
75	80	40	40	150 cm (60")	RAPID R	Fast	Grid

Barium swallow

Enlargement of the aorta or heart produces abnormal impressions on the oesophagus. In the right postero-anterior oblique (RAO) position the anterior wall of the oesophagus is intimately related from above downward to the aortic arch, pulmonary artery, the left atrium, and finally the right ventricle near the diaphragm. However, to show the impressions of these structures on the oesophagus with a barium swallow, the oesophagus must be well filled with barium.

The examination is usually performed using fluoroscopy but can be done without. In the vast majority of cases for cardiac assessment the right postero-anterior oblique position (R.A.O.) is used for the barium swallow, however the postero-anterior and left postero-anterior oblique positions may also be required. In the oblique positions the oesophagus overlies the lung fields and the exposure is similar to that used for oblique plain radiographs (1215, 1219). However in the postero-anterior projection, the exposure must be increased by 10 kVp because the oesophagus overlies the spine.

Method

With the patient correctly positioned for the particular projection required, the exposure selected and the equipment ready for the exposure, the patient is given a mouthful of barium and told to hold it in the mouth. At the instruction 'swallow' watch for the movement of the thyroid cartilage (Adam's apple) and expose the film 3 seconds after the first movement of the thyroid cartilage.

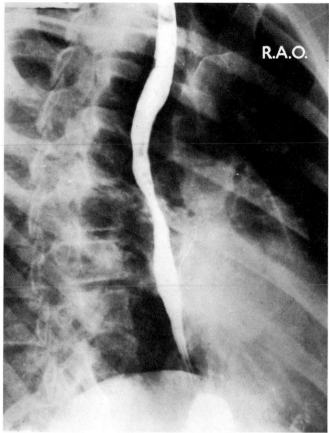

1217(b)

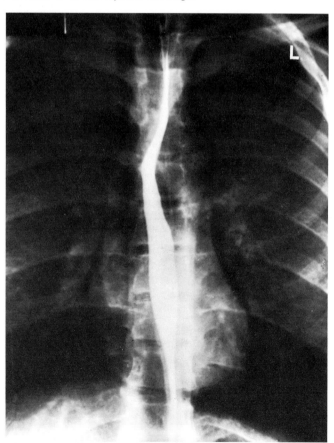

1217(a)

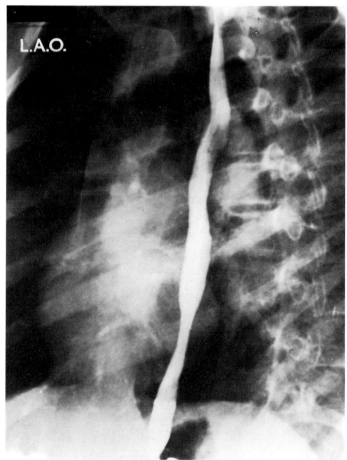

1217(c)

Cardiac angiography

Injection of a water soluble contrast medium, similar to that used for pyelography, into the heart or great vessels is known as cardiac angiography, or angiocardiography and is described and illustrated in Volume II. The tip of a radio opaque catheter is positioned under screen control in the heart or great vessel where contrast medium is to be injected. In adults 40–50 ml of a 70%–80% organic iodine compound is used. A rapid film changer allows 20 to 30 films to be exposed in quick succession and simultaneously from two directions at right angles to each other. Alternatively the examination can be done using cinefluorography.

Two pairs of radiographs selected from an angiocardiographic series of a child taken in the antero-posterior and lateral projections are shown with the catheter in position (1218) and the twelfth exposure at 1½ seconds after the injection of contrast (1219).

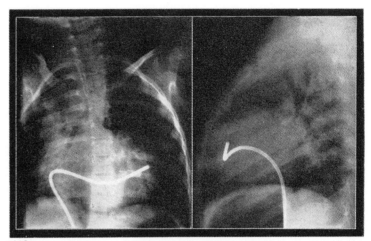

1218

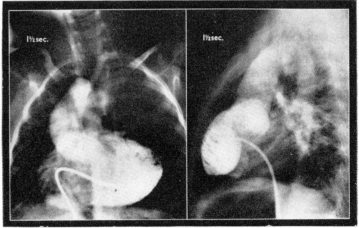

1219

Suspending harness

The photographs (1220a,b,c) show a suspending harness for young children, one of many such accessories used to meet individual requirements. The object of these appliances is to obtain adequate immobilization but allowing free rotation to position a child in the various projections with the minimum of discomfort.

After fitting the harness and seeing the patient is relaxed and breathing quietly the radiographs can be taken. The positions demonstrated (1220a,b,c) are the antero-posterior, right postero-anterior oblique and lateral, but other positions are also readily achieved.

With the child positioned and immobilized no further assistance is required with the examination which can be done at the appropriate stages of respiration by watching the child.

Satisfactory immobilization allows exact positioning, centring of tube, and close collimation of the beam to the smallest dimensions. Appropriately small films can be used and a minimum of repeat exposures should be necessary keeping radiation to both patient and operator down to a minimum.

Radiographs antero-posterior, antero-posterior penetrated with barium, and oblique are shown in (1221a,b,c) for a child of 2 years. The exposure factors were based on the table on this page using a 3 phase unit.

Child
Exposure Factors Child 2 years

Chest	kV	mAS	Sec	FFD	Grid
Antero-posterior	78	4	1/120	72″(180cm)	—
Antero-posterior (penetrated with barium)	95	8	1/140	72″(180cm)	Stat.
Left anterior oblique	100	8	1/140	72″(180cm)	Stat.

Three-phase unit with ILFORD RR film and FT Screens

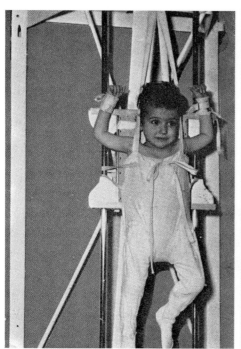

1220a

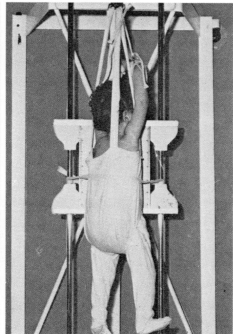

1220b

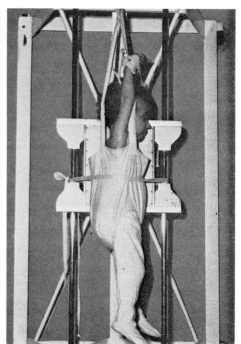

1220c

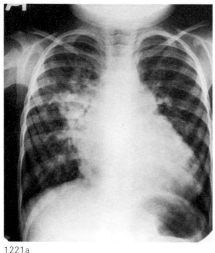

1221a

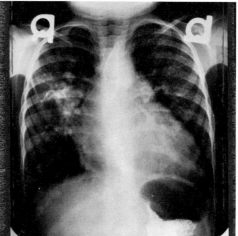

1221b

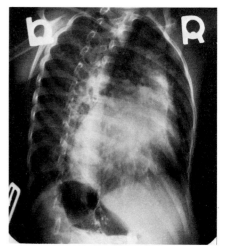

1221c

KYMOGRAPHY

Kymography

Kymography is a radiographic method of recording involuntary movements particularly of the heart and adjacent aorta and pulmonary artery.

A grid is mounted in a frame which has a space for the film cassette (1222). The grid and film are so arranged that the one remains stationary while movement is applied to the other, timing being automatically operated from the X-ray exposure switch.

The grid is made of parallel strips of lead of equal width which are spaced 0·4 millimetre apart and the lead strips are usually 10 millimetres wide.

The range of movement of the grid or film is the same as, or slightly less than, the width of a single grid strip. Time occupied by the movement is equivalent to the X-ray exposure time.

Moving film—Stationary grid

At each instant of the exposure time, a separate image is recorded on the film as it moves over the grid apertures. The resulting 'kymograph' is made up of a series of images following one another in rapid succession and recording the movement of the organ at points 10 millimetres apart in a series of strips on the film. Each 10 millimetre of film showing a number of 0·4 millimetre wide exposures of the margin of the organ and recording its movement during the total exposure period.

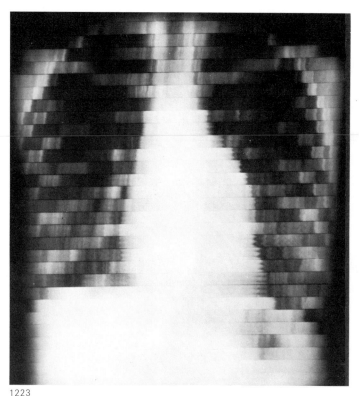

1223

Diagram (1224) shows a small section of heart, grid and film, and also the procession of impressions received by each section of the moving film as it passes the grid apertures through which the X-ray beam projects the shadow of the small section of heart. As will be seen, more than two complete cardiac cycles are recorded during a 2 second exposure. The resulting kymograph is shown in (1223).

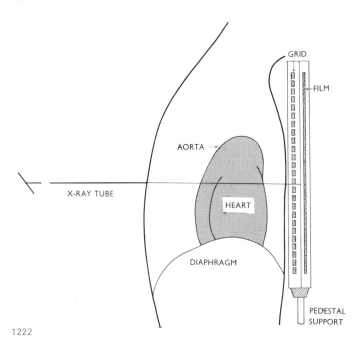

1222

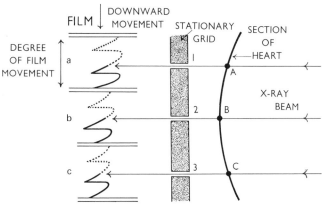

HEART SPOTS A B C ARE
SHOWN THROUGH GRID SLOTS I 2·3
ON CORRESPONDING FILM AREAS
a, b, c

1224

Moving grid—Stationary film

The grid moves relative to the silhouette of the organ, the film receiving a series of images showing transverse movement over areas having the width of the space between the grid apertures, that is 10 millimetres (1225).

Diagram (1226) shows the relationship between a small section of the heart surface and the X-ray beam, moving grid and stationary film.

Illustration (1225) is a typical kymograph of an abnormal subject. It will be seen that the wave-form varies for each section of the heart and great vessels—atria, ventricles, and aorta.

The period occupied by the movement of the heart during the cardiac cycle, from contraction in systole to maximum distention in diastole, occupies a period of 0·6 second in the normal subject, the normal heart beat being 72 per minute, and it will be seen in the kymograph (1225), which was exposed for 2 seconds, that two-and-a-half cardiac cycles are recorded through each grid slot. On joining the troughs of the waves, the heart is seen at its minimum size in systole, the line joining the crests indicating its maximum size in diastole.

The exposure must be done in suspended respiration preferably in inspiration and the phase of respiration must be recorded on the film.

The series of illustrations, kymographs (1223–1225) and the routine chest radiograph (1227), are of a patient with mitral stenosis.

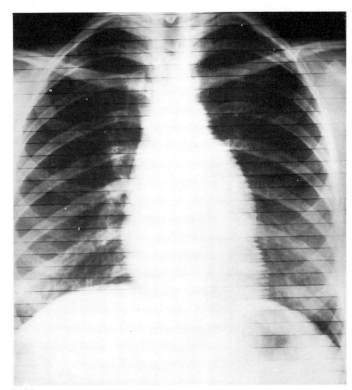

1225

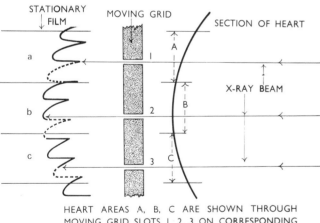

HEART AREAS A, B, C ARE SHOWN THROUGH MOVING GRID SLOTS 1 2 3 ON CORRESPONDING FILM AREAS a, b, c

1226

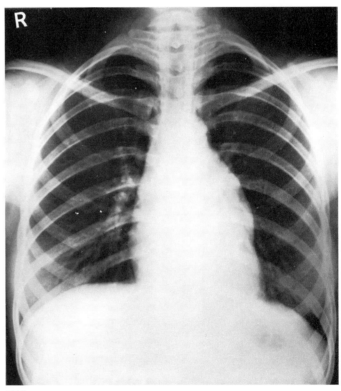

1227

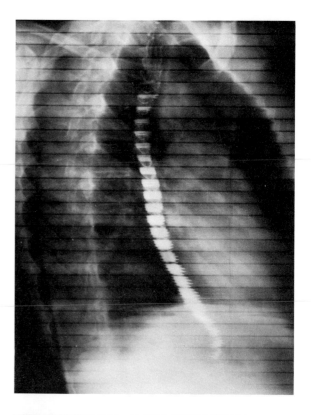

It should be noted that the slower the movement of the organ the longer should be the exposure, the rate of travel of film or grid being correspondingly reduced. Illustration (1228) is a kymograph of the oesophagus with a barium swallow showing transverse movement as seen in the right anterior oblique (R.A.O.) position and taken with a moving grid.

Illustration (1229) shows a foreign body in the heart, the kymograph having been exposed in the antero-posterior position, using the moving film technique.

The aim should be to record at least two but not more than three cardiac cycles. Two-and-a-half cardiac cycles as shown in (1225) is a good average obtained with an exposure of 2 seconds, but in cases of tachycardia the exposure time can, with advantage, be less.

The speed of grid travel must be adjusted so that it travels the full distance during the exposure.

Region	IV-	mA	Sec	FFD	Film ILFORD	Screens ILFORD
Heart PA	80	30	2	36" (90cm)	RAPID R	FT
Heart oblique	90	30	2	36" (90cm)	RAPID R	FT
Oesophagus	90	60	3	36" (90cm)	RAPID R	FT

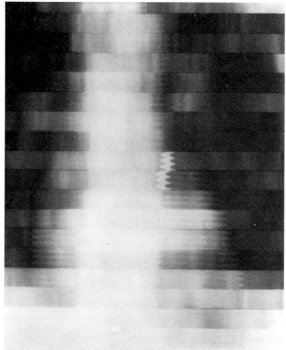

14

RESPIRATORY SYSTEM

RESPIRATORY SYSTEM

The respiratory system consists of the nose, pharynx, larynx, trachea, bronchi, lungs and pleurae. This section deals with the organs of chief radiographic importance, namely, the trachea, bronchi, and lungs and also includes the thymus gland, situated in the anterior part of the mediastinum, as the technique is similar to that for the lungs.

The trachea is a cartilaginous and musculo-membranous tube descending from the larynx to the bronchi, starting at the cricoid cartilage, on a level with the sixth cervical vertebra, and normally ending at the level of the fifth thoracic vertebra where it divides into a right and a left bronchus, at the carina. It lies anterior to the oesophagus in the neck and upper thorax.

The bronchi descend from the termination of the trachea, each toward the hilum of the corresponding lung. The right bronchus is shorter, wider and more vertical than the left, the latter passing beneath the aortic window to reach the hilum of the left lung. The structure of the bronchi is the same as that of the trachea.

On entering the lungs, the bronchi divide and subdivide many times, the smaller branches being termed bronchioles. The bronchioles permeate the lungs, dividing to eventually become the terminal bronchiole which leads in to the alveolar ducts, finally opening out as the pouched air cells called alveoli.

The lungs are the organs of respiration, covered by a serous coat, called pleura. Each lung, the right and left, lies within its pleural cavity. The mediastinum lies between the lungs and contains the heart and great vessels. The right lung is slightly larger than the left and has three lobes; it is also shorter and wider than the left due partly to the bulk of the right lobe of the liver elevating the right hemi-diaphragm which is usually 2 cm (1 in) higher than the left. The heart and pericardium lie a little to the left of the midline and mainly on the left hemi-diaphragm. The left lung has 2 lobes, and anteriorly has the cardiac notch, which lies in contact with the left ventricle of the heart. Each lobe of the lung is subdivided into segments any one of which may be demonstrated radiographically. An accessory lobe may be present particularly in the upper part of the right lung where it is called the azygos lobe.

The mediastinum is the middle space between the lungs, containing the heart and great vessels, the oesophagus, trachea, bronchi, thoracic duct and lymph nodes and extends from the sternum to the vertebrae, and from the upper thorax to the diaphragm.

The diaphragm is a musculo-membranous partition separating the thorax from the abdomen. The superior surface forms the floor of the thoracic cavity and is convex upwards being higher on the right than on the left. The inferior concave surface, forms the roof of the abdominal cavity.

Radiographic appearances

In the frontal view the lung fields, as seen through the ribs, are not homogeneous. The pulmonary vessels both arteries and veins are shown as tapering and branching structures from the hilar regions to the periphery of the lung. The outline of the heart, great vessels, and diaphragm should be sharply defined. The ascending aorta lies to the right of the spine and just behind it the superior vena cava extends upwards towards the apex of the right lung with a well defined lateral margin. The inferior vena cava appears as a small triangular shadow in the right cardiophrenic angle.

The fissures of the lung show as long fine line shadows, the greater fissures being seen on the lateral view and the lesser fissure of the right lung on the frontal view.

Chest films should show the area from the lower cervical spine above to below the costophrenic angles and laterally should include the soft tissues of the axillae. The sterno-clavicular joints should be symmetrical about the midline and the shadows of the scapulae should be away from the lung field.

Respiration

The changes that occur with respiration are of great importance in the appearance of chest radiographs. When the lungs are filled with air they are more transradiant and thus give a brighter picture both on fluoroscopy and on films. On full inspiration the diaphragm is depressed, so that a greater area of lung tissue is visible (1230) but on expiration the diaphragm rises to a higher level making the lungs more radio-opaque (1231) which may then appear abnormal particularly in children. Unless requested otherwise, the X-ray exposure is made at the end of normal inspiration. It is important to have a full normal inspiration and not either a forced or only partial inspiration.

A brief explanation to the patient, with a rehearsal of the procedure, is essential for a satisfactory result. The breathing procedure may need to be repeated several times before it is considered to be satisfactory. With the patient in full inspiration a few moments should be allowed to elapse before the exposure is made to ensure stability. With modern equipment the risk of movement blurring is minimised by using exposures in the region of 0·01 sec.

On inspiration there is a tendency to raise the shoulders, which should be avoided, as the shadows of the clavicles then obscure the lung apices (1232).

Positioning

Chest radiographs are normally done with the patient in the erect position. Only in very ill patients, or those who are immobile are films taken in the horizontal or semi-erect position. Patient positioning is greatly simplified when the patient is erect and it is also easier to see that the film is being exposed in inspiration. The gravity effect on the abdominal organs, particularly the liver, makes the lung fields larger and in the erect position fluid levels are more easily shown.

The postero-anterior position is preferred to the antero-posterior because the scapulae can be projected clear of the lung fields and there is less magnification of the heart and aorta. A considerable part of the lung fields are obscured by the heart and the diaphragm and it is therefore frequently necessary to also take a lateral radiograph of the chest. The additional projections which may be required include antero-posterior, right and left laterals, right and left antero-posterior or postero-anterior obliques, and the view taken in the lordotic position. Special projections for lung apices and in the decubitus position for fluid levels may also be required.

14

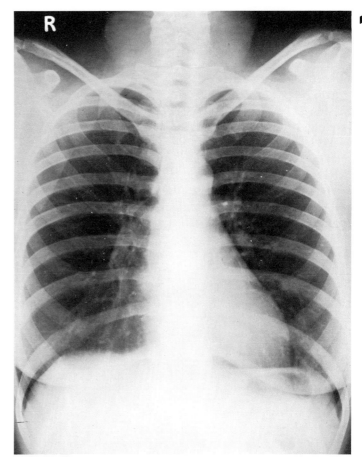

CLAVICLES RAISED
1232

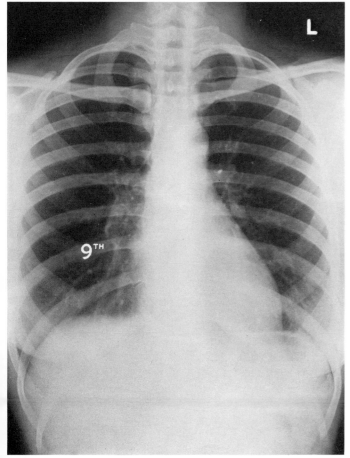

INSPIRATION ERECT
1230

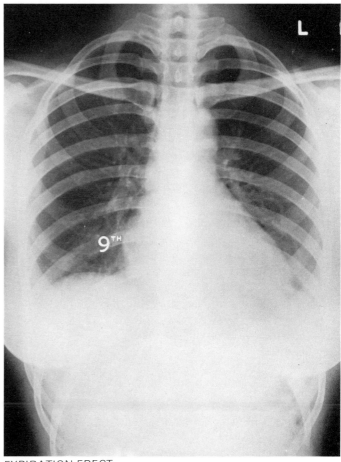

EXPIRATION ERECT
1231

Choice of kilovoltage

There is no single ideal radiographic technique for the respiratory system. Low kilovoltage films (60 to 70 kvp) show the lung fields with maximum contrast needed especially for small soft tissue densities and are best for demonstrating miliary tuberculosis. However, for large patients, and to demonstrate the mediastinum, a high kilovoltage technique (130 to 200 kvp) is preferable. Although high kilovoltage films give good penetration, showing the lung bases, the paravertebral soft tissues, and the lung fields behind the heart, there is loss of inherent contrast in these films. Small lesions of soft tissue density become difficult to see and may even be obliterated entirely.

To show the lung behind the heart, the lung bases posteriorly, and the paravertebral regions with a low kilovoltage technique the exposure factors must be increased and then the film will be relatively over-exposed for the remainder of the lung fields. Some patients will require two postero-anterior radiographs with different exposures for a complete examination of the lung fields.

Maintaining general contrast

The tendency toward the use of higher kilovoltages and the use of grids to reduce the effect of scattered radiation has increased considerably, mainly due to the introduction of very fine-line grids that can be used stationary without the grid lines obscuring lung detail. It is thus no longer necessary to move the grid at a speed for ultra short exposure times, greatly simplifying the use of such grids. A range of kilovoltage 90–120 kVp, mid-way between non-grid and high kilovoltage has developed as a compromise between the advantages and disadvantages of the two techniques.

Alternative methods to the use of grids to eliminate scatter are selective filtration and the use of sheet tin 8/1000 inch thick placed on the front surface of the cassette to improve general contrast up to 100 kVp.

Air-gap Technique

This technique employs an air gap between the subject and the film of approximately 15 cm (6 ins). To accommodate the increased subject-film distance which would otherwise produce more geometric unsharpness the focus-film distance must be increased to 300 cm (10 ft). With the air gap technique the oblique scattered rays from the subject no longer fall on the film. This technique requires a suitable patient support which is 15 cm (6 ins) away from the cassette holder.

Relative exposures at varying kilovoltage

Postero-Anterior
Focus-film distance 180 cm (72 ins)
75 kVp–16mAS
100kVp–5mAS
150kVp–2mAS

Magnification factor
Focus-film distance

For minimal magnification of the intra thoracic structures, especially the heart, chest films are taken in the postero-anterior position at a focus-film distance of 150 cm (60 ins) to 180 cm (72 ins). However the focus-film distance must be kept constant for any particular department to minimize the magnification distortion with minimal variations from day to day. Sharp films are obtained with the use of small foci (0·6 mm) and fast high definition screens provided there is no subject movement. Where very low kilovoltage films are attempted (under 60 kVp) the increased exposure time may cause unsharpness due to movement blurring from cardiac pulsation. Decreasing the focus-film distance in an attempt to decrease exposure time will result in magnification distortion particularly of the heart shadow. A preferred alternative to reducing the FFD is to use rare earth screens which can diminish the exposure by a factor of 4 or 5.

The output of modern mobile units has increased considerably and can now produce chest radiographs which compare favourably with those taken on static departmental units. In modern hospitals patients are moved on mobile beds to the X-ray department where high quality radiographs can be obtained and the use of mobile units should be confined to patients in intensive care or coronary care units (ITU, CCU) or those patients on the ward who are too ill to come to the main department.

Wherever possible, even with mobile units, a postero-anterior projection should be obtained. Frequently in the ITU and CCU unit however the radiograph must be taken in the antero-posterior position.

Exposure time related to subject movement

To avoid movement blurring due to involuntary movements on the part of the patient, especially children, exposure times must be kept as low as possible and should at least be in the millisecond range. Adequate exposures with short exposure times can be obtained with modern 3 phase units using the higher mA settings and taking the film screen speed into account when using conventional kilovoltages (60–70kVp). With high kilovoltage settings short exposure times are no problem provided a unit is used which has accurate timing for short exposures. These units have the added advantage of operating within the rating of smaller foci.

Films taken with a high kilovoltage technique have less contrast and more penetration compared with those done using a low kilovoltage technique.

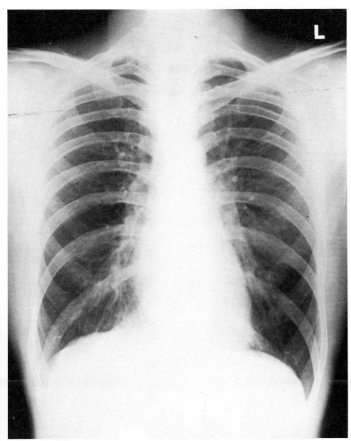

72 INCHES

1233

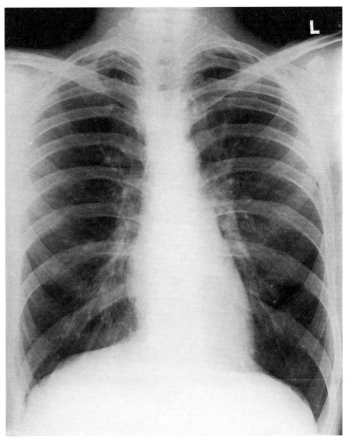

30 INCHES

1234

Uniformity

Using radiographic equipment with automatic exposure control and automatic processing, films of comparable good quality can be obtained for serial examinations and results in the minimum of repeat examinations with a saving in cost and radiation dose to the population at large.

However, even without automatic exposure control, comparable and good quality films can be produced by attention to detail particularly if the postero-anterior diameter of the chest is measured before the exposure factors are chosen. In assessing the exposure factors the variation between men and women is particularly important. A simple method of calculating the required exposure is to relate chest thickness measurement to kilovoltage which produces greater comparability of chest radiographs; for example, if for an average thickness of $22\frac{1}{2}$ cm (9 ins) 67·5 kVp is used at a particular mAs setting then, for each increase of 1 cm, in measured thickness the kilovoltage should be increased by 2·5 kVp.

Radiographic protection

For chest radiography a rectangular adjustable diaphragm is essential and must be used in every case to limit the area of irradiation, taking care however not to exclude any part of the lung fields especially the costophrenic angles. The circular cone has no place in the basic projections of the lung fields because the costophrenic angles are frequently coned off and in the midline the primary beam extends down to the pelvis.

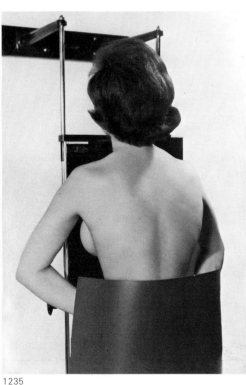

1235

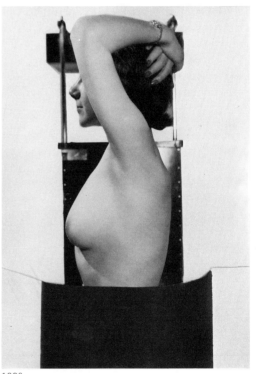

1236

For all projections of the thorax an adjustable mobile lead protective screen should be used to shield the part of the back below the lung fields (1235, 1236).

Intensifying screens

Nearly 90 % of the radographic image is from fluorescence from the intensifying screens and the remainder from direct radiation. The intensifying screens therefore play a major part in the quality of the image. Without intensifying screens it would be impossible to use low enough exposure times to eliminate movement blurring. For the same focal spot size and FFD the faster intensifying screens produce more screen unsharpness. On very fast film/screen systems quantum mottle may occur. However as movement unsharpness due to breathing and heart movement can be a problem when X-raying the chest, the majority of departments use standard film with fast intensifying screens.

With a large focus film distance there will be less penumbra and this can be further reduced by using a small focal spot (0·3–0·6 mm).

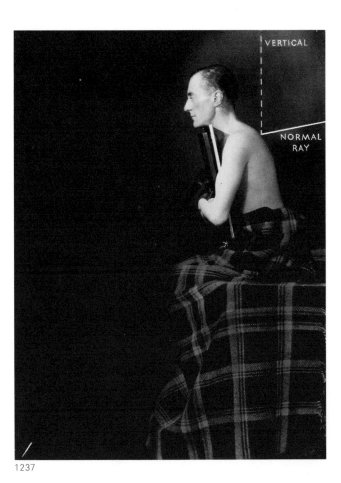

1237

The speed ratio for the different types of intensifying screens are as follows:

Fast Tungstate —3
Standard —1·5
High Definition —1

and this facilitates easy adjustment of the exposure when changing screens.

Where low output units are being used or when patient movement cannot be controlled the use of rare earth screens is an advantage. Rare earth screens are considerably faster than conventional intensifying screens often by a factor of 4 or 5.

When using a high kilovoltage technique it may be an advantage to use only a single back screen which produces a sharper image.

Good film/screen contact is essential, particularly in chest radiography, to eliminate added unsharpness. Cassettes must be regularly tested for contact, inspected for damage which may cause artefacts on the film and cleaned according to the manufacturers instructions.

Identification

Clear and accurate identification labels on chest radiographs are essential. Radiographs must be marked with the patient's name, hospital number, date of examination and also as to right or left sides. Congenital transposition of the organs occurs sufficiently often so that without a correct right or left marker the condition may be misdiagnosed.

Bedside cassette support

A chest-rest, particularly adaptable for examinations in the ward, is of simple design. It consists of a prop 145 cm (56 ins) in length, having a pointed ferrule at one end to prevent slipping. At the opposite end, fixed by means of a hinge, a thin rectangular piece of wood is fitted with an adjustable ledge to hold the cassette (1237).

Pharynx, Larynx, Trachea

Lateral Erect

To radiograph the soft tissues of the neck including the pharynx, larynx, and upper trachea the patient is erect or seated in the lateral position with the cassette at shoulder level. The chin should be comfortably flexed to show the larynx to best advantage. The arms should be in a relaxed position by the side of the body and the patient is asked to say "E" during the exposure to allow air to distent the trachea and larynx. A low kilovoltage, in the region of 75 kVp, should be used to obtain maximum contrast of the soft tissues.

■ Centre to the cricoid cartilage (1238, 1244)

The lateral (thoracic inlet)

To show the whole of the trachea from the lower pharynx to its bifurcation, the patient is placed in the lateral position using a 24 × 30 cm (12 × 10 inch) cassette to include the whole area. The arms are clasped behind the back and the shoulders pulled backward to prevent the densities of the shoulders from overlying the trachea. The film is taken on inspiration.

■ Centre to the sternal notch (1239, 1240)

Anterior-posterior thoracic inlet

With the patient erect or supine on the Bucky couch, the chin is raised to show the soft tissues below the mandible.

■ Centre in the midline to the sternal notch (1241)

Postero-anterior erect thoracic inlet

With the patient erect and facing the cassette the chin is raised so the soft tissues of the neck can be shown.

■ Centre in the midline at the level of the second thoracic vertebra (1242, 1243)

The trachea is shown in all chest radiographs but will be underexposed if the exposure is correct for lung tissue unless a high kV technique is used.

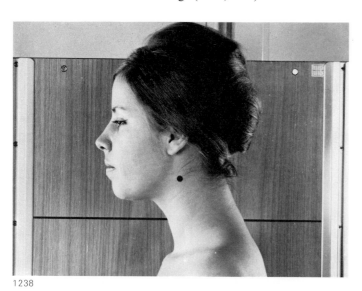

1238

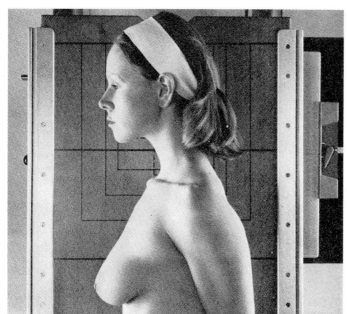

354

1239

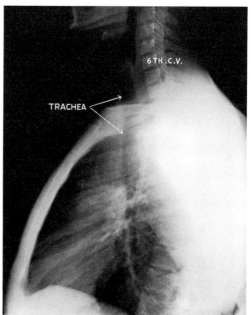

1240

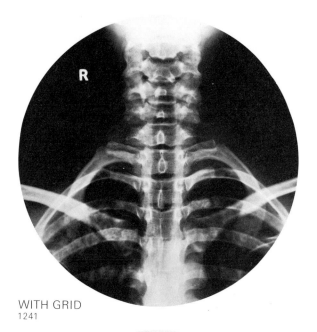

WITH GRID
1241

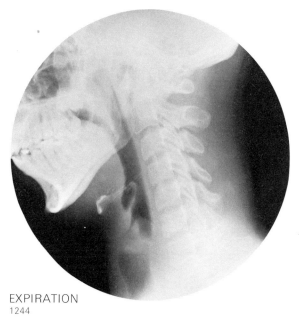

EXPIRATION
1244

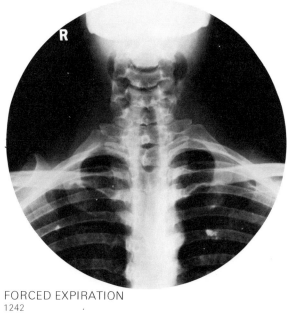

FORCED EXPIRATION
1242

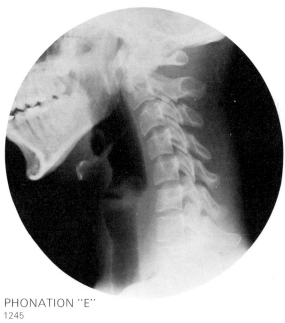

PHONATION "E"
1245

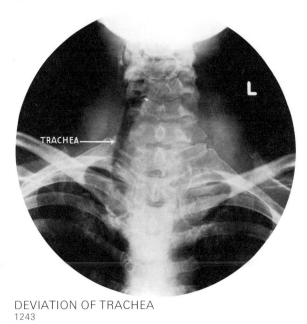

DEVIATION OF TRACHEA
1243

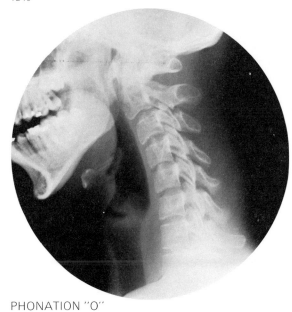

PHONATION "O"
1246

Lungs

Postero-anterior erect

With the patient erect, facing the cassette, and the shoulders level the chin is raised and in the middle of the top of the cassette. The shoulders are rotated forward and pressed downward to make contact with the cassette. This is achieved by either allowing the arms to encircle the cassette (1249), or rotating the arms medially from the shoulder joints bringing the hands and forearms forward against the sides of the chest stand or the buttocks (1250). Either one of these methods will effectively displace the scapulae laterally away from the lung field. The shoulders should not be raised, or the apices will be obscured by the clavicles.

Where the density of the breasts obscure the lower lung their shadow can be removed by the patient raising her breasts in the erect position (1251), or in the prone position by pressure on the breasts causing lateral diffusion of the breast shadows (1252).

■ Centre in the midline to the sternal angle, through the fourth thoracic vertebra. Films are taken on full inspiration (1247, 1249)

Note—films may be required in both inspiration and expiration particularly to distinguish between an opacity in a rib or in the lung or to demonstrate a small pneumothorax. The films should be clearly labelled "inspiration" and "expiration". To maintain similar density on the expiration film, the kilovoltage should be increased by 7 kVp.

Adequate Penetration

In larger patients with increased chest thickness or when the lung is obscured by pathology an increased exposure is required. This is best done by increasing the kilovoltage to obtain the necessary penetration and uniformity rather than by increasing mAs.

Note—2 radiographs of the same subject show (1247) ideal positioning with the shadows of the scapulae displaced outside the lung field whereas in (1248) the scapulae obscure the outer parts of the upper lobes. Obviously the latter positioning technique is unsatisfactory.

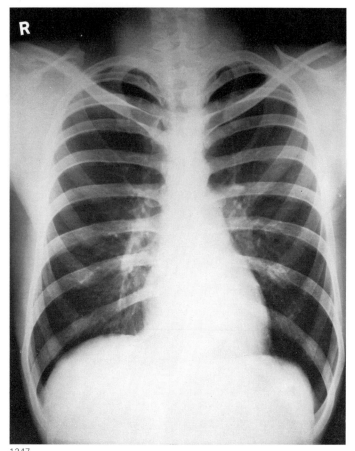

1247

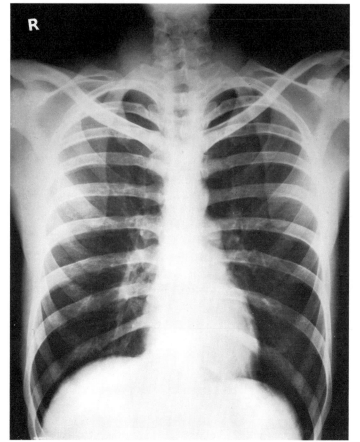

1248

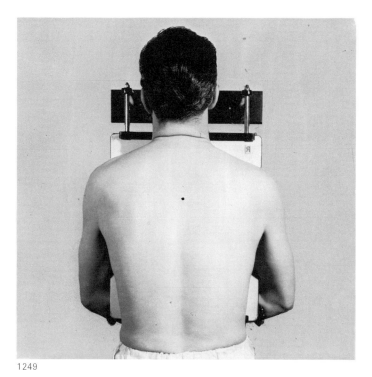

1249

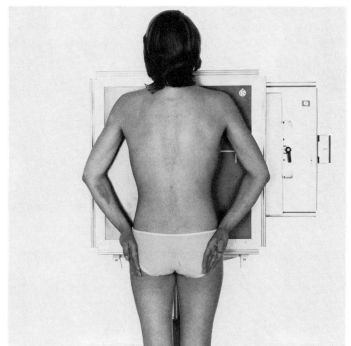

1250

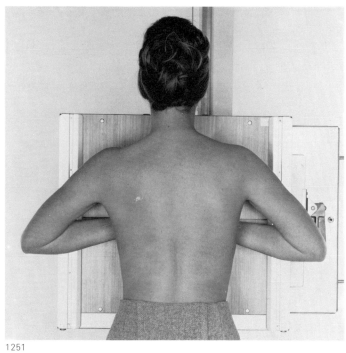

1251

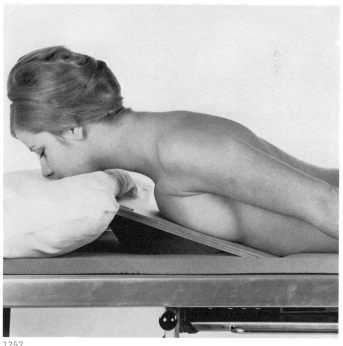

1252

14 Antero-posterior

With the patient erect and facing the tube, the shoulders are level and the chin raised. The shoulders are brought forward and downward, with the backs of the hands below the hips and the elbows well forward.

■ Centre in the midline at the level of the sternal notch and expose on inspiration as previously (1253, 1254, 1255)

For **Exposure Factors** see page 370.

Comparing the antero-posterior view (1255) with the postero-anterior view (1256), on the antero-posterior view the medial ends of the clavicles are at a higher level and the apices of the lungs are shown below and behind the medial half of the clavicles. It is also more difficult to get the spaculae away from the lung fields and the anterior ends of the ribs are magnified.

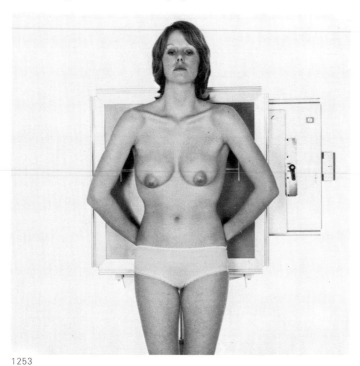

1253

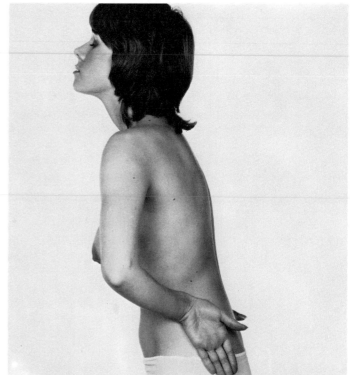

1254

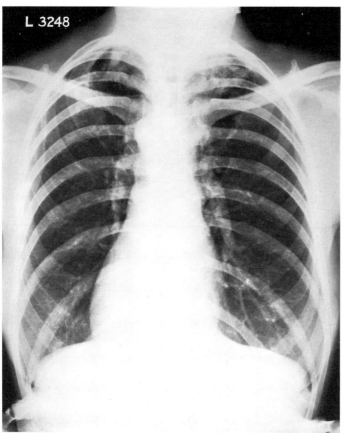

ANTERO-POSTERIOR
1255

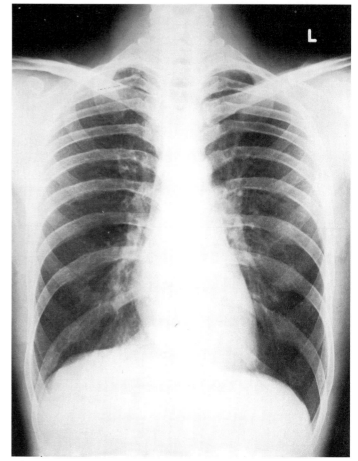

POSTERO-ANTERIOR
1256

The Antero-posterior view is used as an additional projection for the lung fields particularly when a small nodular shadow is being investigated. The nodular shadow is often clear of the ribs on the antero-posterior projection when there is super-imposition on the postero-anterior view.

Apices

For the apices the following projections may be used:

(1) With the patient erect in a postero-anterior position, the tube is angled 40° downward and centred in the midline at the level of the apices (1257, 1260).

(2) With the patient erect in the antero-posterior position, the tube is angled 30° upward and centred in the midline below the level of the clavicles (1258, 1261).

(3) With the patient reclining, the nape of the neck resting on the upper border of the cassette and the upper part of the thorax in contact with the film holder, the tube is centred in the midline at the level of the mid sternum (1259, 1262). This projection is commonly called the lordotic view.

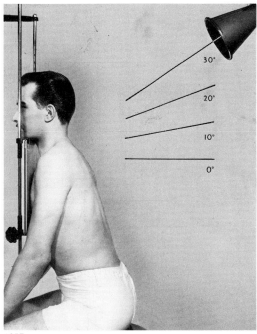

1257

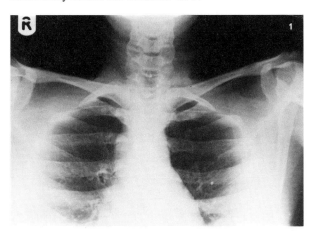

1

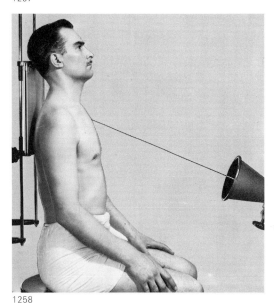

1258

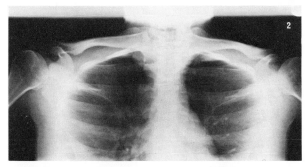

2

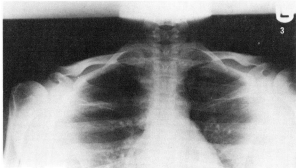

3

1260/1261/1262

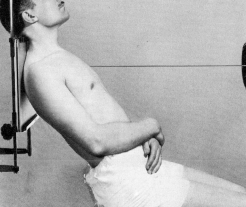

1259

Note—these views must be done with a rectangular collimator to obtain the appropriate exposure field.

Antero-posterior—Arm raised
With the arm raised to lift the clavicle above the apex of the lung, the patient turns slightly toward the affected side.
■ Centre below the clavicle (1263, 1265, 1267)

Two pairs of radiographs taken under standard conditions (1264, 1266) and using the above technique, (1265, 1267) illustrate the value of this projection. It is obvious, however, that for both subjects raising the arm is the important factor. Both lesions were detected originally during a mass chest survey using 35-millimetre film.

Lateral—basic
The lateral projection is essential to localize a lesion to a segment or lobe of the lung (1271, 1272).

It is usually necessary to use a grid for the lateral projection to reduce scattered radiation particularly in large subjects; scattered radiation, which occurs without using a grid, has the effect of obscuring lung detail.

With the patient erect and the arms folded above the head (1268), or brought well forward beside the head (1269), the patient is in the lateral position with the affected side in contact with the cassette. The medial sagittal plane must be parallel to the film, this should be checked from the posterior aspect of the patient.
■ Centre through the lower end of the axilla midway between the front and the back of the chest (1268, 1269)

Lateral radiographs are usually viewed by the radiologist in the position in which they are taken and should be labelled accordingly although many text books including this one are still not consistent in using this convention.

With the above centring the diaphragm is normally shown as two separate distinct shadows lying parallel one above the other (1272).

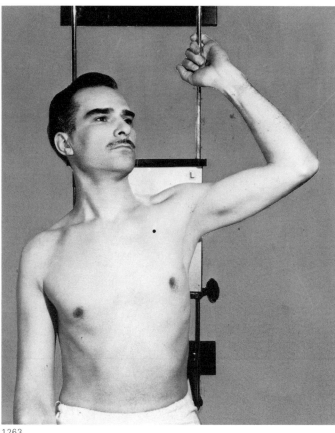

1263

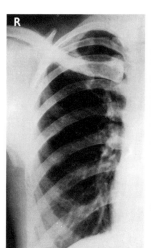
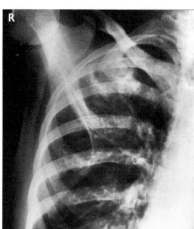

1264/1265

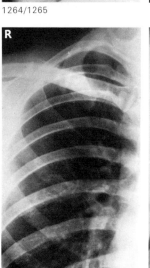
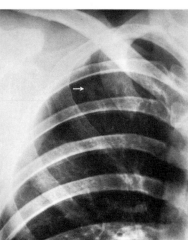

1266/1267

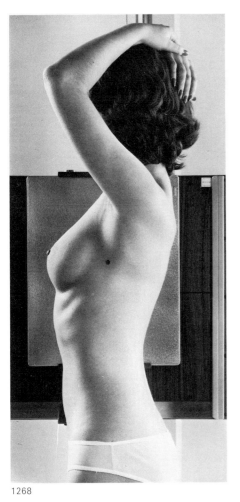

1268

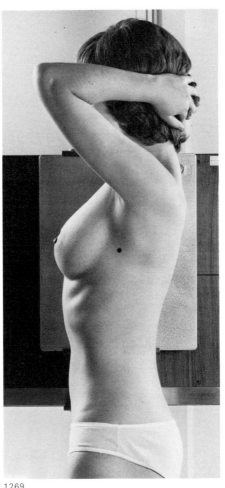

1269

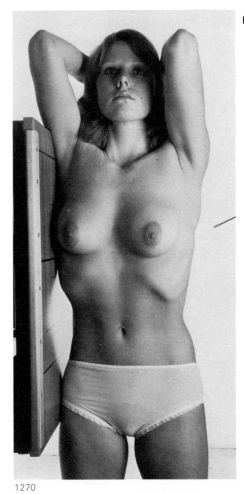

1270

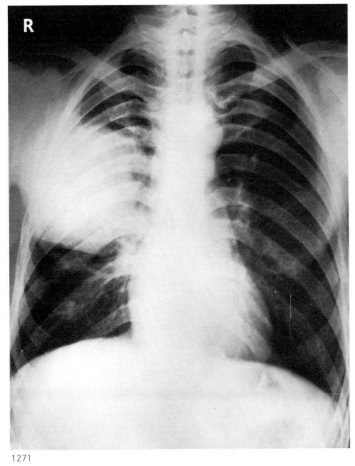

1271

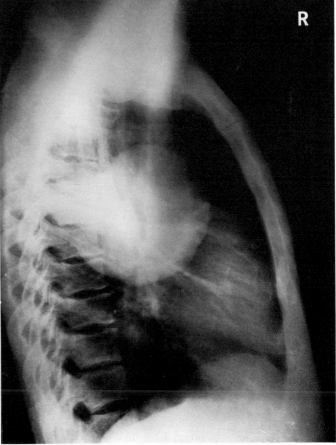

1272

Lateral-apices

With the patient erect in the lateral position, and the axilla of the affected side toward the film, the arm is folded above the head with the opposite arm resting beside the trunk. The trunk is bent slightly at the waist away from the film.

■ Centre above the shoulder of the side nearest the tube with the tube angled 20° toward the feet (1273, 1274a, b)

Lateral for a posterior apical lesion

To show a lesion lying posteriorly in the apex of the lung the following technique can be used.

With the patient erect in the lateral position the arms are rotated internally to bring the scapula well forward with the posterior aspects of the hands touching in front of the patient; the neck should be flexed and there should also be slight flexion of the trunk.

■ Centre behind the shoulders (1275, 1276)

Lateral retro-sternal area (thymus)

To show lesions in the anterior part of the apex of the lung and in the retro-sternal space the following technique can be used.

With the patient erect in the lateral position the shoulders are drawn backward with the arms extended and the hands clasped low down over the buttocks.

■ Centre in the anterior third of the chest behind the sternum (1277, 1278)

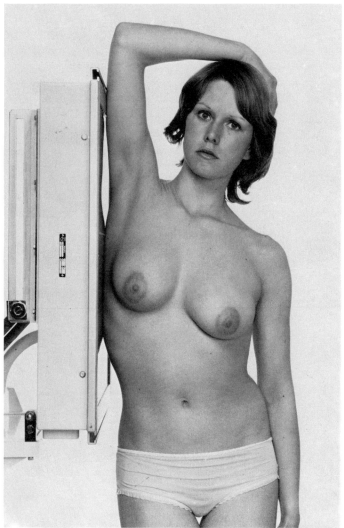

1273

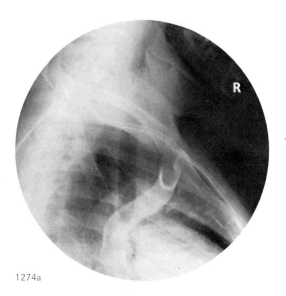

1274a

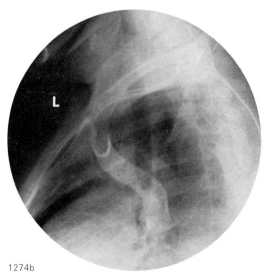

1274b

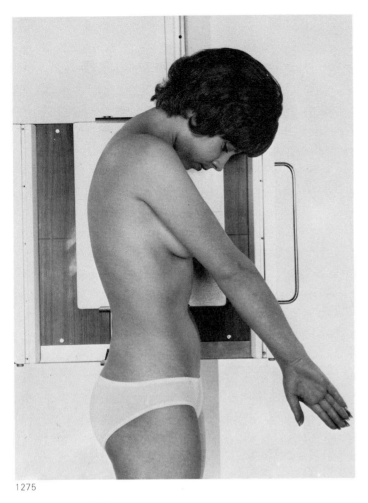

1275

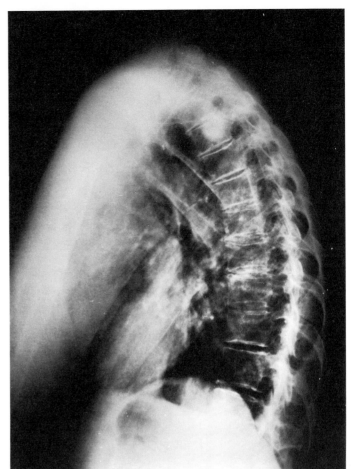

14

1276

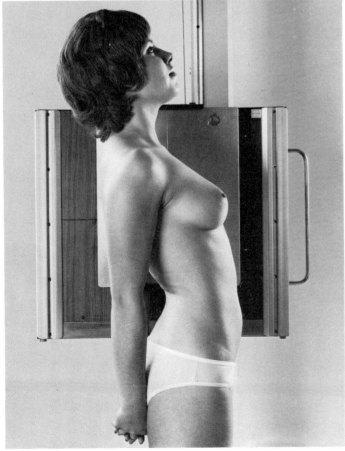

1277

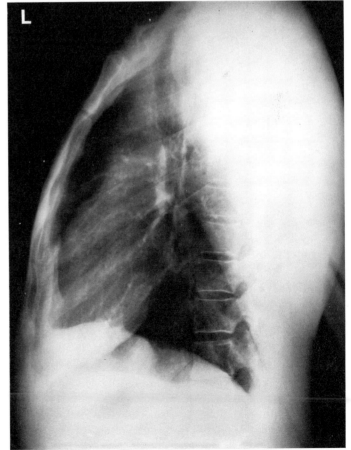

L

1278

363

Bed patients

To examine a patient in bed, usually in the Intensive Therapy Unit (ITU), presents problems both in positioning and exposure. Nevertheless it is essential to obtain radiographs of good quality because serial films are required on these patients. Unless the quality is comparable to departmental films comparison with previous examinations is not possible.

Antero-posterior

Where possible the patient should be semi-erect, support the cassette at the correct level by inserting a sandbag or pillow at the base of the back. Rotate the arms medially to move the scapulae clear of the lung field. Allow the neck to extend over the upper border of the cassette and support the head on a pillow.

■ Centre in the midline at the level of the sternal angle with the tube adjusted to direct the central ray at right angles to the cassette (1279)

Lateral

With the arms raised above the head, place the cassette against the lateral aspect of the chest, supported in position with sandbags and pillows.

■ Centre to the lower end of the axilla with the tube in the horizontal position and directed at right angles to the cassette (1280)

Pleural effusion

For small pleural effusions not readily visible on the erect postero-anterior (basic) projection, the decubitus position (1284), with the patient lying on the affected side, is used.

Large pleural effusions obscure the adjacent lung and pleura. For an adequate view of these regions the fluid must be aspirated but they can be shown to a limited extent by doing a penetrated view or by a decubitus projection. For the lateral chest wall the decubitus position is done with the patient lying on the sound side (1285); to show the lung fields the decubitus view is done with the patient supine (1287); and to show the mediastinal region the patient must have a decubitus view lying on the affected side.

Fluid levels

A horizontal ray is required to show fluid levels and is therefore best done with the patient erect (1281, 1282). However, where the position of the patient does not allow erect projections, films are taken with the patient horizontal using a horizontal ray (1285, 1287).

Both fluid and air may be present in the pleural cavity (hydro-pneumothorax) and can be shown in the erect (1282, 1283) and horizontal (1284, 1285, 1286, 1287) projections. In the erect position the upper part of the pleural cavity will be shown clear of fluid whereas in the lateral decubitus position with the patient lying on the opposite side the whole of the lateral pleural margin will be shown clear of fluid (1285). Similarly to show the anterior aspect of the pleura in its entirety, the patient should be supine using a horizontal ray (1286, 1287).

An abscess cavity with a fluid level is shown in (1281).

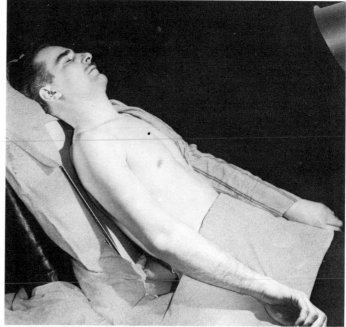
1279

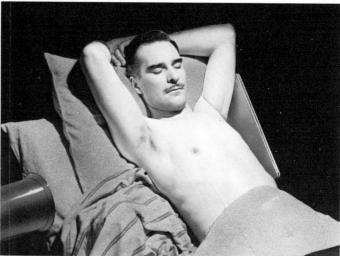
1280

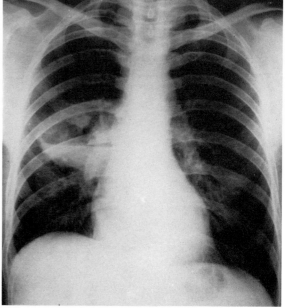
1281

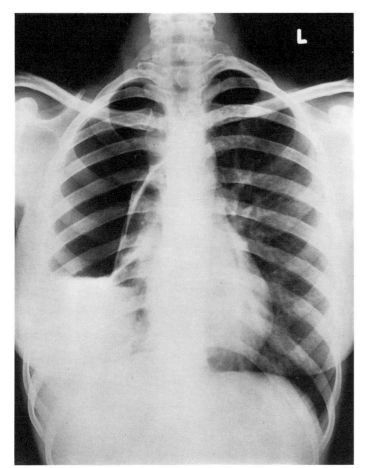

POSTERO-ANTERIOR ERECT
1282

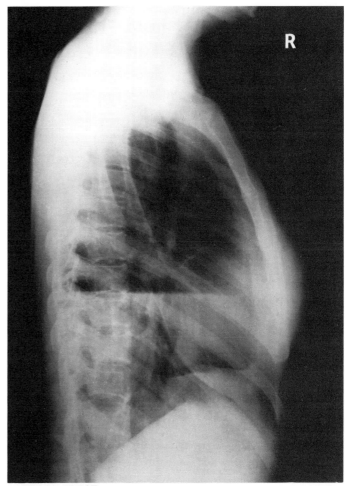

LATERAL ERECT
1283

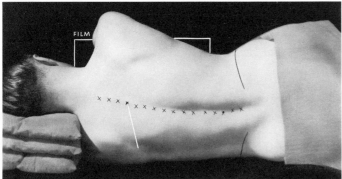

1284

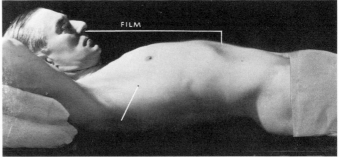

1286

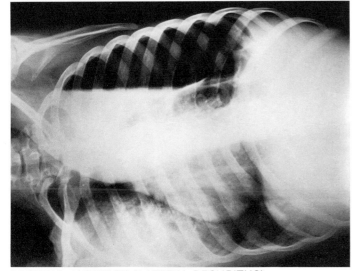

POSTERO-ANTERIOR (LATERAL DECUBITUS)
1285

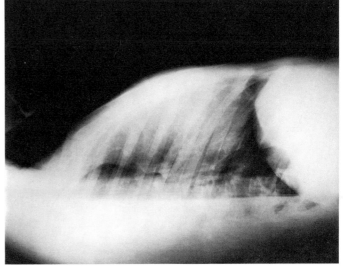

LATERAL (DORSAL DECUBITUS)
1287

Oblique

The right and left oblique projections are taken to show the mediastinum and lung fields. These projections are particularly valuable for the pleural edge and are essential in the diagnosis of asbestosis. For patients with heavy breast shadows the antero-posterior oblique position should be used.

Right anterior (first) oblique

With the patient erect the right shoulder is placed in contact with and the left shoulder rotated away from the cassette until the thorax is at an angle of approximately 45° to the film. The arms are moved away from the trunk not to obscure the lung fields.

■ Centre over the medial margin of the left scapula, at the level of the fifth thoracic vertebra (1288, 1289, 1290, 1291)

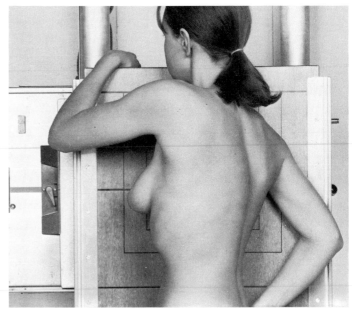

1288

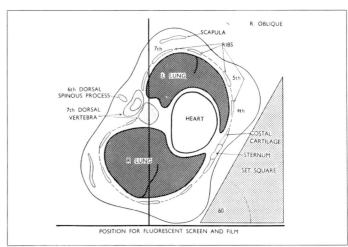

1289

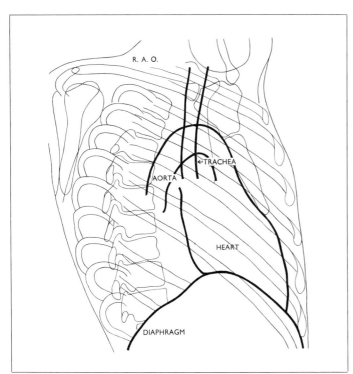

1290

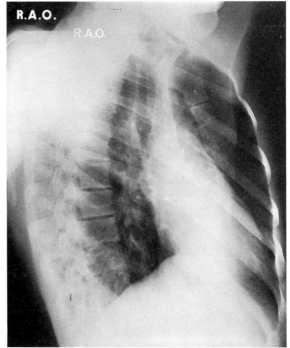

RIGHT ANTERIOR OBLIQUE
1291

Left anterior (second) oblique

With the patient erect the left shoulder is placed in contact with and the right side is rotated away from the cassette until the thorax is at an angle of approximately 45° to the film. Position the arms away from the trunk preferably as in (1292).

■ Centre over the medial border of the right scapula at the level of the fifth thoracic vertebra (1292, 1293, 1294, 1295)

For **Exposure Factors** see page 374.

Use the line diagrams (1290, 1294), for identification of the structures shown on the radiographs (1291, 1295).

Modified oblique

The obliquity of the patient may be modified to show lesions which are at the periphery of the lungs and may vary from 30° to 70°.

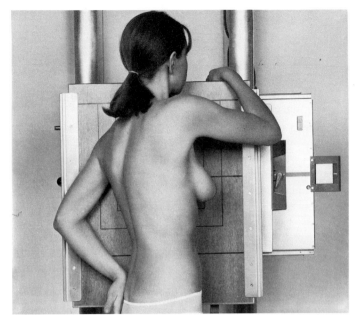

1292

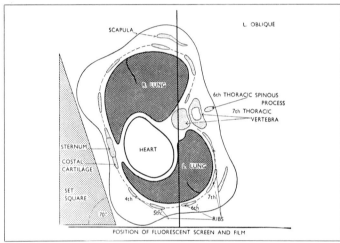

1293

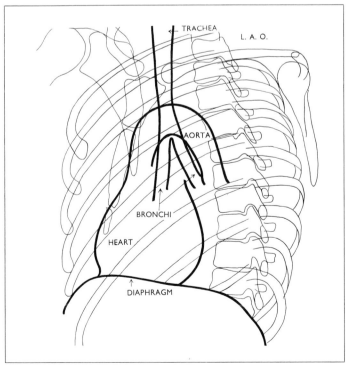

1294

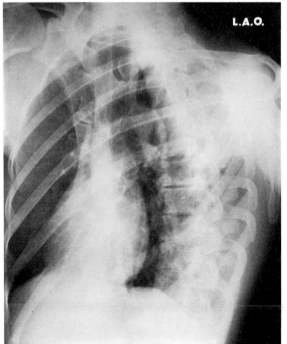

LEFT ANTERIOR OBLIQUE

1295

367

Left and right antero-posterior oblique

The antero-posterior oblique should be used in patients with large breast shadows.

With the patient erect, from the antero-posterior position rotate the patient 45° keeping the affected chest wall in contact with the film holder. The exposure should be made in full inspiration.

■ Centre over the mid sternum (1296)

Lordotic

This view is used to show right middle lobe collapse or an interlobar pleural effusion.

With the patient erect in the postero-anterior position and holding the back of the vertical Bucky, the patient bends backwards from the waist as shown in (1297). The degree of dorsiflexion for each subject varies but in general a 30° inclination is satisfactory. The tube is centred in the midline over the fourth thoracic vertebra (1297, 1299).

Alternative positioning

A similar result can be obtained with the patient in the antero-posterior position and reclining backward to enable the nape of the neck to rest against the upper border of the cassette. The tube is centred 6 cm (3 ins) below the clavicles (1298).

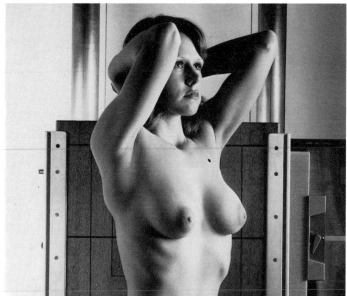

1296

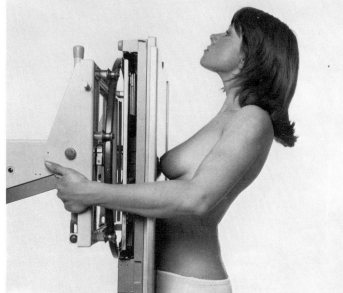

1297

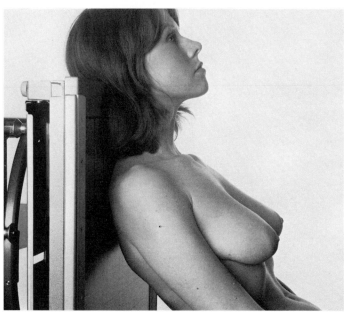

1298

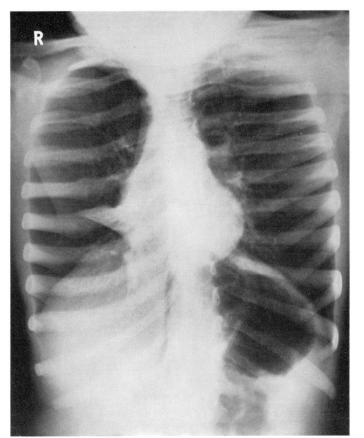

Penetrated views for the mediastinum

The mediastinal structures can only be shown using adequate penetration and is especially required for pericardial calcification and for tumours containing calcium (1300, 1301).

Radiographs (1300, 1301) show a tumour called a Teratoma which contains multiple, not quite fully formed teeth.

LORDOTIC POSITION
1299

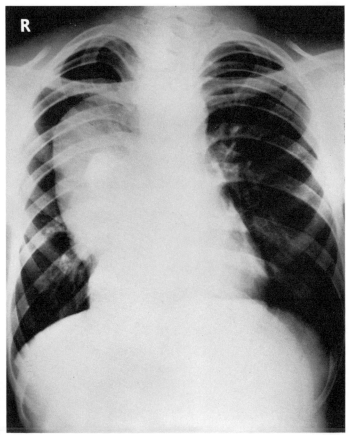

1300

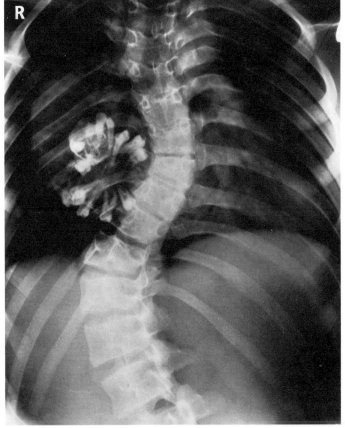

1301

Bronchography

Bronchography is the examination for demonstrating bronchi by contrast medium and is now used to a considerably less extent than in previous years because of the lower incidence of bronchiectasis.

Bronchiectasis is a condition of dilatation of the bronchi associated with infection and accumulation of purulent sputum. The lessened incidence is probably due to the control of childhood infections, particularly whooping-cough.

The contrast medium generally used in bronchography is dionosil which comes in two forms, a water soluble (aqueous) and an oily variety. The oily variety is preferred because it is less irritating. The examination is always preceded by plain films of the thorax, particularly postero-anterior and lateral projections which should be darker than the routine chest radiographs, the kilovoltage being increased by 10 to 15 kVp. A grid is normally used for this examination.

The contrast medium may be introduced either through a tube which is threaded through the nose and pharynx into the trachea and positioned with fluoroscopy to lie in the trachea above the level of the carina or by a needle directly into the trachea through the crico-thyroid ligament

The contrast medium is injected in small amounts with the patient assuming various positions to fill the appropriate bronchi. When a bilateral bronchogram is done the right side is examined first with a postero-anterior and a lateral radiograph. Then the left side is examined using a postero-anterior and an **oblique** radiograph. Before the catheter is positioned in the trachea local anaesthetic is used to anaesthetise the mucosa. The patient must therefore not have anything to swallow for at least 4 hours after the examination or there will be a danger of inhalation of fluid or food into the bronchi. Immediately after the examination the patient is sent to the physiotherapy department for postural drainage to encourage coughing up of the residual contrast medium from the bronchi.

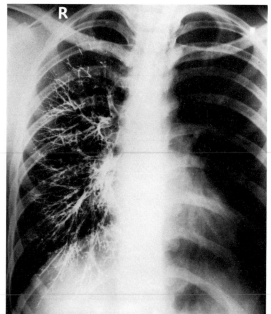

1302

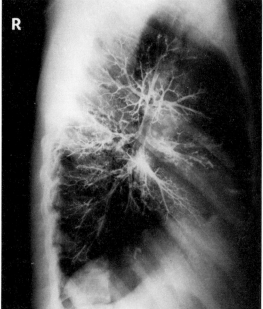

1303

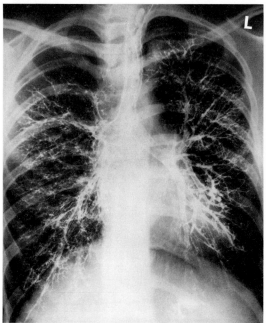

1304

Films are taken on inspiration, usually erect and the patient must not be coughing.

When carrying out bilateral bronchography the following views are taken.
(1) postero-anterior for the right side (1302).
(2) right lateral for the right side (1303).
(3) postero-anterior of both sides (1304).
(4) left antero-posterior oblique for the left side (1305).

With the contrast medium in the bronchi greater penetration is needed; the kilovoltage is increased by 10 to 15 kVp compared with a routine chest radiograph and a grid is normally used.

The radiographer should realize that there is only a limited time in which to take the films before the patient starts to cough up the contrast medium. It is therefore most important to have everything prepared, the cassette in position, a sufficient number of cassettes available, the tube centred correctly and the exposure, based upon the preliminary plain films, noted down.

The procedure is similar in children and an example of a unilateral bronchogram in a child which proved to be normal is shown in the 3 positions for the right lung, postero-anterior (1306), lateral (1307), right antero-posterior oblique (1308).

Important—The patient should be warned against taking either food or fluid for four hours after the examination until the effect of the local anaesthetic has disappeared.

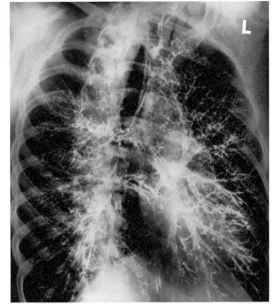

1305

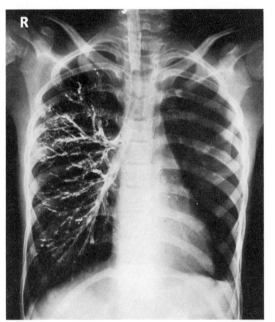

1306

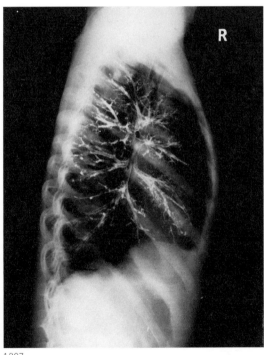

1307

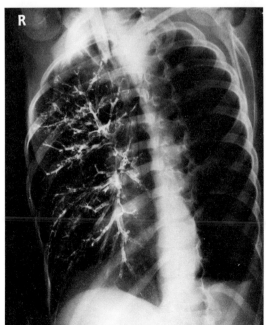

1308

The half-way filter

Although it is possible to use a 3 to 8 millimetre aluminium filter over the normal lung for patients with marked opacification of the abnormal lung, it is more usual to have two separate radiographs; a penetrated view for the hemi-thorax with the large radio density and a normal exposure for the unaffected lung. However radiograph (1309) shows the appearance using a 7 millimetre aluminium filter which produces the line down the centre of the film demarcating the normal side from the abnormal unfiltered side and shows a thoracoplasty done for the treatment of tuberculosis.

Pneumoconiosis

Pneumoconiosis is the term applied to inhalation dust diseases occurring not only in miners but in many other industrial workers as well such as pottery workers and those exposed to asbestos. In the early stages very fine shadowing is seen on the radiograph requiring a film of maximum sharpness and contrast for early detection of the disease. These workers require periodic examinations and a high degree of uniformity in the radiographs is needed for accurate comparison. The fine nodular opacities occurring in pneumoconiosis is shown in the chest radiograph (1310), made more obvious by a macrograph showing a × 1·5 enlargement (1311).

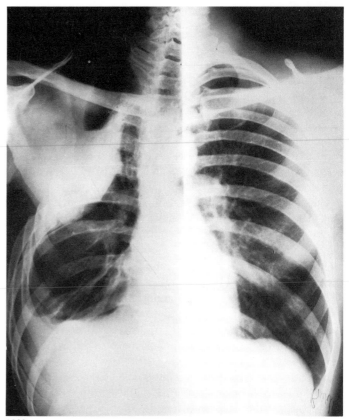

1309

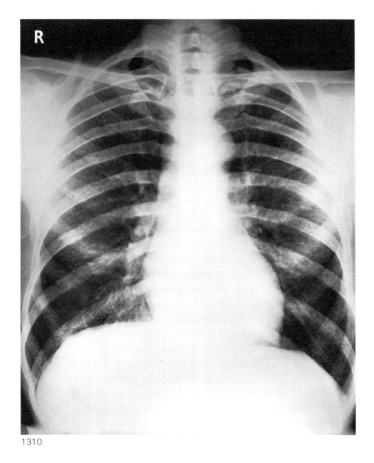

1310

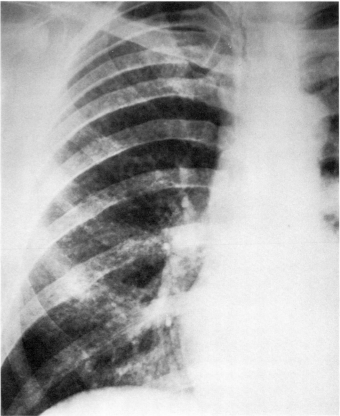

1311

Children

Young children are more easily radiographed in the supine position but the tube must be centred, the exposure factors set for a short exposure time, the tube must be in position and the diaphragm correctly collimated before finally placing the child in the correct position.

The radiographs (1312, 1313) of a child show consolidation in the medial segment of the right middle lobe.

Thymus

In young children the shadow of the thymus produces apparent widening of the superior mediastinum.

The two lobes of the thymus gland extend from the level of the seventh cervical to the sixth thoracic vertebra (1314). Although the thymus increases in size during childhood until puberty, its relative size decreases when compared with the rest of the thorax. After the age of 2 it is no longer as prominent on a chest radiograph. In young children it not infrequently produces a "sail-shaped" shadow on the right side of the mediastinum. When air enters into the mediastinal cavity (pneumomediastinum) the thymus becomes visible in both the frontal and lateral views.

In the adult, the thymus is best shown on fluoroscopy taking spot films in various degrees of obliquity. The thymus lies in the anterior mediastinum and when a lateral projection is done it must be taken with the shoulders drawn backward, the arms extended and the hands clasped behind the buttocks (1277, page 363)

Lateral tomography is also used usually to show thymic tumours.

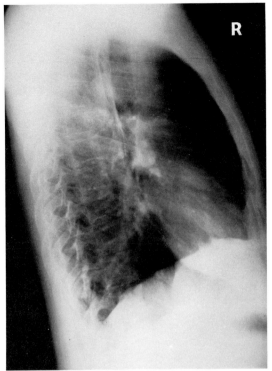

1313

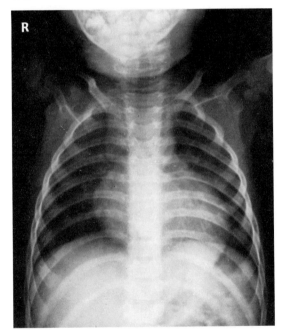

1314

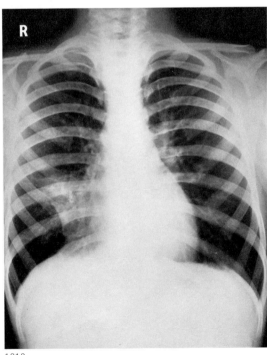

1312

A summary of exposure conditions for the respiratory system suitable for an adult of average physique, with two exposures for a child of six years

Region	Position	kVp	mAS	FFD		Film ILFORD	Screens ILFORD	Grid
Trachea	Postero–anterior	75	12	180 cm	(72")	RAPID R	FT	—
	Antero–posterior	80	30	100 cm	(40")	RAPID R	FT	Grid
	Lateral, upper	65	12	150 cm	(60")	RAPID R	FT	—
	Lateral, general	80	40	150 cm	(60")	RAPID R	FT	Grid
Lungs	Postero–anterior	65	12	180 cm	(72")	RAPID R	FT	—
	Postero–anterior, penetrated	80	25	150 cm	(60")	RAPID R	FT	Grid
	Antero–posterior	65	12	150 cm	(60")	RAPID R	FT	—
Lung apices	30° antero–posterior	65	15	180 cm	(72")	RAPID R	FT	—
	30° postero–anterior	65	15	180 cm	(72")	RAPID R	FT	—
	Lordotic, antero–posterior	65	15	180 cm	(72")	RAPID R	FT	—
	Antero–posterior, arm raised	70	15	180 cm	(72")	RAPID R	FT	—
	Lateral	85	30	150 cm	(60")	RAPID R	FT	—
Lungs	Lateral, general	80	40	150 cm	(60")	RAPID R	FT	Grid
	Lateral, penetrated	90	40	150 cm	(60")	RAPID R	FT	Grid
	Lateral, arms forward	85	40	150 cm	(60")	RAPID R	FT	Grid
	Lateral, arms back	90	40	150 cm	(60")	RAPID R	FT	Grid
	Oblique, RAO	70	24	150 cm	(60")	RAPID R	FT	—
	Oblique, LAO	70	24	150 cm	(60")	RAPID R	FT	—
	Lordotic	65	15	180 cm	(72")	RAPID R	FT	—
	Lateral	80	40	150 cm	(60")	RAPID R	FT	Grid
Mobile Unit	Antero–posterior	65	15	180 cm	(72")	RAPID R	FT	—
	Lateral	80	40	150 cm	(60")	RAPID R	FT	Stat
Bronchogram	Postero–anterior	80	40	150 cm	(60")	RAPID R	FT	—
	Lateral	90	40	150 cm	(60")	RAPID R	FT	Grid
	Oblique	85	40	150 cm	(60")	RAPID R	FT	Grid
Lungs	Postero–anterior half- lter, 7–mm A1	65	12	150 cm	(60")	RAPID R	FT	—
	Macrogram (X2)	80	12	150 cm	(60")	RAPID R	FT	—
Child six years	Postero–anterior	60	8	180 cm	(72")	RAPID R	FT	—
	Lateral	65	12	150 cm	(60")	RAPID R	FT	—

15

ABDOMEN

SECTION 15

ABDOMEN

Plain films of the abdomen are required in several different circumstances, as a preliminary film before a contrast investigation e.g. barium meal, barium enema, choleycystogram, or intravenous pyelogram or to demonstrate perforation of a hollow viscus, obstruction or ileus and in the investigation of mass lesions.

By and large the abdominal organs and muscles have similar X-ray attenuation or "tissue-densities" and are only distinguished from each other because of their surrounding fat planes. In fact the renal outline is seen only because of the surrounding fatty tissue and even after nephrectomy the "renal outline" can still be seen because the perirenal fatty tissue remains behind.

The organ outlines to be noted are shown in radiograph (1315) and include the liver, spleen, kidney and psoas muscle.

Pathological conditions manifest themselves either because of diminished or increased density and the former is usually due to abnormal gas shadows but can be occasionally associated with excessive accumulation of fatty tissue. The commonest cause of increased density is calcification especially of tuberculous lymph nodes (1316, 1317) but hydatid cysts of the liver (1318, 1319) also calcify as well as uterine fibroids (1320), phleboliths and prostatic calcifications. An unusual cause of pelvic calcification is that found in a dermoid cyst (1321) which contains fully formed teeth and often a surrounding halo of fat.

Abnormalities associated with abnormal low tissue attenuation occur with gas in the biliary tree or pelvi-ureteric system, in the retroperitoneal tissues or abnormal accumulations of gas within the bowel.

Technique

Plain films of the abdomen should be taken using a focus-film distance of 100 cm (40 inch) and Potter-Bucky diaphragm. The kilovoltage should be 65–75 kVp to obtain good contrast between adjacent soft tissues. A short exposure time is essential and ideally should not exceed 0·08 second. This can only be obtained when using rare earth intensifying screens or a 3-phase high output generator. Slight movement blur may obscure essential details particularly gallstones.

The size of film to be used will depend on the size of the patient and the area to be examined but for adult patients a 35 × 43 cm (14 × 17 inch) cassette is usually required. With the patient supine the cassette must be positioned with its lower border below the symphysis pubis to allow for the oblique rays which tend to project the symphysis pubis below the cassette. With the patient erect the cassette must be positioned to include the diaphragm particularly to show free peritoneal gas under the diaphragm. It is also essential to take a chest film in all cases of "acute abdomen". Chest disease particularly pneumonia not infrequently presents as abdominal pain and, not infrequently, a subdiaphragmatic abscess is associated with basal pulmonary shadowing.

Abdominal films are usually taken on expiration but for localising opacities to the kidney comparison films in inspiration and expiration are required.

Gonadal protection is important in abdominal radiography (see section 18) but must not be used, however, for patients with bowel obstruction or "acute abdomen" as abnormal radiological signs may be hidden. The most important aspect of radiation protection, in these patients, is to avoid repeat exposures by obtaining an adequate examination initially.

This section deals with the radiography of the acute abdomen and the demonstration of the supra renal glands, spleen, abdominal aorta, pancreas, liver and diaphragm. Pneumoperitoneum and sinography are also included.

Abdomen AP/Lat.

kVp		mAS			Film	Screens	
AP	Lat	AP	Lat	FFD	ILFORD	ILFORD	Grid
70	80	50	80	100 cm	RAPID R	Fast	Grid

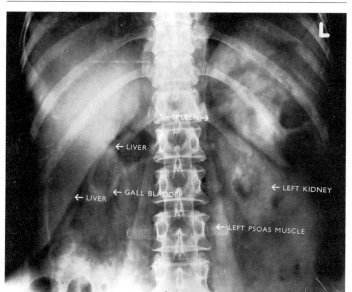

1315

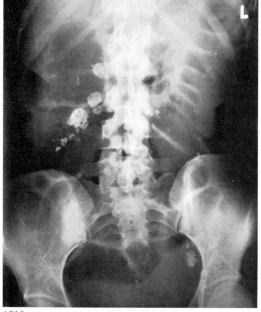

1316

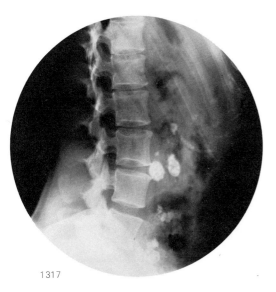

1317

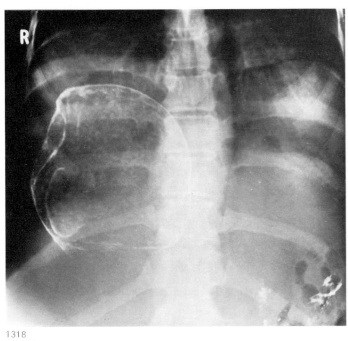

1318

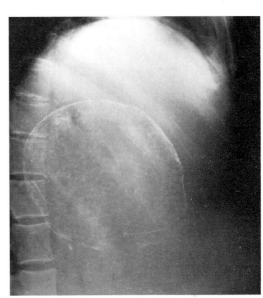

LATERAL
1319

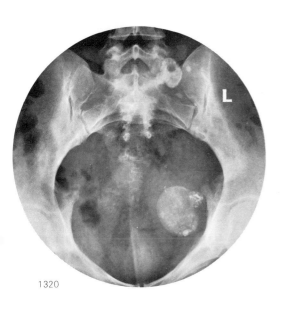

1320

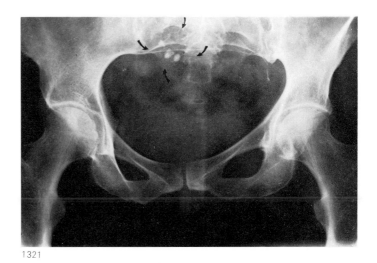

1321

The acute abdomen

Radiography of the acute abdomen is an emergency examination to show whether any of the following conditions are present:

(a) Free gas in the peritoneal cavity.
(b) Retroperitoneal or loculated gas collections.
(c) Extra luminal or extra bowel gas collections.
(d) Gaseous distension of any part of the gastro-intestinal tract.
(e) Free fluid in the peritoneal cavity.
(f) Fluid levels in the intestines.
(g) Evidence of an intra-abdominal mass.
(h) Abnormal calcifications or radio-opaque foreign bodies.

In all cases of acute abdomen a chest film must also be done primarily to exclude consolidation of a basal pneumonia causing upper abdominal pain.

High quality films are essential for diagnosis of these conditions and the examination must therefore be done in the main department and not with a mobile unit on the ward. If radiographs are required on admission the patient should proceed via the radiology department to the ward or if in the hospital should be brought to the department in a bed. A tilting X-ray table with a Potter-Bucky diaphragm is a great advantage as it is possible to obtain erect or semi-erect films without undue effort on the part of the patient. Horizontal ray films are essential for the diagnosis of free peritoneal gas and fluid levels. Sub-diaphragmatic gas is usually obvious on the erect film, but, if there is any doubt a lateral decubitus film with the patient lying on the left side to include the right abdominal margin, is essential. Small amounts of gas are then most easily seen between the lateral margin of the liver and the adjacent abdominal wall. The patient should be allowed to lie on the side for a short while before the film is taken to allow the gas to accumulate in the space between the liver and abdominal wall.

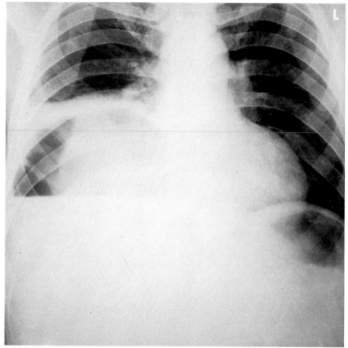

SITTING
1322

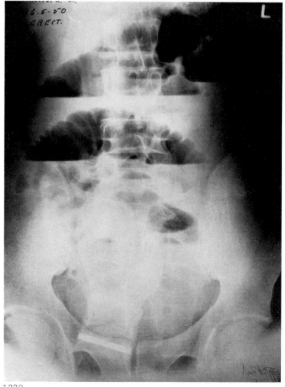

1323

Routine projections

(a) An erect postero-anterior chest radiograph (1322)
(b) An erect antero-posterior or postero-anterior projection of the abdomen to include the diaphragm, (1323,1324)
(c) A supine antero-posterior projection of the abdomen, (1325)
(d) A lateral decubitus film usually with the patient lying on the left side (1326,1327)

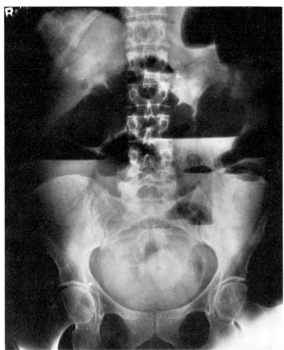

SITTING
1324

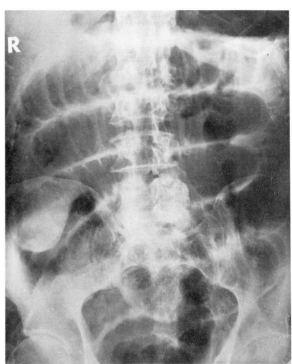

SUPINE
1325

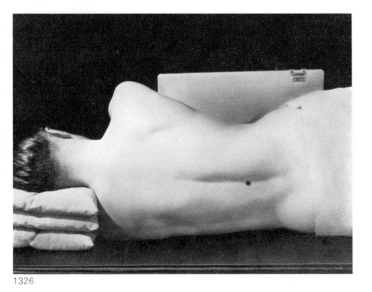

1326

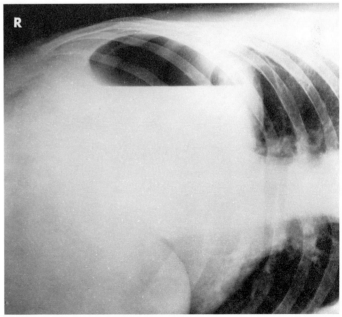

LEFT LATERAL DECUBITUS
1327

Occasionally the patient must be examined in the ward using a mobile unit. Whenever possible a projection with the patient sitting up in bed (1331,1332) should be done as the erect projection but if not possible a lateral decubitus view is required. If the patient cannot even be rolled onto the side a horizontal ray supine must then be taken (1328,1329,1330) to show free gas in the peritoneal cavity or fluid levels.

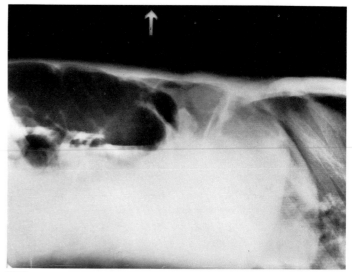

1330

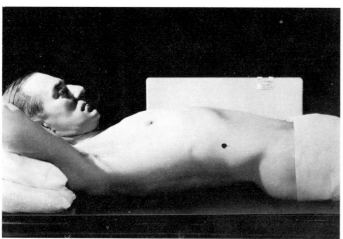

1328

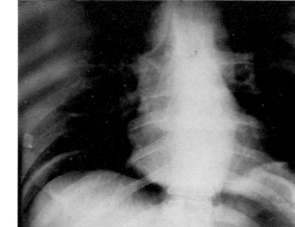

1331

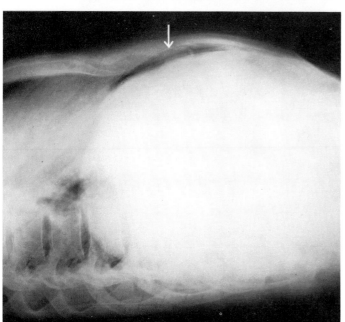

SUPINE
1329

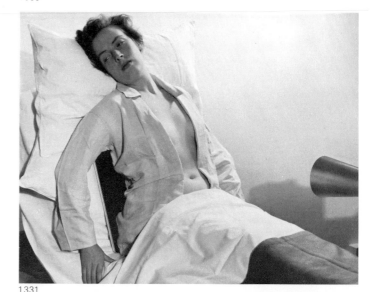

1332

Suprarenal Glands

The right and left suprarenal glands lie above and anterior to the upper poles of the kidneys. The right suprarenal lies behind the inferior vena cava and between the liver and the diaphragm while the left suprarenal lies adjacent to the aorta and medial to the tail of the pancreas. Unless calcified the suprarenal glands are not visible on plain films. In the past retroperitoneal air insuflation (1335), arteriography or venography was required to show the suprarenals but now they can be well shown on computed tomography (1333/4) and ultrasonography. Endocrine tumours of the suprarenals include phaeochromocytoma of the medulla, which causes hypertension, and the cortical adenoma which produces Cushing's syndrome.

Occasionally a non endocrine tumour such as a carcinoma also occurs which can be very large and displace the kidney.

For plain film radiographs of the suprarenals centre to the upper poles of the kidneys which are usually at the level of D12/L1.

Spleen

The spleen lies immediately under the left hemidiaphragm, adjacent to the fundus of the stomach and enlarges downwards and forwards in the line of the lower ribs. The hilum of the spleen is adjacent to the tail of the pancreas and the medial margin is close to the left kidney. (1336)

The splenic outline is often hidden by gas and faeces in the splenic flexure of the colon but is usually well shown in the 'immediate' film taken after injection of urographic contrast medium for the demonstration of the kidneys. To include the spleen, however, a 35 × 35 cm (14 × 14 inch) radiograph of the upper abdomen including the diaphragm must be done. Where calcifications are present in the left hypochondrium and it is suspected that these are intrasplenic an oblique view is required.

Key to 1333/4

A	Aorta	**K**	Kidney
GB	Gall bladder	**L**	Liver
I	Inferior vena cava	**P**	Pancreas
		S	Spleen

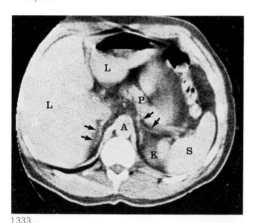

1333

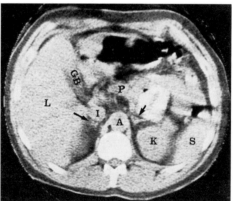

1334

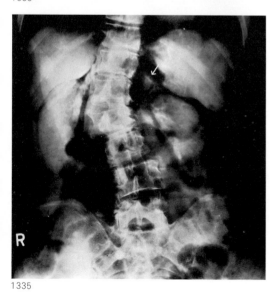

1335

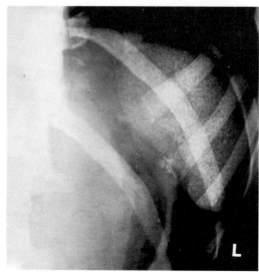

1336

Abdominal aorta

The aorta passes through the diaphragm at the level of the 12th Thoracic Vertebra and continues caudally anterior to the Lumbar Vertebrae and overlying the left side of the vertebral bodies. The Aorta bifurcates at the level of the 4th/5th Lumbar vertebrae to become the common iliac arteries. Calcification of the abdominal Aorta and Iliac arteries is common in the elderly, frequently visible on the frontal radiograph (1337/8) but more easily seen in the lateral view (1339). Even large aneurysms of the aorta may be difficult to demonstrate on plain radiographs but can be shown by Ultrasound (1340) or computed tomography.

Arteriography is required for the detailed demonstration of the aortic lumen and the branches of the aorta.

(1341) shows a normal aorta on ultrasonography.

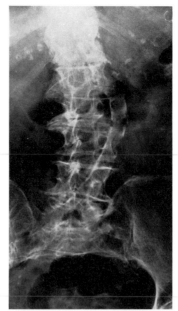

1337

Pancreas

The pancreas is both an exocrine and an endocrine gland which produces important enzymes for the digestion of fat, carbohydrate and protein as well as producing insulin and glucagon.

The pancreas has a head, body and tail. The head is encircled by the 'C' loop of the duodenum at the level of the 1st/2nd lumbar vertebrae and the body and tail are directed upwards and to the left across the spine towards the angle between the left kidney and the spleen (1342). Pancreatic juice of the exocrine pancreatic glands is excreted into the pancreatic duct which joins up with the common bile duct to enter the second part of the duodenum at the papilla of Vater.

Because the tissue attenuation of the pancreas is similar to the adjacent abdominal organs and there is no surrounding fat layer it is not shown on plain films of the abdomen unless calcific pancreatitis is present (1343). However the pancreas can be demonstrated by Ultrasonography and Computed Tomography (1344). The head of the pancreas lies anterior to the Inferior Vena Cava and the curves over the Superior Mesenteric Artery with the body and tail passing posteriorly and to the left.

1338

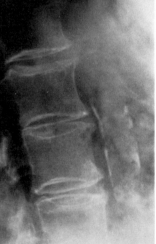

1339

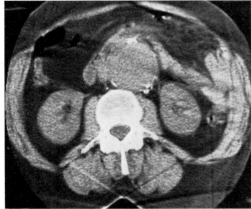

1340

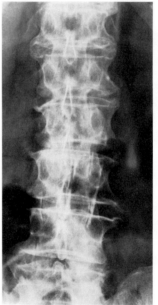

1341

Key to 1341

Ao Aorta
Li Liver
Sp Spleen
St Stomach

The pancreatic duct and its branches are best demonstrated on Endoscopic Regrograde Choleangiopancreatography (ERCP); an endoscope is passed via the osesophagus and stomach into the duodenum and the papilla of Vater is cannulated and injected with a small quantity (1–3 ml) of an anionic water soluble contrast medium such as Metrizamide (1345)

Angiography is also used for pancreatic examinations particularly in the demonstration of endocrine tumours such as an insulinoma. A super selective technique is required using a catheter which passes up the aorta, enters the coeliac axis, then the tip of the catheter is lodged in a pancreatic artery (1346).

Because of the proximity of the pancreas to the duodenal loop, tumours or pseudocysts of the pancreas can impinge on the duodenal loop. A clear view of the duodenal loop is therefore often necessary in the investigation of pancreatic disease and is best achieved with a hypotonic duodenogram (1347).

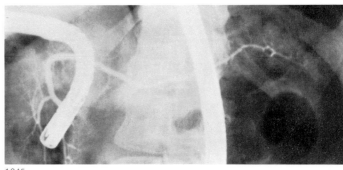

1345

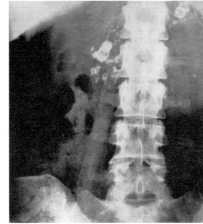

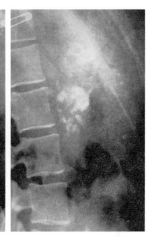

1343

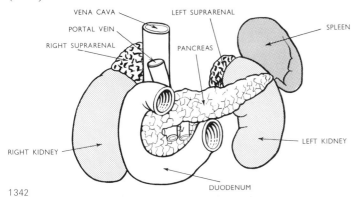

VENA CAVA

PORTAL VEIN

RIGHT SUPRARENAL

LEFT SUPRARENAL

SPLEEN

PANCREAS

RIGHT KIDNEY

LEFT KIDNEY

DUODENUM

1342

Key to 1344

A   Aorta
D   Duodenum
K   Kidney
L   Liver
S   Spleen
V   Vertebral body

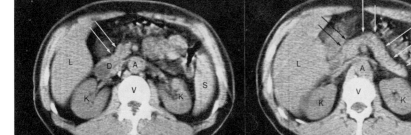

R   L

1344

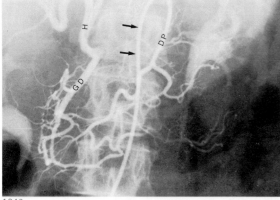

1346

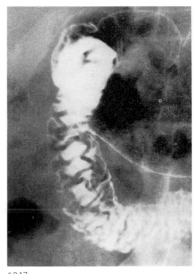

1347

Selective pancreatic arteriogram with catheter tip in the dorsal pancreatic artery (DP). GD-Gastro-duodenal artery H-Hepatic artery (1435). (By kind permission of Dr. H. Herlinger.)

Liver and diaphragm

The liver is a large "biochemical factory" lying in the upper abdomen, mainly on the right side and immediately adjacent to the diaphragm. It is divided into right and left lobes by the falciform ligament which contains the remnant of the umbilical vein. The overall shape of the liver is triangular with its apex towards the left side and its base against the right upper abdominal margin. It is protected from injury by the lower ribs (1348) (1349)

The liver weights approximately 1400 g and measures 20 cm (8 ins) across on the superior surface, 18 cm (7 ins) on the right lateral margin and approximately 16 cm (6 ins) in depth. Bile is formed in the liver and carried in the two hepatic ducts from the right and left lobes to form the common hepatic duct which subsequently joins the cystic duct to form the common bile duct. The gall bladder lies immediately adjacent to and on the inferior surface of the liver. The blood supply to the liver comes mainly from the portal vein which drains the intestine carrying the productions of digestion to the liver.

The liver is also supplied by the hepatic artery which is rich in oxygen.

The soft tissue density of the upper abdomen is due to the liver but in a number of conditions including tropical diseases calcifications occur within the liver. A calcified hydatid cyst is a not uncommon cause of curvilinear liver calcification in sheep rearing countries (1318, 1319)

Key to 1350/1
A   Aorta
Cy   Cyst
Dia Diaphragm
L   Liver

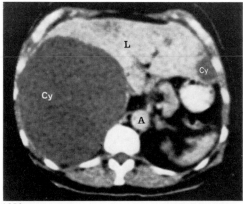

1350

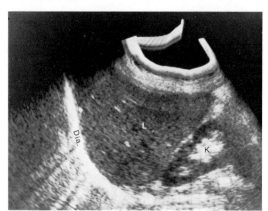

1351

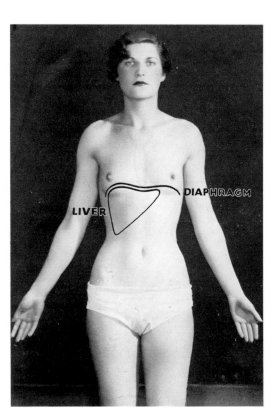

1348

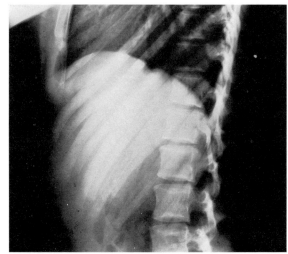

LATERAL
1349

384

Liver, Radiographic procedure

For an average sized patient a 35 × 35 cm (14 × 14 ins) cassette can be used but for a large patient a 43 × 35 cm (17 × 14 ins) cassette should be placed transversely in the Potter-Bucky tray and positioned so that its lower margin is at the iliac crests.

■ Centre to the centre of the cassette.

The exposure should be done in expiration. A relatively low kilo-voltage should be used in the region of 60–80 kVp for maximum soft fissure contrast.

Diaphragm Movement during Respiration

On the chest radiograph the right hemi-diaphragm is usually 2·5 cm (1 inch) higher than on the left. The right hemi-may also be raised because of lung pathology such as collapse of the right lower lobe, because of paralysis of the diaphragm or because of pathology underneath the diaphragm, such as a subphrenic abscess or space occupying lesion of the liver. When the right hemi-diaphragm is raised it is possible to distinguish between paralysis of the diaphragm and inflammatory lesions around the diaphragm by the use of fluoroscopy. When paralysed the diaphragm moves upwards on sniffing (paradoxical movement), compared with the normal diaphragm which moves sharply downwards. With inflammatory lesions, either above or below, the raised hemi-diaphragm shows markedly diminished movement which however, is in a normal direction even on sniffing. The margin of the diaphragm is often obscured by disease in the overlying lung or pleura. Conditions such as pneumonic consolidation or collapse and pleural effusion interfere with visualisation of the diaphragm.

Free gas in the peritoneal cavity accumulates under the diaphragm in the erect position and the erect chest radiograph is the best method for its demonstration, (see page 378).

The movement of a diaphragm can also be demonstrated by taking two exposures on one film, the first in expiration and the second in inspiration. Each exposure should be half of that normally used for a chest radiograph (1358). There is also an obvious difference between inspiration and expiration in the external contour of the body (1352a, 1352b).

The position of the diaphragm varies not only with the phase of respiration, (1353, 1354) but also with a change of position from horizontal to erect; the diaphragm being considerably lower in the erect position than when the patient is horizontal. The outline of the dome of the diaphragm is well shown in the lateral radiograph (1349).

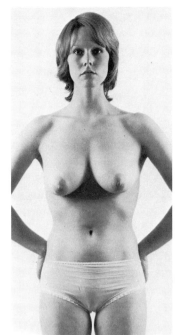
1352a

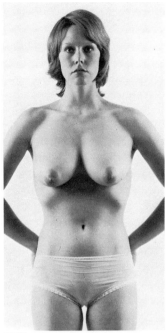
1352b

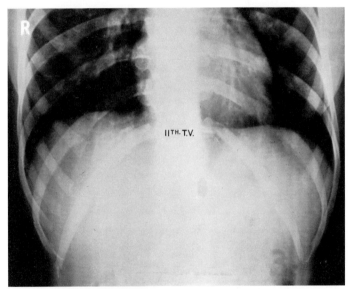
INSPIRATION
1353

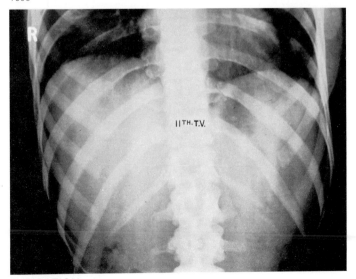
EXPIRATION
1354

Eventration of Diaphragm

Eventration of a hemi-diaphragm is marked weakening associated with replacement of the diaphragmatic muscle by fibrous tissue. As a result, the hemi-diaphragm is markedly raised (1355) and usually has the funds of the stomach immediately below it which can be shown with a barium meal (1356,1357). The inferior margin of the diaphragm can be demonstrated by injecting air into the peritoneal cavity; an investigation known as a diagnostic peneumoperitoneum (1364). The appearances are similar to a spontaneous pneumoperitoneum from a perforated hollow viscus.

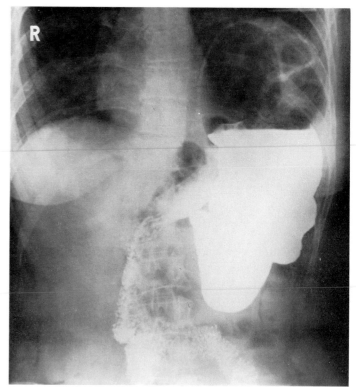

1357

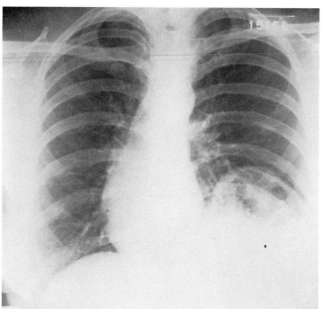

1355

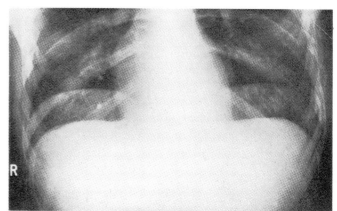

1358

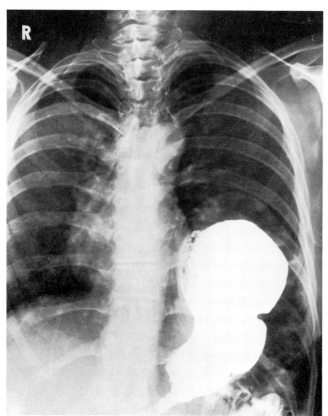

1356

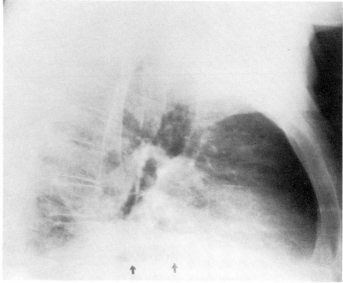

1359

Subphrenic and Intra-hepatic Abscess

A sub-phrenic or intra-hepatic abscess causes a raised right hemi-diaphragm and is often associated with a small right pleural effusion and may produce a fluid level below the right hemi-diaphragm. The extent of the cavity can be demonstrated by taking radiographs with the patient in different positions including the erect and decubitus views (1359,1360). Sub-phrenic and intra-hepatic abscesses are now best demonstrated by using ultrasonography or computed tomography (1361).

Radiographs

The lateral view of the chest demonstrates a fluid level below the diaphragm (arrows) (1359). By taking a decubitus film with the patient lying on the left side the fluid level is demonstrated towards the right lateral abdominal wall (1360) indicating that there is a large subphrenic space due to a subphrenic abscess; however a subphrenic abscess is much more readily demonstrated on computed tomography (1361) and easily distinguished from an intra-hepatic abscess (1362).

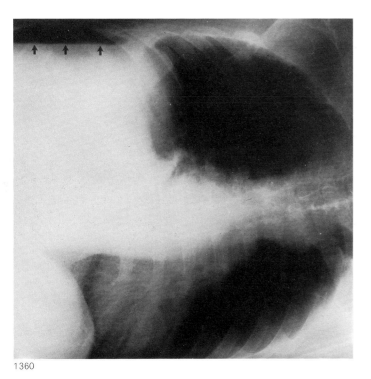

1360

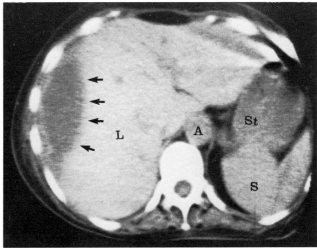

1361

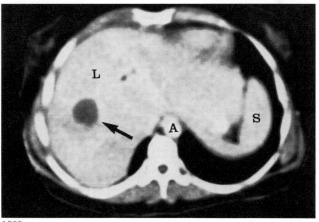

1362

Key to 1361
A   Aorta
L   Liver
S   Spleen
St   Stomach

Key to 1362
arrow   Intra-hepatic abscess
A   Aorta
L   Liver
S   Spleen

Free gas in the peritoneal cavity (pneumoperitoneum) can also occur spontaneously due to perforation of a hollow viscus as occurs with a perforated peptic ulcer of the stomach or duodenum.

A pneumoperitoneum is best shown by an erect film of the lower chest which in ill patients must be done in bed, either with a mobile unit (1363) or by transporting the patient in the bed to the main X-ray department. In the erect position the gas collects under the diaphragm which becomes visible as narrow curved lines because it lies between the gas below the diaphragm and the air in the lungs above, (1364).

When there is doubt about the visualisation of a very small collection of a gas, a *left* lateral decubitus film should be taken in which the air will be shown between the liver and the lateral abdominal wall. In a decubitus view with the patient lying on the *right* side (1365) the gas overlies the spleen (1366) which is well outlined by this manouvre. However, for an examination to exclude a small pneumoperitoneum a decubitus view must be taken with the patient lying on the *left* side.

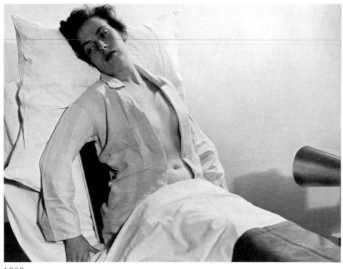

1363

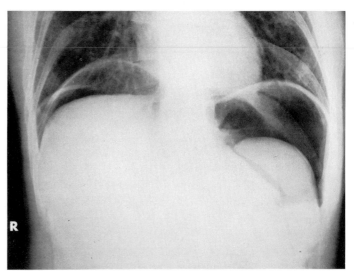

1364

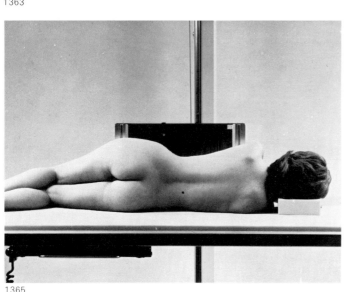

1365

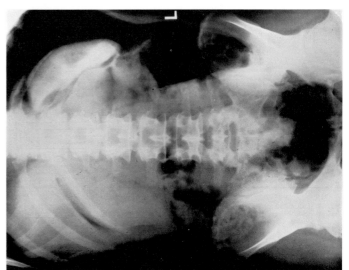

1366

Retroperitoneal gas

In the past retroperitoneal gas insufflation was used to demonstrate the suprarenals. This is now best done using Computed tomography but can also be achieved with ultrasonography.

However, a perforation of a hollow viscus may occur into the retroperitoneal tissues forming a gas collection around the kidneys and suprarenals and often shows as multiple small gas bubbles in the retroperitoneal tissues (1335).

Sinogram

A persistent fistulous tract may occur following operation but is occasionally spontaneous in association with tumours or inflammatory bowel disease.

A sinogram is the examination for a fistulous tract and is carried out in the X-ray department using fluoroscopy. A water soluble contrast medium such as Meglumine diatrozoate (Conray "280") is injected along the fistula in one of a variety of ways, using a cannula, catheter, a nozzle type introducer or by balloon catheter. Gentle pressure is used on the introducer or on the skin opening of the fistulous tract to prevent backflow of the contrast medium during the injection. It is essential to obtain two radiographs at right angles to each other, preferably in the antero-posterior and true lateral positions to accurately demonstrate the position of the fistula.

These fistulous tracts may communicate with the stomach, bowel, ureter, or may end blindly in an abscess cavity. Radiographs (1367, 1368) show a fistulous tract extending posteriorly into the sub-phrenic region on the left side from a right sided opening on the skin.

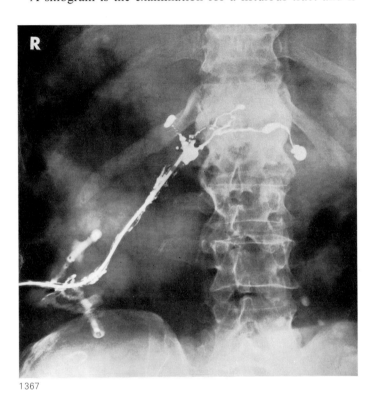

1367

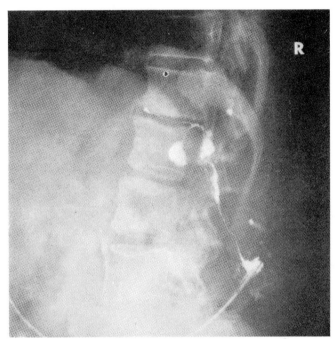

1368

389

16

ALIMENTARY TRACT

ALIMENTARY TRACT

The alimentary tract extends from the mouth to the anus with the various parts having different functions and varying in length and calibre but forming a continuous tube. The chief parts are the mouth, pharynx, oesophagus, stomach, small intestine, large intestine, rectum and anus.

The pharynx or throat cavity lies between the mouth and oesophagus, extending from the base of the skull to the 6th thoracic vertebra. Only the lower part (oro-pharynx) below the level of the soft palate serves as a passage for food. The part above the soft palate is the naso-pharynx lying behind the nasal cavity. The oro-pharynx lies below the soft palate in front of the pre-vertebral soft tissues and extends from the 1st cervical vertebra to the 6th cervical vertebra, below the naso-pharynx (1369).

The oesophagus extends from the termination of the pharynx at the lower border of the cricoid cartilage, usually at the level of the 6th cervical vertebra, to the cardiac sphincter lying between the oesophagus and the stomach about the level of the 11th

thoracic vertebra. The oesophagus passes through a hole in the diaphragm called the oesophageal hiatus which is approximately at the level of the 10th thoracic vertebra (1370).

The stomach is the widest part of the alimentary tract acting as a reservoir for food and drink with a capacity of approximately 2 pints (1371). It lies between the oesophagus and the small intestine, mostly to the left of the spine, but varies in position, particularly with different subject types. In long thin subjects and in the elderly the lower part of the stomach may reach below the level of the iliac crest. The stomach is quite mobile changing its position with different positions of the body especially from erect to supine.

The food enters the stomach through the cardiac orifice and leaves by the pyloric canal, to go into the duodenum. The medial margin of the stomach is known as the lesser curvature and the lateral and inferior margin as the greater curvature. The fundus lies beneath the left hemi-diaphragm and the antrum immediately adjacent to the pyloric canal with the body of the stomach between the fundus and gastric antrum. The fundus actually lies above the level of the entry of the oesophagus into the stomach, being closely approximated to the inferior surface of the curved left hemi-diaphragm. Gas collects in the fundus of the stomach in the erect position, but is in the gastric antrum when the patient is supine, with food or barium then moving into the fundus (1372).

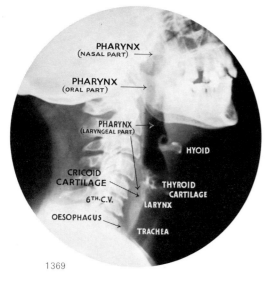

1369

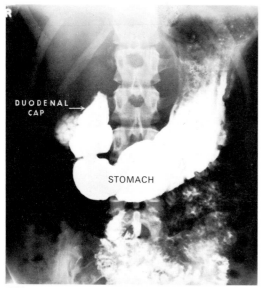

1371

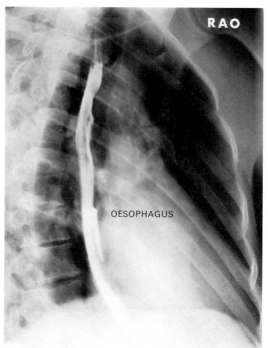

1370

The small intestine, approximately 6·5 m (22 ft) in length and from 2–4 cm (1–2 ins), in diameter, extends from the pyloric canal to the ilio-caecal valve, (1373) and is a long coiled tube which connects the stomach with the colon. The small intestine (1372) is divided into three parts; the Duodenum 30 cm (12 ins) long, the Jejunum 2·5 m (8 ft) and the Ileum which is 4 m (12 ft) long. Immediately after the pyloric canal the duodenum opens out into a triangular shape called the duodenal cap (1371) and then passes backwards and turns downwards, on the right side of the upper, lumbar spine, before crossing to the left of the abdomen at the level of the second lumbar vertebra. It then passes upwards and to the left behind the stomach to form the duodeno-jejunal flexure at the ligament of Treitz. The jejunum lies between the duodenum and the ileum below the level of the stomach within the margins of the colon. The ileum is frequently found in the pelvic cavity particularly when the bladder is empty. A full bladder will displace the ileum out of the pelvic cavity.

The large intestine or colon is approximately 1·5 m (5 ft) in length and from 3–9 cm (1½–4 ins) in diameter (1374).

The caecum, or blind end of the colon, lies in the right iliac fossa extending slightly, 6 cm (2½ ins), below the ileo-caecal valve.

The appendix which is a blind ended tube 3–12 cm (2–5 ins) long projects from the inferior and medial end of the caecum (1374).

The ascending colon passes upwards from the ileo-caecal valve to the under surface of the liver, where it bends to form the right colic or hepatic flexure continuing as the transverse colon, which passes across the upper abdomen from the right to the left side along the under surface of the liver. On the left side the transverse colon passes upwards and backward towards the left hemi-diaphragm to form the left colic or splenic flexure which then bends downward becoming the descending colon. The descending colon passes downwards on the left side of the abdomen to the iliac crest where it bends toward the midline to form the sigmoid colon, curving posteriorly in front of the sacrum, and then ends in the rectum beyond which is the anus, the distal orifice of the alimentary canal (1375).

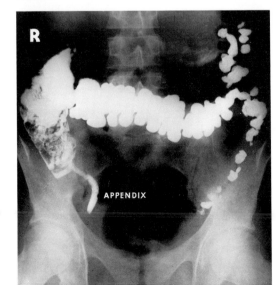

SMALL

INTESTINE

1372

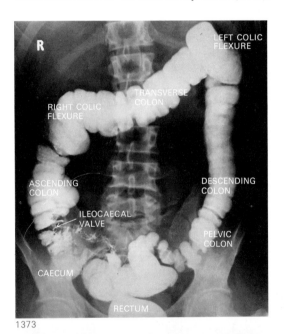

LEFT COLIC FLEXURE

TRANSVERSE COLON

RIGHT COLIC FLEXURE

ASCENDING COLON

DESCENDING COLON

ILEOCAECAL VALVE

PELVIC COLON

CAECUM

RECTUM

1373

APPENDIX

1374

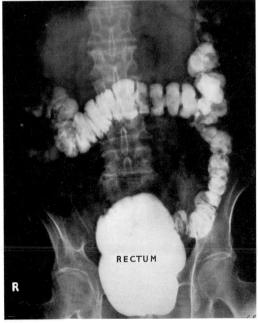

RECTUM

1375

Regions

The abdomen is, for descriptive purposes, divided into 9 regions by two vertical and two transverse lines (1376). The vertical lines which are parallel to the median plane of the trunk, are midway between the anterior superior iliac spines and the symphysis pubis. The upper transverse line, the transpyloric line, is at the level of the 1st lumbar vertebra and the lower, or transtubercular line, is at the level of the 5th lumbar vertebra. The 9 regions defined by these lines are named from above downward, the epigastric, umbilical and hypo gastric medially, and the hypochondriac, lumbar and iliac laterally (1376). Additionally there is a sub-costal line lying at the level of the 3rd lumbar vertebra which is usually associated with the natural depression at the waist line.

The relative positions of the intra-abdominal organs, vary according to subject type as discussed previously (page 330, 331) and shown in diagrammatic form for the asthenic and hypersthenic types (1377).

Respiration

The position of the intra-abdominal organs varies on respiration. Radiographs of the abdomen are usually done on arrested expiration. There must be a short delay after the patient stops breathing and before the exposure to prevent blurring from the continuing movement of the intra-abdominal organs. On deep inspiration, the upper abdominal organs including the kidneys, liver and spleen are moved caudally. Respiration does not however, affect the organs lying in the pelvis.

The patient

For patients requiring contrast examinations, such as a barium meal, enema or a cholecystogram there should be a printed proforma giving details of the preparation including diet and laxatives. For example before a barium meal it is most important for the patient to have nothing to eat or drink for 6 hours prior to the examination. The patient should also be told what to expect from the examination, how long the procedure will take and the time of the appointment. At all times, kindly reassurance is essential; similarly during the examination the patient should be told what to expect before it actually happens.

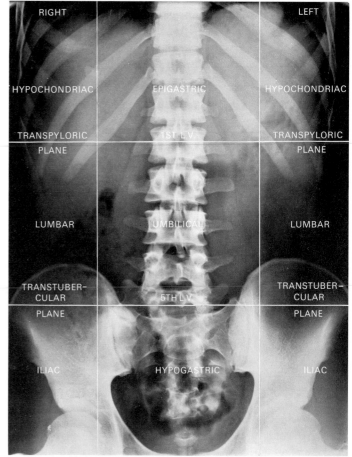

1376

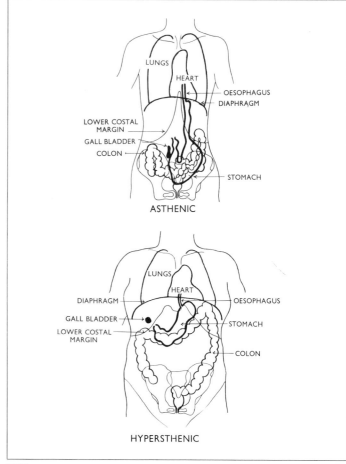

1377

Opaque medium

Very little of the gastro-intestinal tract is shown on the plain abdominal film in normal patients. Air shadows and opacities due to stones are visible, but contrast medium is needed to show the stomach, small intestine, and colon.

For the gastro-intestinal tract, barium suspensions are the most commonly used contrast agents and are supplied by the manufacturers ready for use although they usually need to be shaken immediately before the examination. Some barium suspensions should be put on an automatic mixer prior to use. Barium preparations also come in powder form which are readily suspended in water by mixing or shaking and made up shortly before use. For infants a water soluble contrast medium may be used, but there is a danger of causing dehydration by its high osmolarity. Therefore a non-ionic water soluble contrast agent should be used in these circumstances.

Modern methods include the use of both gas and barium to produce a double contrast examination whether for the stomach or colon. Double contrast barium meals and enemas require much lower exposures than those performed with barium only. For double contrast examinations relatively under-exposed radiographs are needed whereas a well penetrated exposure must be used for examinations using barium only. The appropriate radiographic techniques for the different parts of the alimentary tract will be considered separately under Pharynx and Oesophagus, Barium Swallow, Stomach and Intestines, Colon and Rectum.

Current developments

It is now accepted practice that these contrast examinations are all performed with image intensification and television monitoring. In some centres remote control equipment is used and automatic exposure devices are now commonly found in fluoroscopic rooms. The fluoroscopic exposure has been considerably reduced with image intensification, particularly with caesium iodide intensifier tubes, which give a particularly fine image. However, an even more important factor in reducing patient exposure has been the introduction of rare earth screens together with the use of double contrast techniques.

Exposures are now only 20–25 % of those previously used. A further reduction in patient exposure can be obtained by using 100 mm film which takes direct exposures from the output phosphor of the image intensifier (fluorography) and not directly (radiography).

Screening and filming

The exposure factors are individual for each patient and for each position during an examination. Where automatic exposure devices are not available a measurement of the antero-posterior diameter of the patient at the level of the epigastrium is a guide for each individual exposure and should be routinely done on every patient before starting a barium examination. The antero-posterior diameter must be related to the kilovoltage chosen for a particular patient and then the milliampere seconds varied according to the obliquity of the patient.

Most modern fluoroscopic rooms also have a television monitor close to the control panel for the radiographer. Any change in the position of the patient can immediately be assessed by watching the monitor and listening to the instructions given by the radiologist to the patient.

The films of each patient should be checked immediately after the examination to ensure that tube output and processing are being kept constant and that the radiographer's choice of exposure factors is correct. If the spleen or liver are enlarged or if ascites is present an increased exposure will be needed to produce the correct film density.

It is the duty of the radiographer to ensure that the apparatus is in working order, that all the accessories such as pads and protective devices are to hand, that the fluoroscopic equipment is kept clean and particularly that there is no barium on the table top and explorator. The radiographer should also ensure that there is a minimum of personnel movement in the room during the examination so that there should be no unnecessary distractions. Patients who are ill should not be left unattended.

Identification of radiographs

All radiographs must be carefully labelled as to the name of the patient, name of the hospital, hospital number and date. Special identifications are also occasionally required, such as the timing of a follow-through radiograph or the position of the patient.

Exposure conditions

For consistently good results the exposure time must be kept to a minimum, preferably in the range of 0·04–0·05 of a second and can now easily be achieved in double contrast examinations in the vast majority of patients by using rare earth screens. However, where the exposure is made using barium only it must be immediately altered to a high kilovoltage to achieve the necessary penetration. The radiographer can quite easily assess this by watching the dedicated TV monitor on the control panel.

Barium examinations are carried out using a grid to reduce scattered radiation thereby producing a sharper image. Two radiographs (1378, 1379) taken of the same subject show the difference between using a grid (1378), and no grid (1399). The film taken without the grid has less contrast and definition.

Coning and diaphragm control

During fluoroscopic examination of the gastro-intestinal tract varying sized areas are viewed and radiographed with spot films using cassettes of various sizes. The fluoroscopic field is coned to the smallest area and, when a film is taken, the diaphragms are similarly collimated to show only the required region However, with most modern equipment there is automatic control of the diaphragms to correspond to the size of the cassette being used. These methods result in a considerable reduction in radiation to the patient and also increased detail on the films due to a reduction in scattered radiation.

An equally important feature in producing consistently good results with films taken during a fluoroscopic barium examination (spot film) is to have the fluoroscopic screen as close to the patient as possible. This considerably decreases the magnification factor as well as the required exposure. The exposure factors can then be accurately assessed for the size of each patient. The use of compression while taking spot films considerably reduces intervening soft tissue thickness and also results in a considerable reduction in the exposure factors required.

Positioning

During a fluoroscopic barium examination the stomach or colon are examined with the patient in many different positions including erect, horizontal, oblique, lateral, supine and prone. The exposure factors will need to be altered for each position of the patient as well as for the amount of intervening barium, particularly when using the double contrast technique for the barium meal or enema.

Protection

Radiation is kept to a minimum by undertaking only those examinations which are indicated clinically and not performing unnecessary repeat investigations. During the course of the examination the number of exposures, the fluoroscopy time, and the field of view must be kept to a minimum. These precautions are particularly important for children and for women of child bearing age. With barium examinations it is mandatory to enforce the 'ten day rule' ensuring that no examinations are done during very early pregnancy. For women of child bearing age, contrast examinations are performed, apart from emergency situations, only in the first ten days of the menstrual cycle.

All fluoroscopy should now only be done using an image intensifier with television because of the reduction in radiation.

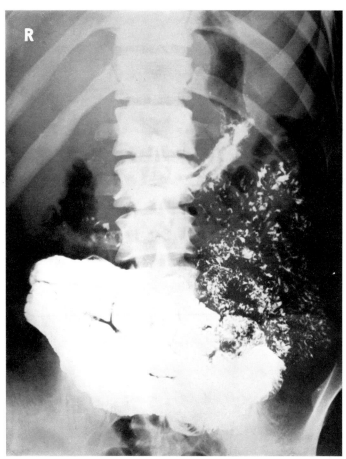

WITH GRID
1378

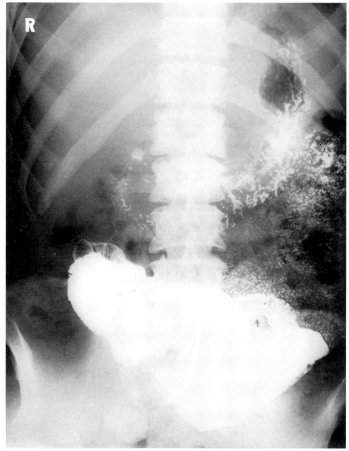

WITHOUT GRID
1379

Note—A plain film of the abdomen is usually taken as a preliminary to a contrast examination of the gastro-intestinal tract.

Pharynx and Oesophagus

Barium Swallow

For the pharynx, or throat cavity plain films are usually all that are required. However, if there is difficulty in swallowing (dysphagia), the examination must show the oro-pharynx and oesophagus and requires the use of barium.

In adults the most common reason for examining the pharynx is for a foreign body, when a relatively under exposed lateral view should be taken.

No special preparation is required for a barium swallow examination which is performed using fluoroscopy while the patient drinks the barium (1381, 1382). An exposure immediately after the patient has swallowed is needed to show the uppermost part of the oesophagus filled with barium and is achieved by accurately timing the swallow (see page 340).

For the mid and lower oesophagus, films are taken during swallowing to show the full oesophagus, the oesophagus in double contrast, and if necessary, the "collapsed" oesophagus. The oesophagus is best seen in the right postero-anterior oblique view but films are often taken in the frontal and in both oblique positions.

Note—Barium should not be used as the contrast medium where a tracheo-oesophageal fistula is suspected, particularly in babies. A non-ionic contrast agent must then be used and the examination carried out using cine-fluorography.

Radiographs (1383a, 1383b) show a pharyngeal diverticulum which occurs at the uppermost part of the oesophagus. The diverticulum retains the barium for a little while after the barium swallow.

Occasionally in patients who have difficulty in swallowing the barium may pass into the trachea—"tracheal spill" (1381)—outlining the inner margin of the trachea and sometimes even the major bronchi.

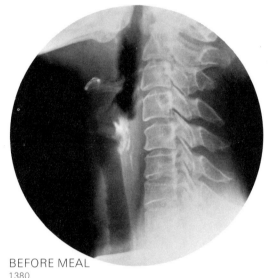

BEFORE MEAL
1380

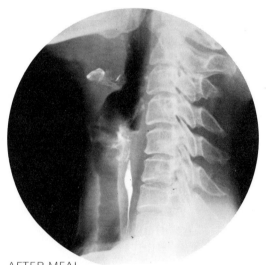

AFTER MEAL
1382

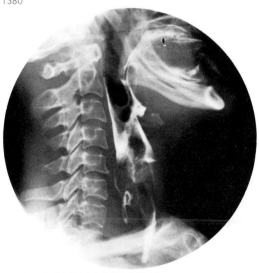

DURING PASSAGE OF MEAL
1381

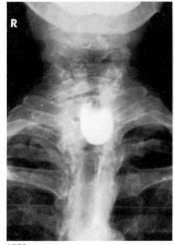
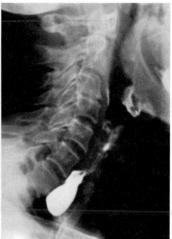

1383a   1383b

Films of the oesophagus may also be taken without fluoroscopy, usually to show residual barium, either in a diverticulum or proximal to a stricture.

Postero-anterior
The patient faces the film with the chin slightly raised and, using accurate collimation, the exposure is made during breath holding.
■ Centre in the midline at the level of second thoracic vertebra (1383a, 1384)

Lateral Neck
With the patient lateral and the chin slightly raised to show the soft tissue in profile the arms should be beside the trunk with the shoulders depressed to show the maximum area of soft tissue above the density of the shoulders.
■ Centre in the middle of the neck at the level of the fifth cervical vertebra (1383b, 1385)

Lateral radiograph (1386) shows a small fishbone in the pharynx, (a) before and (b) after a drink of barium.

Lower Oesophagus
The preparation of a patient for an examination of the lower oesophagus is similar to that for a barium meal. No food or fluid is taken for six hours before the examination and is essentially similar to that described on the previous page, with films being taken during fluoroscopy.

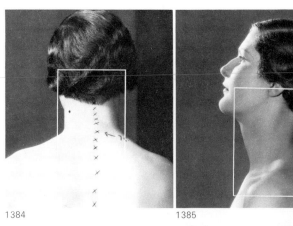

1384   1385

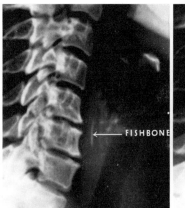 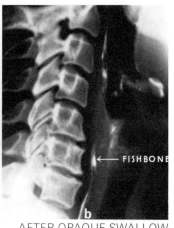

← FISHBONE

← FISHBONE

a

b

BEFORE OPAQUE SWALLOW   AFTER OPAQUE SWALLOW
1386a   1386b

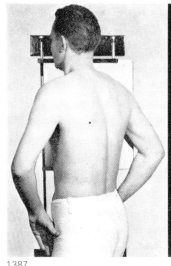 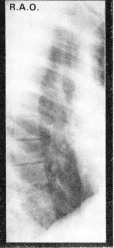

R.A.O.

1387

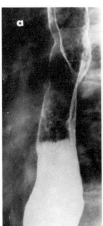 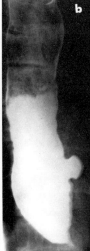 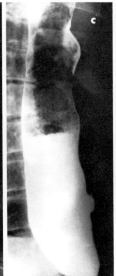 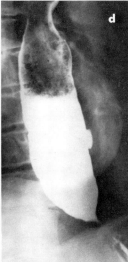 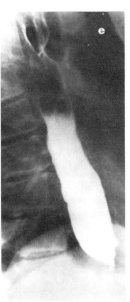

a   b   c   d   e

1388

Barium Swallow (Fluoroscopy)
Right Postero-anterior oblique (RAO)

With the patient erect and facing the fluoroscopic screen and radiologist the patient is turned towards the left to bring the right shoulder forward. The left shoulder is backward and nearer the table top, making an angle of approximately 50° to 60° with the fluoroscopic screen. After a swallow of barium the oesophagus can be seen to pass in front of the spine and behind the aorta and heart (1389). As the barium moves down the oesophagus it is immediately followed by air producing a double contrast view of the oesophagus (1391). Subsequently there is a stripping wave which empties the oesophagus of both air and barium producing the "collapsed" appearance of the oesophagus.

In Radiograph (1388) the oesophagus is shown in different projections.
(a) Left postero-anterior oblique (LAO).
(b) Postero-anterior (PA).
(c) }
(d) } Right postero-anterior oblique (RAO).
(e) Right lateral (RLat).

Radiograph (1390) shows an irregular narrowing of the lower end of the oesophagus with the barium held up proximal to it.

Radiograph (1391) are double contrast views of a normal
Radiographs (1391) are double contrast views of a normal oesophagus and (1392) views of the oesophagus showing a peptic ulcer (arrow).

Diagram (1393) is of an axial section of the thorax in the R.A.O. position showing the oesophagus projected between the spine and heart.

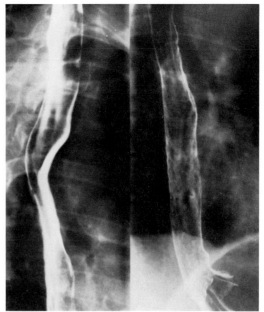

1391

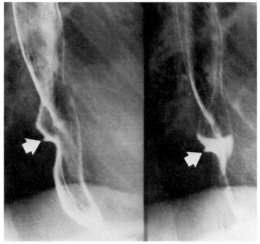

1392

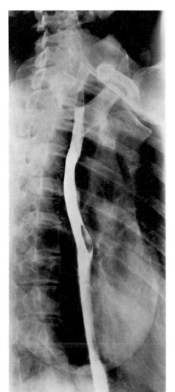

1389

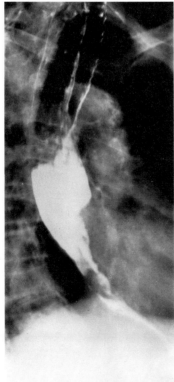

1390

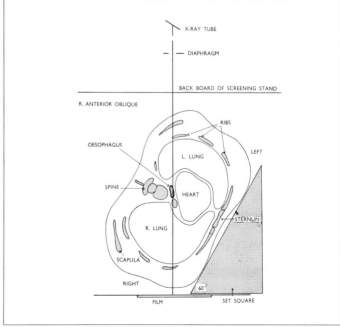

1393

399

Stomach and Intestines

Stomach and intestines

As a preliminary to a barium meal examination a full length plain film of the abdomen should be taken. Opacities such as gall stones or pancreatic calcification might otherwise be hidden by contrast medium. Should the clinical history suggest that gall bladder disease is a possibility a preliminary localised oblique view of the right hypocondrium should also be taken before the barium meal.

The usual barium meal examination includes the oesophagus, stomach and duodenum. In the barium meal follow-through examination the small bowel including the terminal ilium, is also examined.

Opaque medium

The vast majority of examinations are performed using barium sulphate, either in suspension from a pharmaceutical company or in powder form and then prepared in the department prior to the investigation. A double contrast barium meal technique is now the usual practice. Gas tablets or granules are swallowed by the patient with a minimal amount of water (5 ml) and then a muscle relaxant such as Buscopan or glucagon is given intravenously.

The patient then swallows 50 ml of barium sulphate for views of the oesophagus and for a prone film of the stomach and is followed by a further 100 ml of barium. Films are taken in the supine and supine-oblique positions after "coating" the stomach with the air/barium mixture. If barium and air have entered the duodenum spot films are taken at this stage followed by semi-erect and erect views of the gastric fundus after which spot films with compression of the lesser curve and duodenum (1394, 1395, 1396) are taken.

In special circumstances a water soluble organic iodine compound, such as gastrografin may be used particularly when there is the possibility of a perforation of a hollow viscus. In infants a non-ionic organic iodine compound is preferred.

Radiographs

In (1394) a prone film shows a polypoid lesion in the gastric antrum while in (1395) a double contrast view with the patient supine shows a fine network pattern of arae gastricae. Multiple small polyps are demonstrated in the fundus on the semi-erect oblique view of the fundus (1396).

Preparation

In women of child bearing age the "ten day" rule must be applied. The barium meal must be done within the first 10 days from the first day of bleeding in the menstrual cycle unless there are over-riding clinical indications. The referring clinician must then over-ride the 10 day rule by a signed cancellation on the request form.

When the appointment is made a written pro-forma of instructions is given to the patient who is told to fast, taking neither solids nor fluids for a minimum of 6 hours before the barium meal examination.

It is also advisable to explain the procedure to the patient at this stage and to ascertain whether the patient is a diabetic or suffers from migraine. If so the examination must be done first on the list. In migraine patients, starvation often provokes a headache which may cause marked "pylorospasm".

On the day of the examination the procedure should again be explained to the patient and a suitable x-ray gown provided which is comfortable and warm but without opaque fasteners.

Although the patient must undress "completely", briefs or panties should be worn for the barium meal provided there are no opacities on these garments. Patients should have a warm dressing gown, suitable changing rooms, readily available toilet facilities and a comfortable waiting room. Larger cubicles must also be available for patients having follow-through examinations as they need to lie on their right sides.

Patients must be warned that they may be in the department for some time, even though the actual barium meal examination usually only takes 10 to 20 minutes. Most of the period spent in the department will be taken up with waiting for the examination.

For patients with haematemesis an emergency barium meal may be required, although in a large number of centres endoscopy is performed within the first 24 hours. The barium meal examination is modified because these patients are often having intravenous fluid or blood and are in no condition to stand up.

Barium Swallow and Meal examinations are almost invariably done by a radiologist with fluoroscopy. A set sequence of films including views of the oesophagus and then of the stomach, in prone, supine, and erect positions using double contrast and also with compression are taken and viewed immediately after processing for correct exposure and whether the examination has been adequate. If no further films are required then the patient can leave the department.

Those patients requiring a follow-through examination are given a further 300 ml of barium. They should then lie on the right side to encourage the barium to flow into the duodenum. Further films are taken at intervals to outline the small bowel until the terminal ileum is reached when spot films are taken. In some patients with gastric outlet disease, or pyloric obstruction, delayed films up to six hours will be needed to see the amount of barium remaining in the stomach. Occasionally a late film to show the colon is also needed.

A different examination, such as a Cholecystogram may subsequently also be required. An appointment should then be made before the patient leaves the department.

Radiographs

Radiograph (1394) is a prone view showing a "polypoid" filling defect in the gastric antrum. In this position the barium fills the body and antrum of the stomach.

Radiograph (1395) is a supine view of a normal stomach showing the areae gastricae which give the appearance of a small net-like pattern. If the double contrast barium meal technique is carried out correctly the areae gastricae will frequently be seen.

Radiograph (1396) is a semi-erect oblique view with gas in the fundus of the stomach showing multiple small polyps.

Note—Patients should be warned that barium can be extremely constipating, particularly in the elderly. Plenty of fluids should be taken as well as a laxative whenever constipation is likely to be a problem.

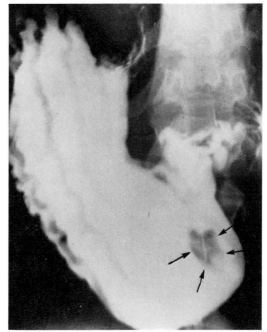

1394

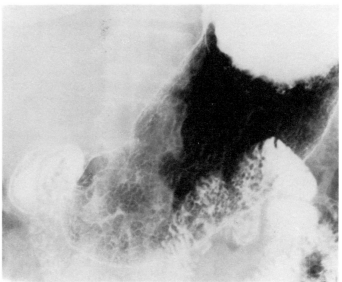

1395

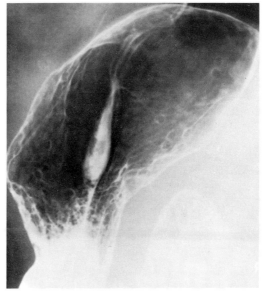

1396

Positioning

During the barium meal, positioning of the patient is extremely important, not only to show the various parts of the oesophagus, stomach and duodenum, but also to control the barium and gas. With the patient in the supine postion the barium is in the fundus of the stomach and gas in the body and antrum (1397). To keep the barium in the stomach now allowing it to enter the duodenum the patient should be turned with the left side down. In the prone position the barium is in the body and antrum of the stomach and the gas is in the fundus (1394). To empty the stomach the patient should be turned with the right side down. In the erect position the barium falls to the gastric antrum and its weight elongates the stomach with the gas distending the fundus, and a clear air/fluid level appears at the gas/barium interface (1398).

Radiograph

(1397) is of the stomach with the patient supine and barium in the fundus (1398) shows the fundus in the erect position and (1399) the fundus in the semi-erect oblique view.

Overcouch Films

In some centres, barium meal examinations are performed with the minimum amount of screening and spot films. The examination is then completed with overcouch views. These are almost invariably done with the patient horizontal in supine and prone positions. With extremely careful positioning it is possible to use a 24 × 30 cm (10 × 12 inch cassette), but in the vast majority of cases, 35 × 35 cm (14 × 14 inch) will be needed with the lower margin of the cassette at the level of the anterior, superior iliac spine and the middle of the cassette slightly to the left of the midline of the patient. For the postero-anterior projection centre 4 cm to the left of the midline at the lower costal margin.

Radiographs 1400–1407 on page 403 is a sequence of overcouch films taken over 48 hours showing stomach, duodenum, jejunum, ileum and colon. (1408) is the colon and terminal ileum during a single contrast barium enema.

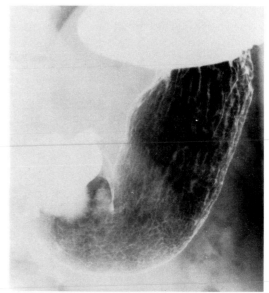

1397

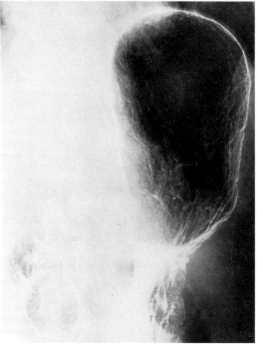

1398

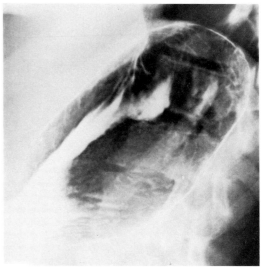

1399

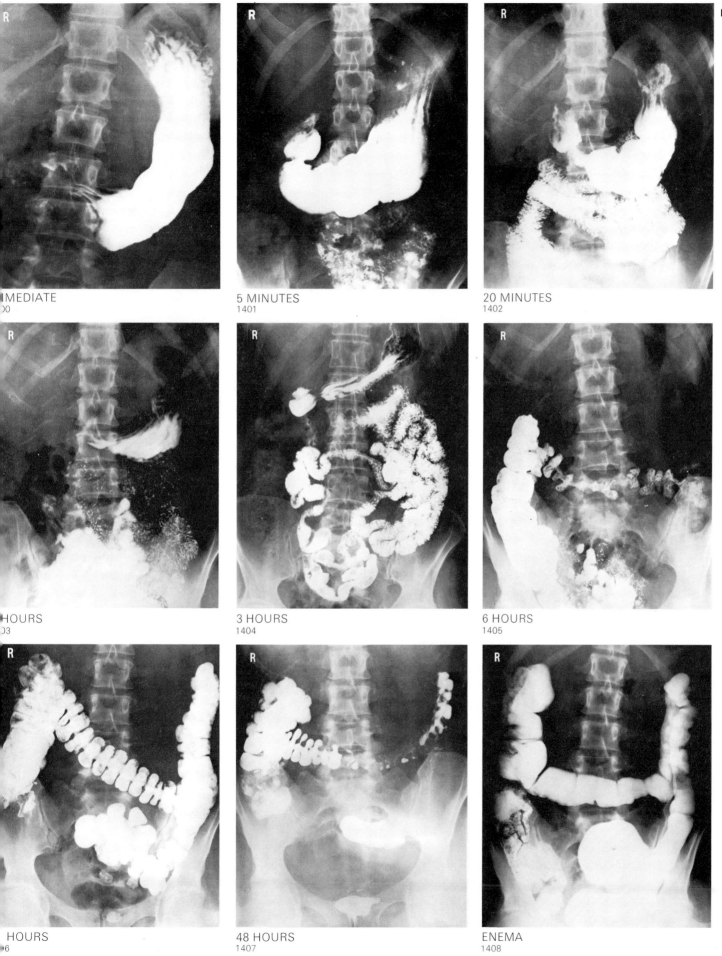

IMEDIATE
00

5 MINUTES
1401

20 MINUTES
1402

HOURS
03

3 HOURS
1404

6 HOURS
1405

HOURS
6

48 HOURS
1407

ENEMA
1408

16

403

Overcouch Films
Stomach—Patient Supine
Most views of the stomach will be done with the patient supine (antero-posterior).

Left (antero-Posterior) Oblique
This view is equivalent to the right anterior oblique (R.A.O.) when the film is taken during fluoroscopy with an undercouch tube. In the supine position rotate the patient 45° to the left by raising the right side. The right arm should be above the head of the patient with the left arm well in front.

■ Centre in the midline at the level of the lower costal margin.

Right (antero-Posterior) Oblique
This view is equivalent to the left anterior oblique (L.A.O.) when the film is taken during fluoroscopy with an undercouch tube. From the supine position rotate the patient 45° to the right by raising the left side. The left arm is above the head of the patient with the right arm well forward.

■ Centre in the midline at the lower costal margin.

Right Lateral
With the patient lying on the right side and the median plane parallel to the film the arms are held forward away from the abdomen.

■ Centre midway between the front and back of the patient at the level of the lower costal margin.

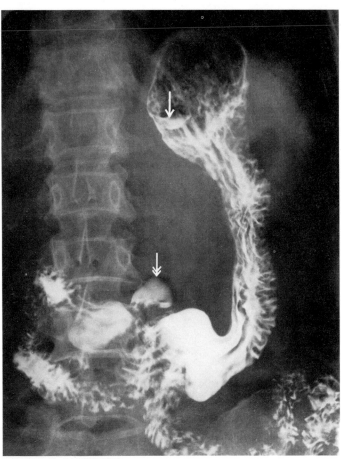

POSTERO-ANTERIOR
1409

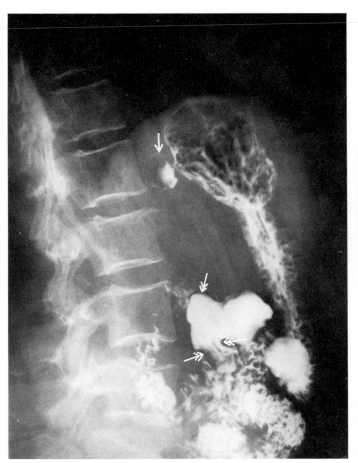

LATERAL
1410

Radiograph (1409) is a postero-anterior overcouch view of the stomach and duodenum showing a duodenal diverticulum (arrow) and (1410) is a right lateral view in the same patient.

Duodenum

The duodenum must be examined during fluoroscopy because of the variable position of the duodenal cap and loop (and, in the vast majority of cases, using compression). Spot films are taken during fluoroscopy in varying degrees of obliquity and with varying degrees of compression.

A double contrast examination of the duodenum is usually performed using a muscle relaxant with the duodenum well filled with barium and then allowing gas to enter from the stomach through the pylorus. A double contrast examination of the duodenum is done in both prone and supine positions with varying degrees of rotation of the patient towards the left.

Tube Duodenogram

For maximum detail of the duodenum the examination is carried out with a oesophago-gastro-duodenal tube and the barium and gas are injected into the duodenum via the tube.

When the duodenum is filled with barium use a high kilo-voltage exposure, but for double contrast duodenography use a medium kilo-voltage, between 60/80 kVp.

Gastric surface pattern—mucosal relief

There are two quite distinct appearances of the stomach surface obtained with a thin coating of barium.

When the stomach is not distended its surface is thrown into marked mucosal folds, which are seen in the barium meal as longitudinal and nearly parallel lines stretching from the fundus to the gastric antrum (1411, 1412, 1413).

However when the surface of the stomach is examined with adequate gastric distention, the gastric folds are flattened. If a correct technique is used including the proper barium and a relatively under-exposed radiograph taken with a medium kilo-voltage (60/80 kVp), a fine network pattern becomes visible in the majority of patients. The network pattern is due to barium entering the tiny grooves which lie between the small raised area of the stomach (arae gastricae) measuring 3–5 mm in diameter. If the technique is defective the areae gastricae will not be shown on double contrast barium meal examination.

An essential part of the double contrast barium meal technique is therefore adequate gas distension of the barium, a hypotonic stomach using a myorelaxant, the correct barium which has been well shaken or mixed, rare earth or fast intensifying screens, and a medium kilovoltage technique (60/80 kVp) but using the shortest possible time (0·04–0·06 sec).

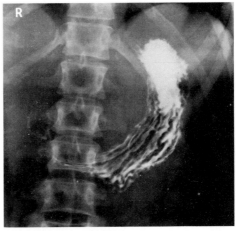

SEMI-RECUMBENT
1411

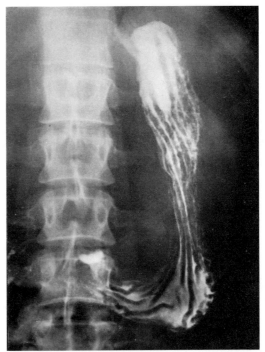

GASTRIC MUCOSA 1412   ERECT

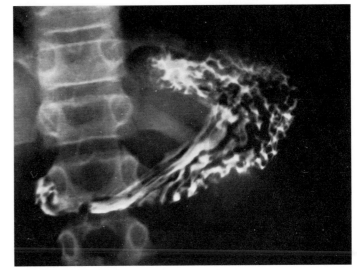

GASTRIC MUCOSA
1413

Duodenal cap projections

Because of the lie of the duodenal cap it is usually best seen in a frontal projection when the patient is in the right anterior oblique (R.A.O.) position during fluoroscopy. In this position the duodenal cap is at its longest and is positioned in such a way as to be free of the adjacent stomach and duodenal loop shadows for the exposure. Compression is often required to demonstrate a duodenal ulcer (1415a, b, c). The duodenal cap is seen in the "lateral" view when the patient is in the steep left anterior oblique position (L.A.O.) during fluoroscopy. Ulcers are then visible as a niche either on its anterior or posterior margin (1415c). Compression of the normal duodenal cap produces a parallel longitudinal mucosal fold pattern (1414b, c).

Small Intestine

The small bowel may be examined either as a follow through, immediately after the barium meal or as a separate examination using oesophago-gastro-duodenal intubation, with the tip of the tube lying well into the third part of the duodenum.

Barium Meal/follow through examination

Where a rapid but not very detailed examination of the small bowel is required a further 300 ml of barium is given after the barium meal examination of the stomach and duodenum has been completed. A hydrophilic non-flocculating barium should be used for the small bowel, together with a hurrying agent, such as a small dose of glucagon (0·1 to 0·2 mg intravenously), or metaclopramide (20 mg orally). Films are taken at regular intervals, either with fluoroscopic control or as overcouch exposures. Using a hurrying agent two to three films are usually sufficient to show the full length of the small bowel from duodenum to terminal ilium, with films taken at 15–20 minute intervals. The terminal ileum is then examined using fluoroscopy and localised compression.

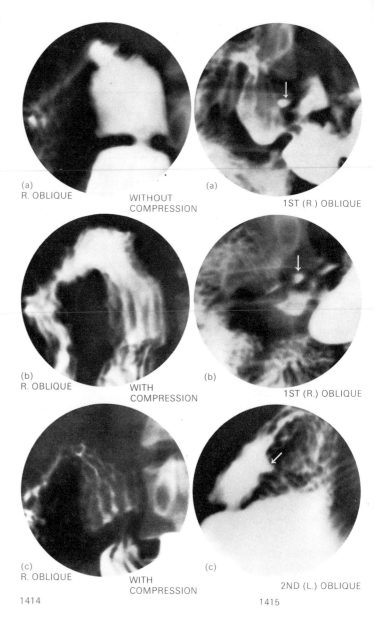

(a) R. OBLIQUE — WITHOUT COMPRESSION

(a) 1ST (R.) OBLIQUE

(b) R. OBLIQUE — WITH COMPRESSION

(b) 1ST (R.) OBLIQUE

(c) R. OBLIQUE — WITH COMPRESSION

(c) 2ND (L.) OBLIQUE

1414

1415

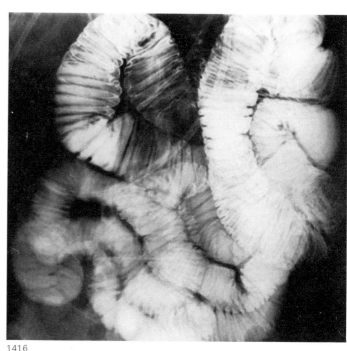

1416

Small Intestine—Small bowel enema

Following oesophago-gastro-duodenal intubation under fluoroscopic control, the tip of the tube is positioned in the third part of the duodenum. A guided tube such as a Dotter tube is usually preferred, 150 ml of barium being injected into the duodenum via the indwelling duodenal tube to be followed by the injection of water or a methyl cellulose suspension. In some centres a fixed specific gravity barium suspension is injected. The examination is performed using fluoroscopy and large 'spot films', 24 × 18 cm (10 × 18 ins), 30 × 24 cm (12 × 10 ins), or 35 × 35 cm (14 × 14 ins) films. Filming continues until the terminal ilium has been visualised. The examination needs to be done rapidly before there is precipitation of barium and it is not usually possible to repeat films due to poor exposure technique because the barium settles out spoiling the demonstration of the small bowel.

The appearances on follow-through examination and the small bowel enema examination are quite different. With the follow through examination, the small bowel has a longitudinal feathery pattern (1417), whereas using the small bowel technique the valvulae conniventes are demonstrated giving the small bowel a distended transverse band pattern (1416).

Terminal Ileum

The terminal ileum is frequently involved by disease, particularly Crohn's granulomatous enteritis, small bowel tuberculosis and as a "backwash ileitis" in ulcerative colitis. The terminal ileum may be shown either as part of the small bowel examination or by reflux from a barium enema (1418).

Compression with varying degrees of obliquity are usually required to show the terminal ileum and is best done under fluoroscopic control. It also helps considerably if the patient has a full bladder which displaces the small bowel out of the bony pelvis. The exposure factors for the compression views of the terminal ileum must be reduced considerably compared with non-compression views.

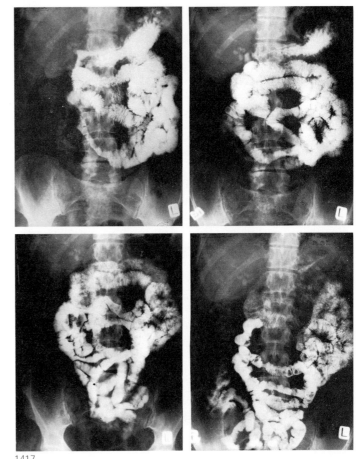

16

1417

Radiograph (1419) shows the appendix and colon on a film taken 24 hours after a barium meal examination.

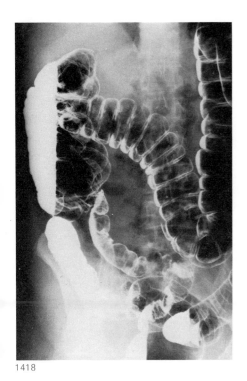

1418

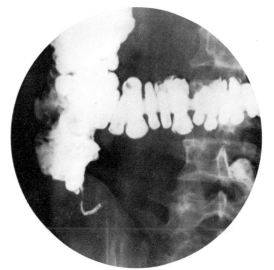

24 HOURS AFTER 1ST MEAL

1419

Colon or Large Intestine

Six hours after a barium meal examination barium is present in the caecum and often in the ascending colon, while at 12 hours contrast will be seen in the caecum, ascending colon and transverse colon. At 24 hours barium is usually present in the whole of the colon from the caecum to rectum. Thereafter it is evacuated and the colon may be entirely empty of barium by 48 hours apart from minimal residual mucosal coating but there is great variation between individuals in the rate of filling and emptying of the gastro-intestinal tract. The speed of filling and emptying has, by and large, no clinical significance.

Diverticula, associated with diverticular disease of the colon (1420, 1421) retain barium for a considerable time. Not infrequently barium may be present in colonic diverticula 10 days or even 3 weeks after a barium meal.

A barium enema however, is mandatory for the demonstration of colonic disease and not a barium follow through examination. Occasionally however the caecum can be adequately demonstrated when barium has reached the terminal ileum and ascending colon, by distending the colon with air by insufflation from the rectum. A double contrast view of the caecum is then possible.

Radiograph (1424) was taken 48 hours after a barium meal examination and shows barium in the caecum, ascending colon, transverse colon and descending colon. Diverticular disease of the colon is present. After 72 hours, (1425) the diverticula have filled with barium while most of the barium from the lumen of the colon has been evacuated. Barium is present in the rectum.

Radiograph (1420) shows a film following evacuation after a barium enema and (1421, 1422, 1423) show varying stages of the filling phase of a barium enema with barium in the rectum and sigmoid colon.

Radiograph (1426) is the filling phase of a barium enema with poor patient preparation. The ascending colon and transverse colon have multiple filling defects due to faeces and in the after evacuation film (1427), faeces is still present in the transverse colon.

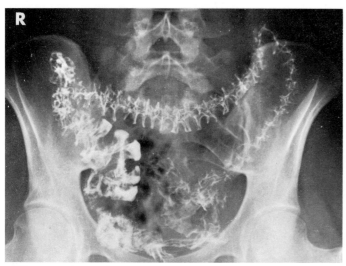

AFTER EVACUATION
1420

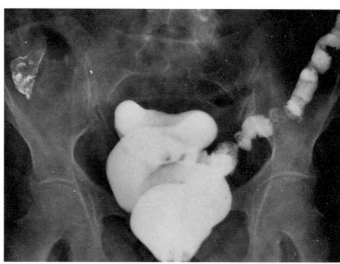

1421

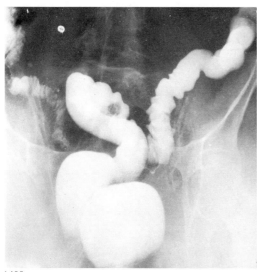

1422

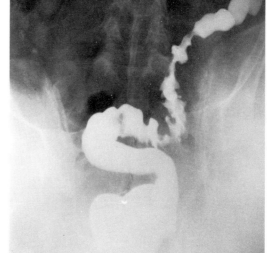

1423

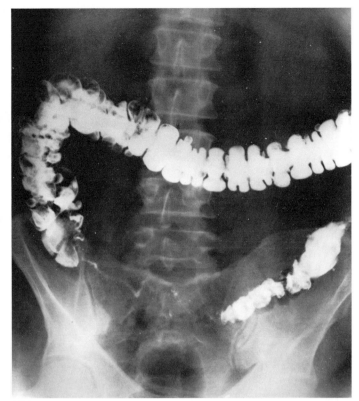

1424

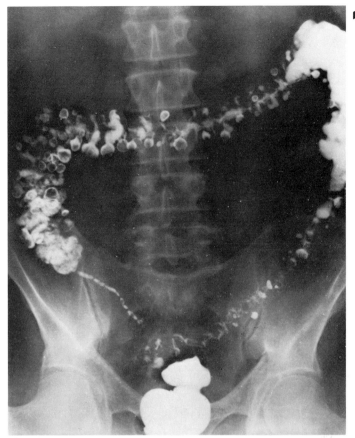

1425

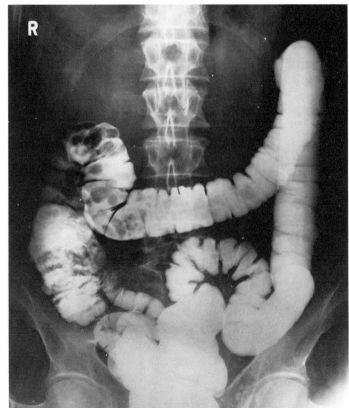

R

1426

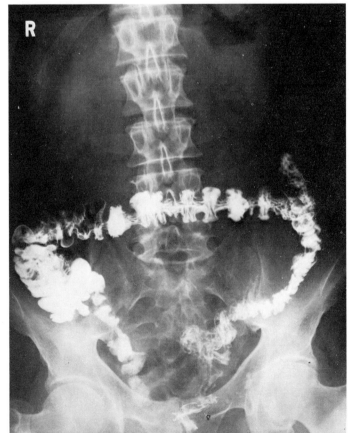

R

1427

Colon double contrast enema

In many centres, immediately prior to the examination, the patient has a cleansing enema. However in patients with ulcerative colitis and children with Hirschsprung's disease, no preparation must be given. These patients have an "instant" enema. An "instant" enema is also done in patients suspected of having a volvulus of the sigmoid colon.

Preparation of the patient
At the time the appointment for the examination is made the patient receives written instructions of the preparation required together with a simple explanation of the examination. The patient must be told that the examination including waiting time may take approximately 2–3 hours. Fluid diet starts 48 hours before the examination consisting of fruit juices, jelly, thin soup, milk, ice cream, tea, coffee and water. The patient must under no circumstances have food containing roughage; fruits and vegetables are expressly excluded. The patient should take at least 4 pints of fluid on each of the two days preceding the examination. An effective laxative such as dulcados or castor oil is given for two nights prior to the examination.

The patient should arrive in the department for the morning examination at 8.30 to 9.00 am, for a plain film of the abdomen which is assessed for residual faeces. If the colon appears to be reasonably clear on the preliminary plain film a colon wash out is performed, after the patient takes 30 mg of propantheline orally to relax the colon.

For the colonic wash out 2 g of Veripaque are dissolved in 2 litres of warm (not hot) tap water and run into the patient via a rectal tube over a period of 15 minutes. The patient is then asked to retain the enema for 5 minutes before evacuation in the toilet.

The patient then waits for a minimum of one hour during which time the colon should be evacuated completely.

Filling Technique
The tube is inserted with the patient in the left lateral position and after being turned prone the barium is allowed to run in under fluoroscopic control using image intensification and a television monitor. The barium is stopped when it reaches the proximal part of the splenic flexure and then the barium is evacuated from the rectum by lowering the plastic barium enema bag below the level of the table top and allowing the barium to drain out by gravity.

With the patient in the right lateral position air is then insufflated to push the barium around to the caecum. Films of the rectum in the true lateral position (1431) are taken and when there is adequate double contrast coating of the colon the patient is brought into the erect position for oblique views of the hepatic and splenic flexures. These films must be relatively under-exposed to show the details of the mucosal pattern (1428, 1429, 1430).

The patient is then moved onto a Bucky table with an overcouch tube which can be moved to take horizontal beam films in the decubitus positions.

A prone film (1432) of the abdomen is taken, using the Potter Bucky and a 43 × 35 cm (17 × 14 ins) cassette.

The patient remains in the prone position and a view of the sigmoid colon (Hampton's view), is then taken. The tube is angled 45° towards the feet with the central ray passing in the midline midway between the anterior, superior iliac spines, displacing the cassette accordingly so that the central ray passes through the centre of 35 × 35 cm (14 × 14 ins) film (1433).

The patient is then turned onto the right side for a right lateral decubitus view and using a 43 × 35 cm (17 × 14 ins) cassette and a fine line stationary grid a frontal radiograph is taken.

The patient is then turned onto the left side and a similar frontal view obtained the; left lateral decubitis view.

The cassette and grid must be positioned from the anus upwards and centred to the anterior superior iliac spine. The central ray must always be at right angles to the grid to avoid grid cut-off.

Radiographs
(1428, 1429) are oblique erect views during fluoroscopy to show the hepatic flexure and (1430) the splenic flexure with an erect lateral view of the recto-sigmoid region in (1431).

In (1379) multiple polyps are shown (curved arrows) and a carcinoma (straight arrows) on a prone view and in (1432).

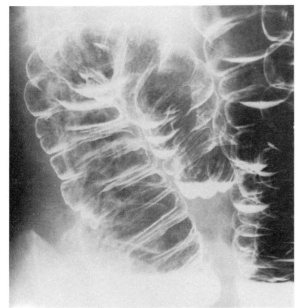

1428

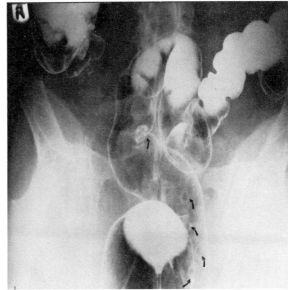

1429

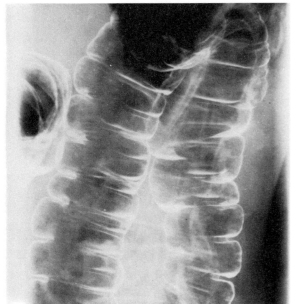

1430

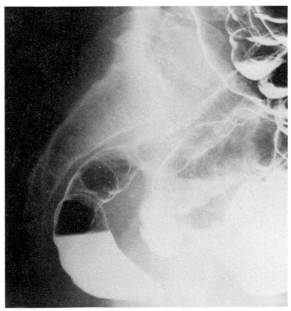

1431

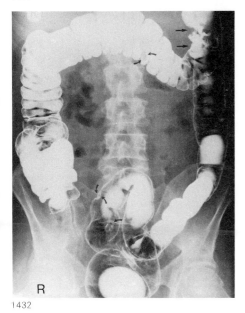

1432

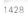

1433

Single contrast enema

For the single contrast enema either a much more dilute barium is used or a high kilovoltage technique to penetrate the barium.

Barium is run in slowly with he patient in the left lateral position; a lateral film of the recto-sigmoid region is taken followed by an oblique view of the sigmoid colon (1423). Undercouch, either 24 × 30 cm (10 × 12 inch) or 35 × 35 cm (14 × 14 inch) films are taken in the most appropriate positions to avoid overlapping of the transverse and descending colon on the left side and transverse and ascending colon on the right. Filming is continued until there is adequate filling of the caecum (1440) and preferably reflux into the terminal ileum.

Following the filling phase of the barium enema the patient evacuates as much of the barium as possible and a prone overcouch, after evacuation film is taken on a 35 × 43 cm (14 × 17 inch (film (1438).

Radiograph (1434) shows the appearance of the colon after air insufflation following evacuation of barium.

A double contrast barium enema (1435) shows a malignant polyp (arrow).

(1436 and 1438) are filled and after evacuation films of a single contrast enema.

In (1437 and 1440) the colon is filled with barium up to the caecum.

(1439 and 1441) are views of a double contrast enema, a supine and right lateral decubitus respectively.

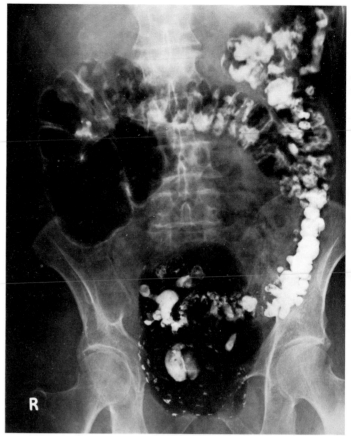

POSTERO-ANTERIOR
1434

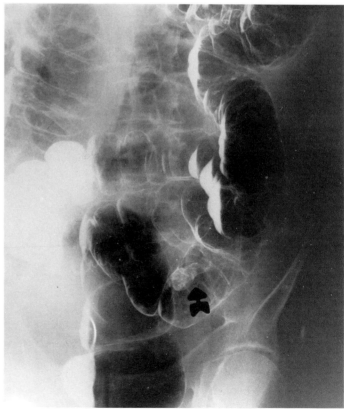

1435

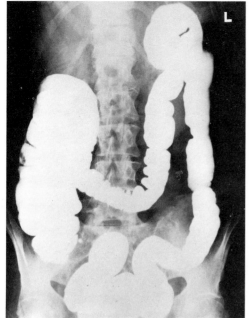

1436

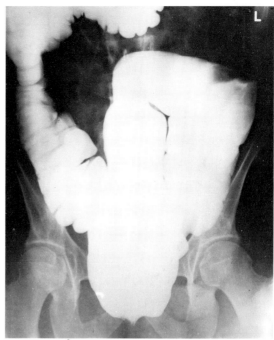

DISTENDED COLON
1437

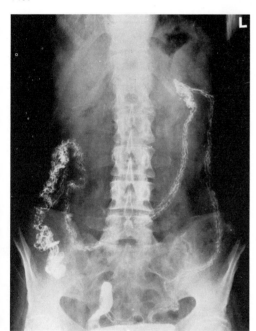

1438

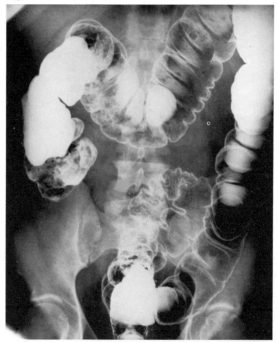

1439

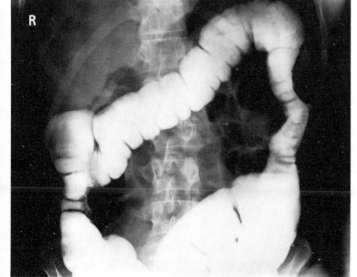

DISTENDED COLON
1440

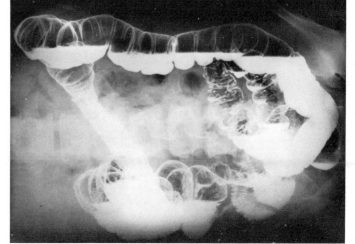

1441

Air inflation

Air inflation of the colon is not infrequently done following a single contrast examination and performed after the patient has been to the toilet to evacuate the barium (1447, 1448).

Air inflation through a rectal catheter is also done for a double contrast examination of the caecum as part of a follow through examination where there is any doubt about the distensibility of or filling defect in the caecum. Reflux of air into the terminal ilium can similarly be used to show the terminal ilium in double contrast.

Radiographs (1442, 1443, 1444) show a carcinoma of the transverse colon.

(1445–1448) are of a single contrast enema in the filled phase, after evacuation and then air insufflation. (1448) is a supine oblique view with the left shoulder raised (L.A.O.).

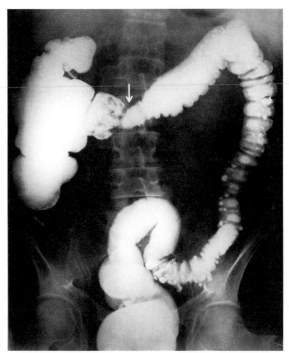

DISTENSION BY BARIUM ENEMA
1442

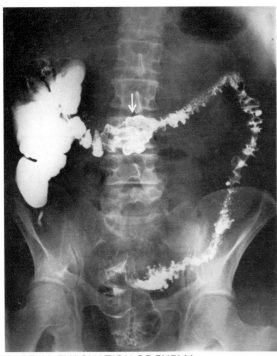

PARTIAL EVACUATION OF ENEMA
1443

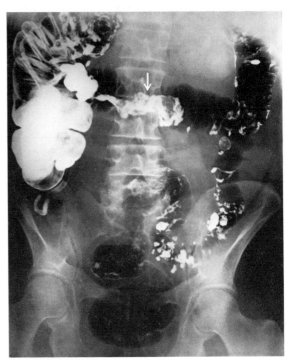

AIR INFLATION
1444

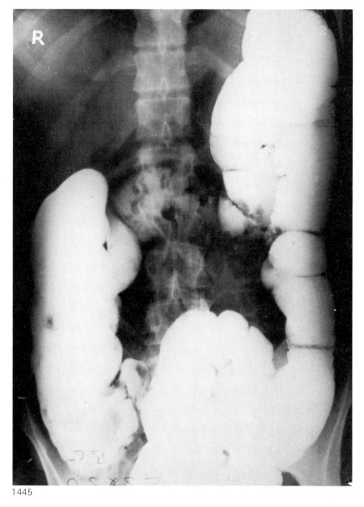

1445

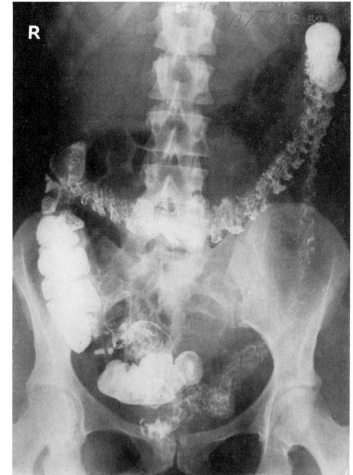

1446

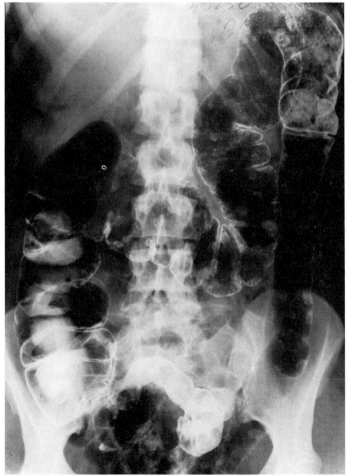

1447

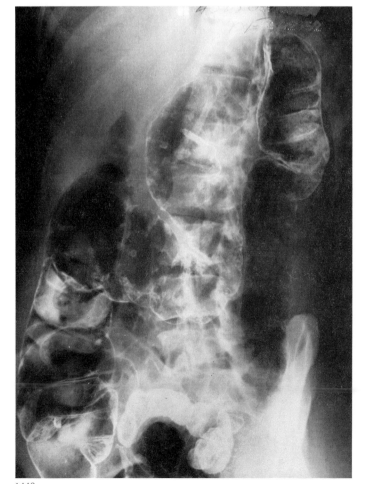

1448

In babies and infants the pyloric canal and duodenal cap are usually hidden by the gastric antrum but can be shown with the child horizontal, lying on the right side, with slight forward rotation, that is, in a slightly prone position. The pyloric canal and duodenum then appear behind the stomach towards the spine. This position is also advantageous by allowing the barium to accumulate in the gastric antrum against the pyloric canal which helps barium to pass from the stomach into the duodenum.

Oesophagus

For the diagnosis of oesophageal atresia a soft rubber catheter is passed and a film taken with the tube at the site of holdup. If contrast is used only a minimal amount must be given, approximately 0·5–1 ml. A non-ionic contrast agent, such as metrizimide, may be used or lipiodol. Other water soluble contrast agents should not be used because tracheal spill may occur.

For the diagnosis of a tracheo-oesophogeal fistula an oesophogeal tube is used and, while injecting barium into the oesophagus, it is slowly withdrawn. With the child horizontal films are taken in the Right Anterior Oblique (R.A.O.) position The examination, is best done using cine-fluorography.

Opaque meal

For young babies the contrast examination replaces the normal feed so that the child has not been fed for 3–4 hours before the examination. A feeding bottle containing a warm 50% suspension of barium sulphate which excludes foodstuffs should be used. The child is given the bottle when lying horizontally on the right side. After observing the oesophagus the child is turned slightly forwards while feeding continues. When there is sufficient barium in the gastric antrum the feeding bottle is turned horizontal so that sucking of the teat can continue without taking in more barium. Air swallowing helps to fill the stomach and to produce a double contrast examination. The diagnosis of pyloric stenosis is made on the elongated appearance of the pyloric canal and not by taking repeated films to assess gastric emptying.

A summary of exposure conditions for the alimentary tract suitable for an adult subject of average physique (over couch)

Region	Position	kVp	mAS	FFD	Film ILFORD	Screens ILFORD	Grid
Pharynx	Antero–posterior	65	30	(40")—100 cm	RAPID R	FT	
		75	15	(40")—100 cm	RAPID R	FT	Grid
	Lateral	65	10	(40")—100 cm	RAPID R	FT	Grid
		75	6	(40")—100 cm	RAPID R	FT	Grid
							Grid
Oesophagus	Oblique	75	15	(40")—100 cm	RAPID R	FT	
		85	8	(40")—100 cm	RAPID R	FT	Grid
							Grid
Stomach	Postero–anterior	85	20	(40")—100 cm	RAPID R	FT	
		90	10	(40")—100 cm	RAPID R	FT	Grid
	Oblique	85	20	(40")—100 cm	RAPID R	FT	Grid
		90	10	(40")—100 cm	RAPID R	FT	Grid
	Lateral	95	40	(40")—100 cm	RAPID R	FT	Grid
Duodenum (localized)	Postero–anterior	85	15	(40")—100 cm	RAPID R	FT	—
		85	30	(40")—100 cm	RAPID R	FT	Grid
	Lateral	90	20	(40")—100 cm	RAPID R	FT	Grid
Colon (meal)	Postero–anterior Antero–posterior	85	40	(40")—100 cm	RAPID R	FT	Grid
	Oblique	90	40	(40")—100 cm	RAPID R	FT	Grid
	Lateral	95	50	(40")—100 cm	RAPID R	FT	Grid
Colon (enema)	Postero–anterior	90	35	(40")—100 cm	RAPID R	FT	Grid
	Oblique	90	45	(40")—100 cm	RAPID R	FT	Grid
	Lateral	90	60	(40")—100 cm	RAPID R	FT	Grid

Radiographs (1449a–f) are a series of films of a barium meal and follow-through examination of a child taken over a 24 hour period. The stomach and small intestine is shown up to 6 hours and the colon at 24 hours.

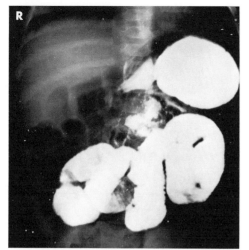

IMMEDIATE
1449a

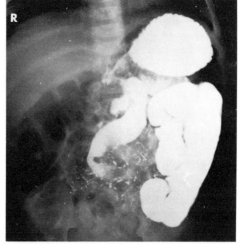

½ HOUR
1449b

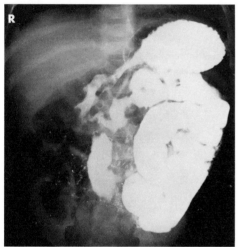

2½ HOURS
1449c

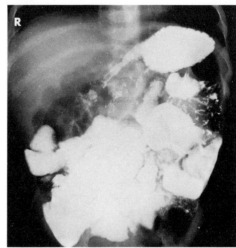

1 HOUR
1449d

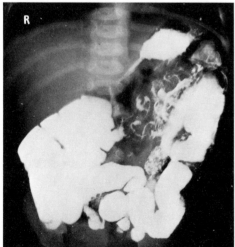

6 HOURS
1449e

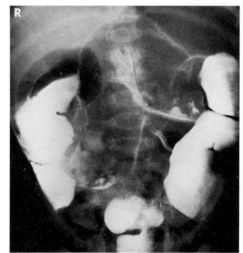

24 HOURS
1449f

16 Opaque enema

In infants and children the opaque enema may demonstrate intussusception, meconium ileus or Hirschsprung's disease. Preliminary bowel washout is both unnecessary and dangerous. In Hirschsprung's disease water intoxication could occur after a colon washout.

A soft rubber tube is used for a barium enema in infants and children and the buttocks are firmly strapped together with adhesive tape. The use of a self-retaining or a rigid catheter must be avoided. In Hirschsprung's disease the barium inflow is stopped after showing the narrowed segment. The whole colon should not be filled in this examination.

In intussusception a low pressure system is advised particularly when the enema is being performed for its reduction. The enema bag must not be elevated more than 1 m (3 ft) above the level of the child.

Radiograph (1450a) shows barium in the colon up to the hepatic flexure and (1450b) the colonic pattern after evacuation.

Radiograph (1451a) is a spot film of the filled rectum and sigmoid in the frontal view and (1451b) in the lateral view, whereas (1452a, 1452b) shows the rectum and sigmoid in frontal and oblique positions.

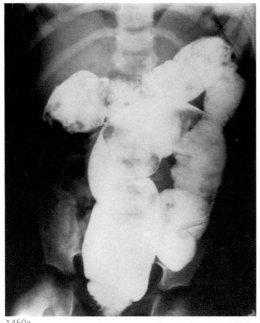

1450a

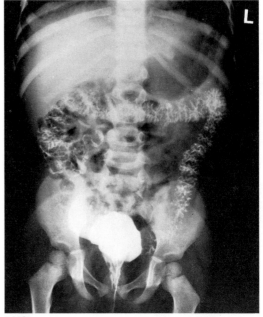

1450b

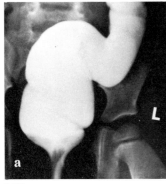

1451

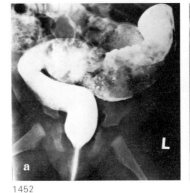

1452

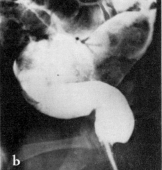

17

BILIARY TRACT

BILIARY TRACT

The gall bladder is a pear shaped, hollow structure lying anterior and inferior to the lower margin of the liver and contains bile which is manufactured in the liver. It is divided into the fundus, body and neck (1453a) and is normally 7–10 cm (2½–4 ins) in length while the fundus is approximately 3 cm (1 inch) wide. The gall bladder normally has a capacity of 30–50 ml. The neck of the gall bladder communicates with the cystic duct which has a spiral valve (of Heister) producing an irregular margin when shown with contrast medium. Bile is secreted in the liver and then passes into the biliary system collecting in the right and left hepatic ducts which join together to form the common hepatic duct. The common hepatic duct joins the cystic duct to form the common bile duct which passes behind the first part of the duodenum and along the lateral margin of the head of the pancreas being close to the medial wall of the second part of the duodenum. It finally joins with the pancreatic duct and then empties into the duodenum forming a small mound on the mucosa called the papilla of Vater. The opening of the combined pancreatic and common bile duct is known as the sphincter of Oddi.

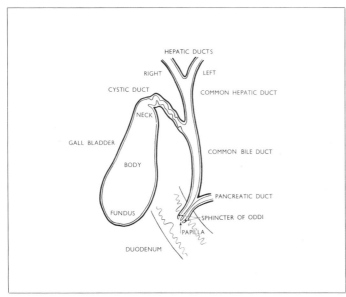

1453a

Varying position and shape

There is considerable variation in the size, shape and position of the gall bladder. In the vast majority of cases, it lies close to the lower margin of the right lobe of the liver. Radiographically it usually appears pear shaped, but may be rounded depending on its relationship to the direction of the central ray (1453b).

Its position can vary from the level of the 11th rib to the first sacral segment and from close to the lateral wall of the abdomen to near the spine. Very rarely the gall bladder is even left sided.

From front to back it may be at the level of the anterior margin of the vertebral bodies or close to the anterior abdominal wall. There is considerable variation in the position of the gall bladder with postural variation particularly with a change from the horizontal to erect position, especially in elderly patients. The gall bladder also moves downwards on inspiration and is often close to the outer margin of the duodenal loop and close to the duodenal bulb. Gas and faeces in the hepatic flexure of the colon are not infrequently superimposed on the gall bladder region.

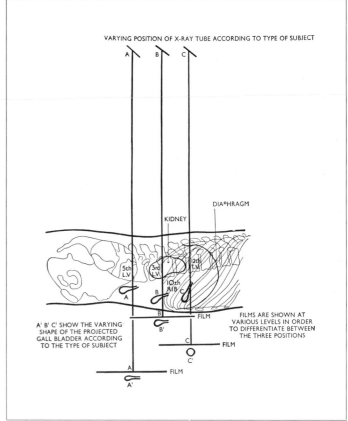

1453b

In some patients many different positions may be needed to project the gall bladder free of overlying colonic shadow or to distinguish between opacities in the kidney and the gall bladder.

The diagram of a body in the prone position in longitudinal section (1453b) shows the gall bladder in three different positions as seen from the lateral aspect.

In persons of average physique (sthenic, hyposthenic) the gall bladder is shown as pear shaped opposite the 3rd lumbar vertebra approximately 5 cm (3 inch) from the spinous process and towards the right side of the abdomen. [1454) and (B1) in illustration (1453b)].

Less commonly in larger subjects (hypersthenic) the gall bladder is horizontal and appears circular at the level of the 1st lumbar vertebra [(1455) and (C) and (C1) in illustration 1453b).]

In a small group who are tall thin subjects (asthenic) the gall bladder is elongated and at a lower level, nearer the midline, often overshadowing the 4th and 5th lumbar vertebrae. [(1456) and (A) and (A1) in (1453b)].

Summary of procedures

Radiographic techniques for the gall bladder are discussed under the following headings:

Preliminary Examination (Plain film)

A plain film of the gall bladder region is always done prior to a contrast examination to exclude the presence of opacities or transradiancies in the gall bladder or biliary region. This oblique view of the right hypochondrium shows the position of gas and faeces in the colon or opacities such as costal cartilage calcifications and renal calculi. If an opacity is noted in the right hypochondrium on an antero-posterior film of the abdomen taken prior to a barium meal or enema then a postero-anterior oblique view of the right hypochondrium should be done to show whether the opacity can be related to the gall-bladder region.

Oral Cholecystography

A contrast medium is used which when taken orally is absorbed by the bowel, excreted by the liver and accumulates in the gall bladder. This examination is used to show gall stones, adenomyomatosis of the gall bladder or a 'non-functioning' gall bladder.

Intravenous Cholangiography

This procedure demonstrates the hepatic and common bile ducts and is used in patients who have had a cholecystectomy.

Ultrasonography

The gall bladder and gall stones are well shown with ultrasound as well as dilated intra-hepatic bile ducts.

Percutaneous Cholangiogram

A long thin needle or fine catheter is introduced into the liver by passing it through the overlying skin and sub-cutaneous tissue either from the front or the side of the patient. The tip of the needle or catheter is positioned in an intra-hepatic bile duct and contrast medium injected. This examination is used in patients with obstructive jaundice to show the size of the ducts and the point of obstruction.

Endoscopic Retrograde Cholangio—Pancreatography (ERCP)

A gastro-duodenal endoscope is positioned to view the papilla of Vater and a fine catheter is passed through the sphincter of Oddi after which a water soluble contrast medium is injected into the common-bile duct and the pancreatic duct.

Operative Cholangiography

During gall bladder surgery prior to removal of the gall bladder, contrast medium is injected into the cystic duct to outline the common bile duct and hepatic ducts. Films are taken which are viewed during the operation to exclude the presence of stones in the common bile duct.

Post-operative Cholangiography (T-Tube Cholangiography)

Following cholecystectomy a T-tube is left in position to splint the common hepatic and bile ducts. Approximately 10 days later contrast medium is injected into the free end of the T-tube which emerges at the skin surface. Contrast medium outlines the T-tube, the common hepatic and bile ducts and flows into the duodenum. This procedure is used to exclude residual stones following cholecystectomy.

17

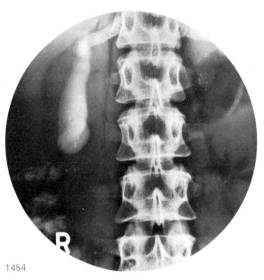

1454

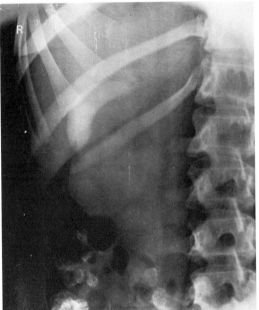

1455

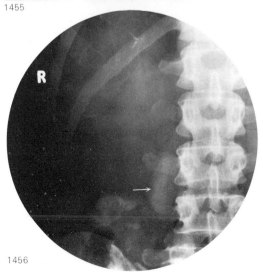

1456

POSTERO-ANTERIOR

421

Gall stones may be large or small, single or multiple, opaque or transradiant. When a gall stone passes into the cystic or common bile duct it can cause pain or can obstruct the cystic duct producing a "non-functioning" gall bladder or lodge in the common bile duct and can then cause jaundice. Pure cholesterol stones are often large and transradiant. Opacities in the right hypochondrium are considered to be gall stones when multiple, laminated, faceted, related to the line of the liver edge and outside the renal margin on the oblique film. However, the vast majority of gall stones are transradiant and are shown only after oral cholecystography (1471) or ultrasonography.

(1460) Many small stones with crenellated margins.
(1461) Circular laminated stones.
(1462) Multiple laminated and faceted gall stones.
(1463) Multiple gall stones in the gall bladder. A single stone has been passed into the common bile duct at its distal end (arrow).
(1464) Multiple gall stones and barium in the colon.
(1465) Multiple large laminated stones.
(1466) Multiple less dense calculi in the gall bladder with one stone stuck in Hartmann's pouch.
(1467) Three densely laminated and faceted gall stones.
(1468) Oval shaped laminated gall stone.
(1469) Large laminated oval gall stone.
(1470) Small stone in gall bladder containing contrast medium lying adjacent to the duodenal cap. The gastric antrum contains barium.
(1471) Multiple calculi within contrast medium in the gall bladder.

A short exposure time is essential because even large gall stones can become invisible with slight movement blurring. Accurate centring and careful collimation is equally essential.

Although greater contrast is achieved with lower kilovoltages there must be sufficient penetration of the contrast medium in the gall bladder as well as the shortest possible exposure time to eliminate movement blurring and produce sharp outlines.

Careful labelling of each radiograph is essential to identify the patient, the preliminary film, the time of the exposure after contrast medium and after fatty meal (or an equivalent) to produce contraction of the gall bladder.

Films of the gall bladder are always taken with a grid and definition can be further improved with compression (1457, 1458, 1459).

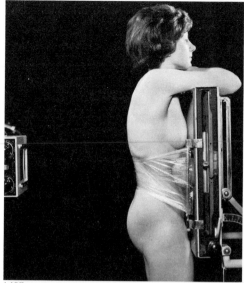

1457

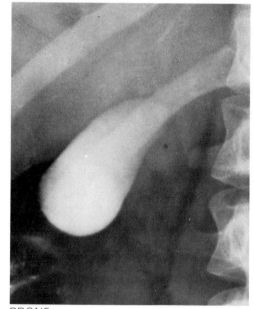

PRONE
1458

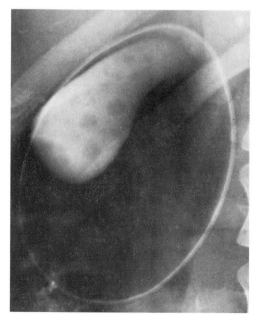

COMPRESSION
1459

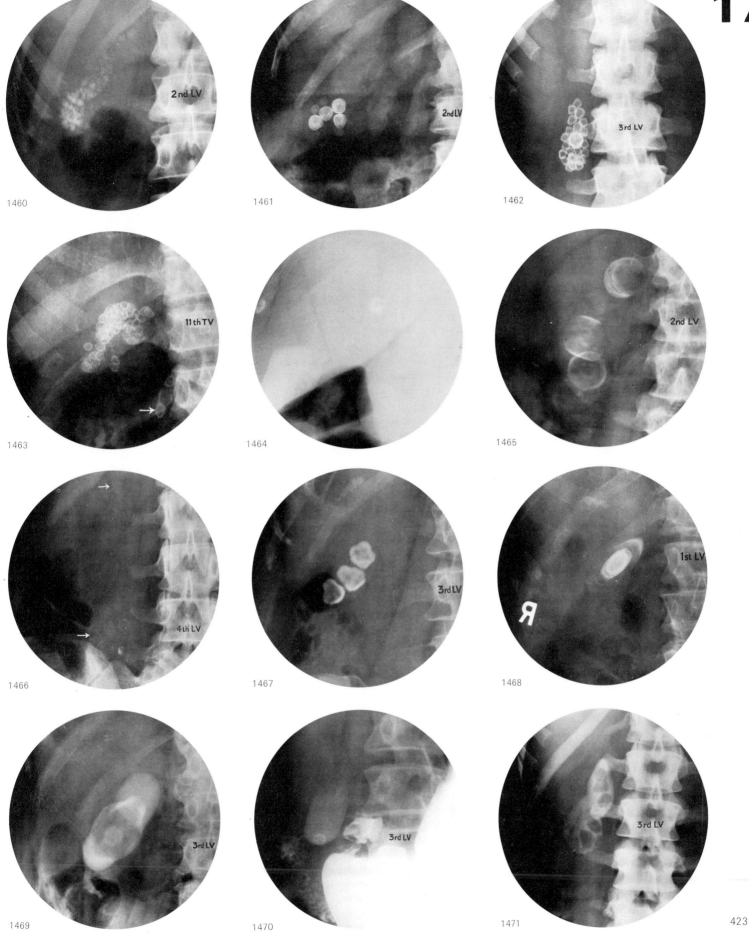

1460

1461

1462

1463

1464

1465

1466

1467

1468

1469

1470

1471

Preliminary examination

A contrast examination of the gall bladder or biliary system is always preceded by a plain film. The patient may have had a full length plain film of the abdomen for a barium meal or pyelogram which showed opacities in the right hypochondrium. However a prelminary film of the gall bladder area prior to giving contrast is often the only initial examination.

The preliminary examination of the gall bladder region taken of the right hypochondrium is in the oblique position and can be done either antero-posterior or postero-anterior. The antero-posterior projection (right AP oblique) is easier for both the patient and the radiographer. A medium kilovoltage in the region of 60 to 80 kVp is preferred for maximum soft tissue contrast. The exposure time must be as short as possible and should not exceed 0·04 of a second, which can be achieved with most units with rare earth screens or by using a 3 phase high output generator. Compression and immobilisation with a Bucky band helps to achieve a better result.

The preliminary films should be done at the patient's initial visit to the department when the appointment for the contrast examination is made. The patient is given written instructions on a pro-forma sheet which includes the amount of contrast agent and the date and time on which to take each dose. The procedure should also be explained at this stage and the patient informed as to the time that will be required to be spent in the X-ray department when the contrast examination is carried out.

If the patient inadvertently has contrast medium in the alimentary tract because of a previous barium examination a repeat preliminary examination will usually be needed after a few days.

Cholecystography

Cholecystography is the visualisation of the gall bladder after taking an oral contrast medium (1481, 1482). Oral Cholecystographic contrast agents including Telepaque, Biliodyl, Biloptin, and Solubiloptin are organic iodine compounds which are absorbed from the bowel, excreted by the liver into the bile ducts and concentrated in the gall bladder. Although these compounds are relatively non-toxic they not infrequently cause mild diarrhoea and may cause vomiting. Often diarrhoea or vomiting is a cause of non-visualisation of the gall bladder which is also caused by gastric retention of contrast medium, due either to pylorospasm or pyloric stenosis. This examination is not performed in the presence of jaundice because again the gall bladder will not be demonstrated. Compounds such as Telepaque, Biliodyl, and Biloptin take at least 14 hours to show the gall bladder whereas with Solubiloptin the gall bladder will be shown after 2 to 4 hours.

The preparation varies from one department to another, but a common method now used is to have the patient take 4 tablets (2 g) of Telepaque 38 hours before the examination and then to have a fat free diet for the following day, with a light meal that evening, after which a further 4 tablets (2 g) of Telepaque is taken. Thereafter the patient must have only water to drink until the examination the following morning.

If the gall bladder is well demonstrated on routine views the examination can be completed, with compression spot films if necessary and then after fatty meal films. However, if the gall bladder shows poor concentration of contrast medium or no gall bladder is visible a dose of Solubiloptin (2 g, one sachet) is then given and further films of the gall bladder region are taken three to four hours later. If at this stage no gall bladder is seen a film of the whole upper abdomen should be taken to exclude a left sided gall bladder.

There is also considerable variation in the "fatty meal" used to obtain contraction of the gall bladder. The fatty meal can consist of an "egg nog", a milk chocolate drink, a chocolate bar, or a commercial preparation such as prosparol or biloptin fatty meal. A "fatty meal" is used to contract the gall bladder which then fills the common bile duct with contrast medium and can be shown on films taken 10 to 20 minutes after the fatty meal.

The gall bladder must be shown free of gas shadows in the colon or duodenum and a horizontal beam radiograph must also be done to exclude "floating" stones. The common routine for the demonstration of a contrast filled gall bladder is to do supine and erect oblique radiographs which are then viewed. If the gall bladder is free of overlying gas and the necessary information has been obtained a further film is taken 10 to 20 minutes later. However, to avoid unnecessary delay both a prone and supine oblique radiograph can be done in addition to the erect which will help to show the gall bladder clear of gas shadows in the vast majority of cases. If overlying gas shadows are however present then fluoroscopy must be carried out with spot films taken in the optimum degree of rotation to throw the gall bladder away from the gas shadows.

Intravenous cholangiography

A preliminary film of the gall bladder is done in the same way as for oral cholecystography. Contrast medium used for intravenous cholangiography is at present the most toxic of the injected water soluble contrast agents used in radiology. Biligrafin Forte or Biligram may be used but must be given extremely slowly and is now usually administered in an intravenous drip infusion of 200 ml in 5 % glucose over a period of 15 to 30 minutes. Not more than 10 g of iodine equivalent (20 ml of Biligrafin forte) should be used.

A film is taken at 30 and 45 minutes after the injection but tomography at 45 to 60 minutes is essential to show the details of the common bile duct. Later films at 90 and 120 minutes will demonstrate whether there is any evidence of increasing density in the common bile duct indicating obstruction at the papilla of Vater. The films of the common bile duct are best done in the supine oblique position to throw it clear of the lumbar spine. Tomography should also be carried out in the supine oblique position at levels between 12 to 15 cm from the table top depending on patient's build. Intravenous Cholangiography is used for cholecystectomised patients who have symptoms suggesting the presence of stones in the biliary system, but is not recommended in patients with jaundice.

The fundus of the gall bladder lies more caudal and anterior than its neck. In the supine position gall stones will tend to run away from the fundus towards the neck of the gall bladder being shown as a narrow file of small opacities (1472, 1474) However, in the prone position gall stones will collect in a small group in the fundus of the gall bladder which is then in a more dependent position (1473, 1475).

Radiographs (1472, 1474) show multiple small gall stones strung out in a long line in the supine position whereas in Radiographs (1473, 1475) the gall stones have collected in a group in the fundus of the gall bladder in the prone films.

Where there is gas in the colon overlying the gall bladder a change from the prone to supine position often helps to show the gall bladder free of gas shadows.

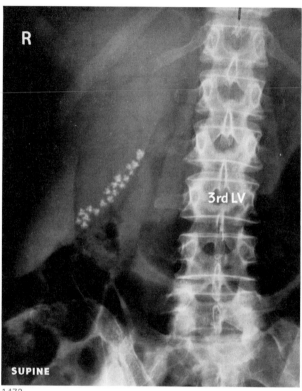

SUPINE
1472

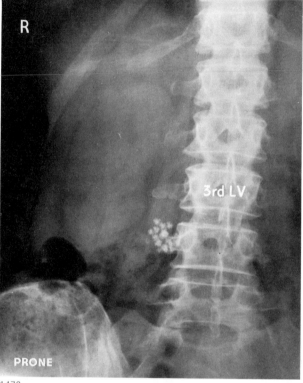

PRONE
1473

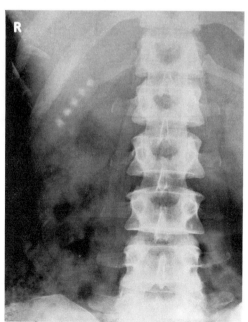

SUPINE
1474

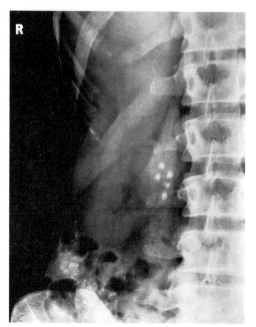

PRONE
1475

Right Antero-Posterior Oblique
With the patient supine the left side is raised from the table top by approximately 20° to 30° and supported by foam pads under the hip joint and lower thorax; the arms are raised and the hands folded behind the head. The gall bladder is then displaced towards the right, usually away from overlying colonic shadows to lie over the liver region. The common bile duct then lies clear of the vertebral column.

■ Centre just below the costal margin midway between the umbilicus and right abdominal wall (1476, 1477).

The initial film must include an area from the anterior superior iliac spine to the 11th rib and transversely from the vertebral column to the right abdominal wall.

This projection is also used for showing the common bile duct particularly during intravenous cholangiography and tomography. The common bile duct can frequently be shown with oral cholecystography on radiographs taken between 10 and 30 minutes after a fatty meal (1479).

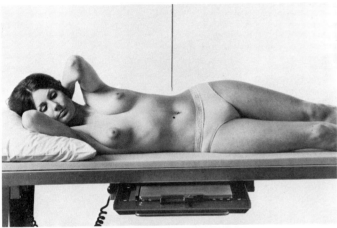

1476

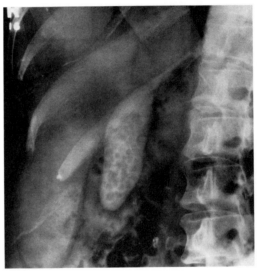

1477

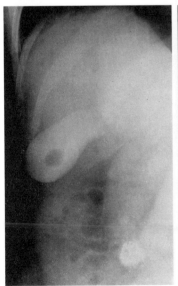

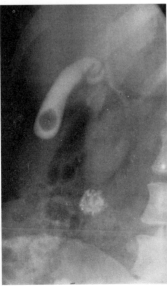

OBLIQUE INSPIRATION
1478　　　　14 HOURS

OBLIQUE AFM
1479

An alternative method for positioning the gall bladder over the liver and the common bile duct away from the spine is the left postero-anterior oblique (prone oblique) position.

If in the supine position there are overlying gas shadows, particularly of the hepatic flexure of the colon then the gall bladder may be shown clear of interfering shadows by turning the patient into the prone oblique position.

Left Postero-anterior Oblique (Prone oblique)

With the patient prone the right side is raised approximately 20° to 30° from the table top and supported by foam pads under the hip joint and upper abdomen. The head is turned towards the right and the right hand is raised above the head with the arm resting on the couch. The right knee is flexed and rests on the couch for support. In the average patient an obliquity of 20° is usually sufficient but this may need to be decreased in the heavily built patient and increased to 30° in the long thin patient. Although the gall bladder is nearer the front of the body than the back, by raising the right side of the abdomen from

the table, it is displaced some 5 to 10 cm (2–4 ins) further from the table top, whereas in the supine position raising the left side of the patient tends to bring the gall bladder nearer the film. In practice there is very little difference in distance of the gall bladder from the film in the prone oblique and supine oblique positions. The supine oblique position however, is more comfortable for the patient.

■ Centre midway between the lower costal margin and iliac crest and midway between the vertebral column and the right abdominal wall (1480, 1481, 1482)

The Centering for the gall bladder in the prone position is approximately 4 cm (1½ ins) more caudal than in the supine oblique position.

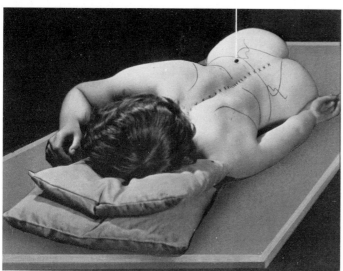

1480

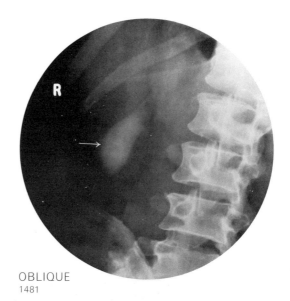

OBLIQUE
1481

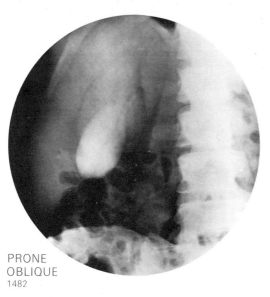

PRONE
OBLIQUE
1482

Erect Left Postero-Anterior Oblique
Erect Right Antero-Posterior Oblique
(Modified)

The examination of the gall bladder must include a horizontal beam radiograph which is most easily done in the erect position (1483). The postero-anterior view is easier for the patient if the right arm can rest on the top of the Bucky. The horizontal ray film is essential in gall bladder examinations to show "floating" gall stones. Not infrequently gall stones are multiple small and transradiant and hidden by the dense contrast medium when the film is taken with the patient horizontal. However, on a horizontal ray film small transradiant gall stones become visible usually just above the line of dense contrast medium (1484, 1485, 1486) as "floating gall stones".

With the patient erect and facing the Potter-Bucky diaphragm the right side is rotated away from the Bucky by 20°–30° with the left hand on the hip and the arm resting against the side of the Bucky platform and the right arm resting on the top of the Bucky (1483).

The erect antero-posterior oblique position can be used as an alternative projection. The patient is then erect and facing the tube and the back of the patient rotated away from the Bucky by 20° to 30°.

■ Centre 2 cm (1 in) above the iliac crest midway between the midline and right abdominal wall.

The centering point in the erect oblique position is approximately 4 cm (1½ ins) more caudal than in the supine position. Better definition is obtained by using a small localising cone, particularly if there is also compression and adequate immobilisation.

Radiographs (1484, 1485, 1486), shows the appearance of transradiant gall stones just above the level of the dense contrast medium. Radiograph (1487) shows a filled gall bladder and (1488) gall stones shown on a film using compression.

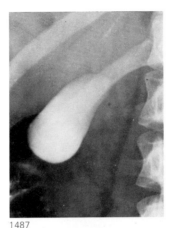

1487

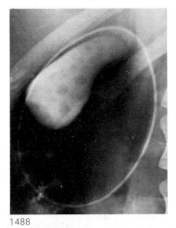

1488

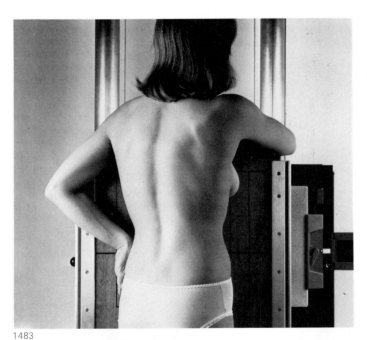

1483

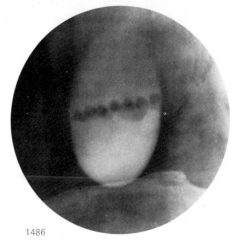

1489

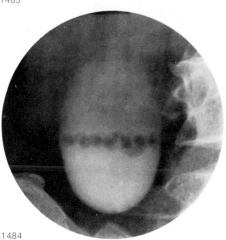

1484

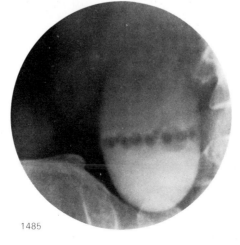

1485

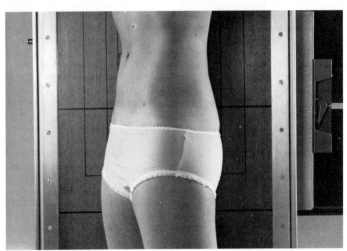

1486

Lateral

Occasionally the gall bladder or small gall stones can be seen free of overlying bowel shadows only in the lateral position. The patient lies on the right side in the true lateral position with the spine parallel to the couch top, the left arm raised above the head, and the legs flexed at the hips and knees with a foam pad between the knees.

■ Centre midway between the lower costal margin and iliac crest, anterior to the third lumbar vertebra, midway between the front and back of the patient (1490, 1493)

A short exposure time is absolutely essential to show opaque gall stones as even the slightest movement blurr may make them invisible.

Radiograph (1491) shows multiple gall stones on the frontal view. In the lateral view of the same subject (1492) even such large gall stones (arrows) become barely visible due to movement blurring.

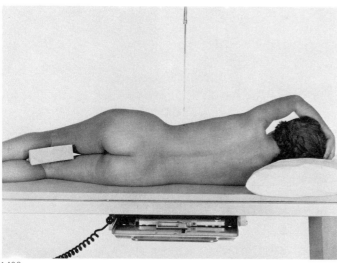

1490

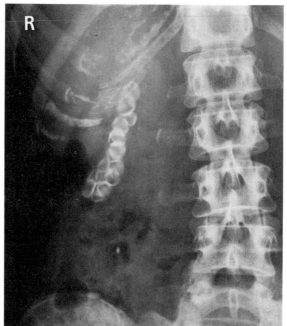

1491

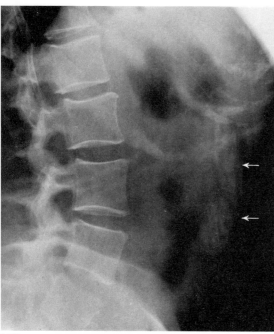

1492

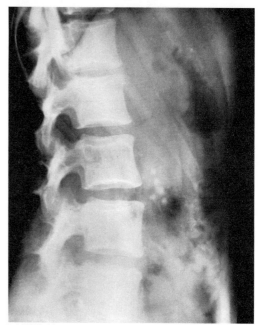

LATERAL
1493

A horizontal beam film can also be obtained with the patient in the right lateral decubitus position.

With the patient lying on the right side and the spine parallel to the table top, the front of the patient must be pressed against the vertical Potter-Bucky diaphragm or grid cassette.

■ Centre at the level of the lower costal margin midway between the spine and right abdominal wall (1494, 1495).

This position is used occasionally when in all other views colonic shadows still overlie the gall bladder. Floating gall stones may be shown with this projection as with the erect horizontal ray projection.

Radiographs

(1495) shows a gall stone in the gall bladder in the lateral decubitus position which is not easily seen on the prone oblique radiograph (1496).

In (1497, 1498, 1499) three projections show multiple small transradiant gall stones which lie below the contrast medium on the erect and decubitus (1499) radiographs.

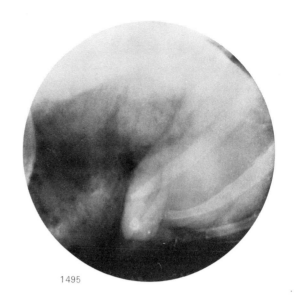

1495

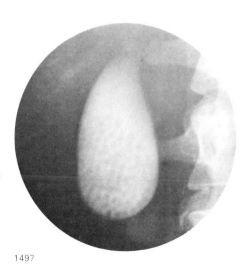

1494

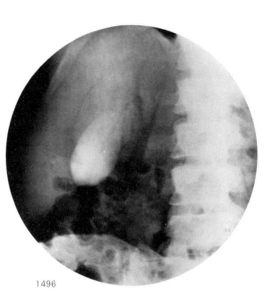

1496

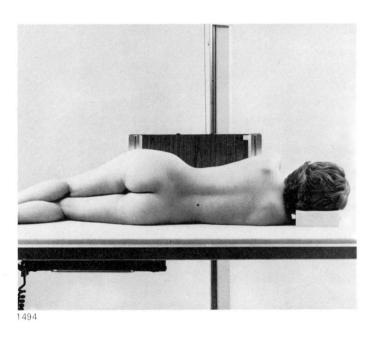

1497

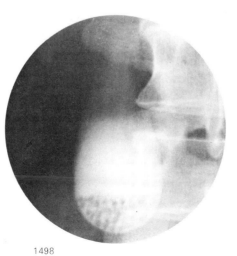

1498

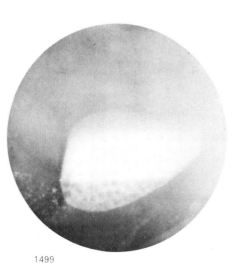

1499

431

The cystic, common hepatic and common bile ducts are often shown on radiographs taken between 10 and 30 minutes after a fatty meal (1501, 1502). Following a fatty meal the gall bladder contracts and contrast medium passes into the hepatic and common bile ducts which become visible. Films for the bile ducts must be done in the oblique position to throw the common bile duct clear of the vertebral column.

Intravenous cholangiogram

Intravenous cholangiography is recommended in the investigation of non-jaundiced patients with biliary symptoms who have had a previous cholecystectomy. Contrast medium is given by slow intravenous infusion and films are taken at 30, 45, 60, and 120 minutes. Tomography is carried out in the supine oblique position usually at 45 minutes after the infusion of the contrast medium. To show the common bile duct the tomographic cuts are approximately 12 cm from the table top in a thin and 16 cm in a large patient.

Radiographs (1500 to 1502) show the gall bladder, cystic and common bile duct at 8, 15, and 25 minutes after a fatty meal with the patient in the supine oblique position. Contrast medium is also present in the caecum which is frequently seen with oral cholecystographic contrast agents.

(1503 to 1505) show multiple small gall stones in the gall bladder at 8 hours after ingestion of contrast medium and 30 and 90 minutes after fatty meal. There has been no significant contraction of the gall bladder on the after fatty meal films.

(1506 to 1508) show a dense gall bladder two hours after intravenous injection of contrast medium with an area of adenomyomatosis at the fundus of the gall bladder and is well shown on the radiograph taken 10 minutes AFM.

(1509 to 1511) show radiographs taken during intravenous cholangiography. There are multiple stones in the gall bladder and a dilated common bile duct with a stone at its lower end.

(1512 to 1514) show a dense gall bladder after oral cholecystography. After a fatty meal the cystic and common hepatic ducts have been demonstrated in the prone and supine positions. The irregular beaded appearance of the cystic duct is normal and is produced by the valve of Heister. (1514)

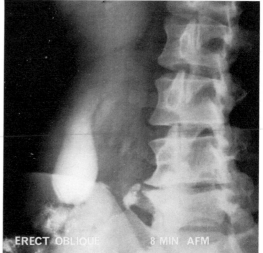

ERECT OBLIQUE   8 MIN AFM
1500

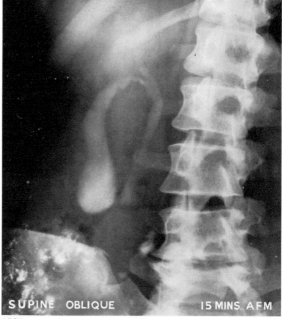

SUPINE OBLIQUE   15 MINS AFM
1501

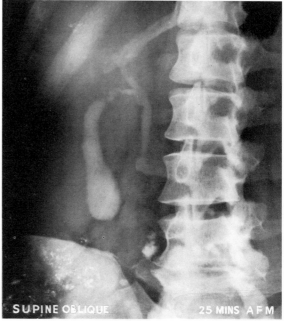

SUPINE OBLIQUE   25 MINS AFM
1502

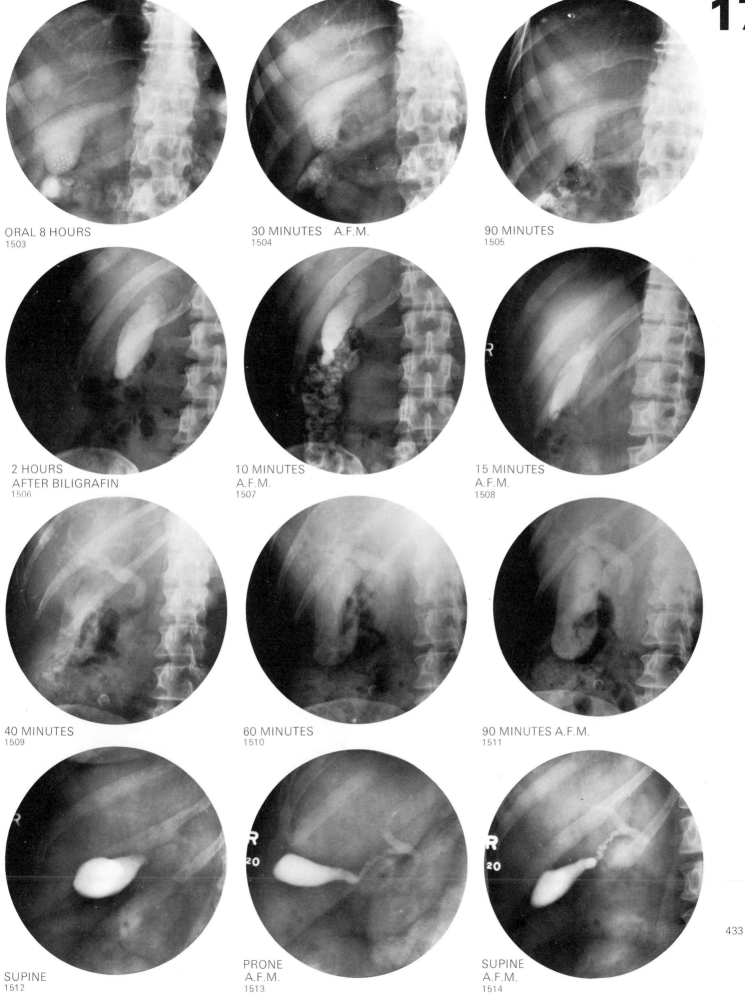

ORAL 8 HOURS
1503

30 MINUTES   A.F.M.
1504

90 MINUTES
1505

2 HOURS
AFTER BILIGRAFIN
1506

10 MINUTES
A.F.M.
1507

15 MINUTES
A.F.M.
1508

40 MINUTES
1509

60 MINUTES
1510

90 MINUTES A.F.M.
1511

SUPINE
1512

PRONE
A.F.M.
1513

SUPINE
A.F.M.
1514

Cholecystography—Choledochography

Ultrasonography

Scanning with ultrasound will show the gall bladder and dilated intrahepatic bile ducts. The gall bladder shows as a well defined echo-free area immediately beneath the right lobe of the liver in the right hypochondrium. When stones are present they produce high level echoes with acoustic shadowing below. Dilated intrahepatic bile ducts produce multiple linear or rounded low level defects within the liver. If the common bile duct is dilated it may also be shown.

Percutaneous Transhepatic Cholangiography

In jaundiced patients it is possible to inject contrast medium into the intra-hepatic biliary system either through a catheter passed into the liver or by using a "fine" needle ("Chiba" skinny needle).

Percutaneous Transhepatic Cholangiography is performed under fluoroscopic control in the radiology department. After injection of a local anaesthetic into the skin, either in the subcostal region of the right hypochondrium or into a lateral intercostal space overlying the liver, the needle or "catheter over the needle" system is passed into the liver and a water soluble contrast medium is then injected while the needle or catheter is withdrawn slowly. As soon as contrast medium is seen to enter the biliary system, withdrawal of the needle or catheter stops and 20 to 50 ml of water soluble contrast medium is injected to show the biliary system up to the site of obstruction (1518, 1519).

Positioning of the patient including tilting into the semi-erect position may be required to show the biliary system. If a normal biliary system is shown the fine "Chiba" needle is withdrawn and the patient can be returned to the ward, being monitored for vital signs. However, if a dilated biliary system is demonstrated the patient proceeds either to theatre or percutaneous biliary drainage is instituted. It is now also possible to guide the catheter down the dilated biliary system and past the site of obstruction to provide catheter drainage of the dilated intra-hepatic biliary system into the duodenum.

Endoscopic Retrograde Cholangiopancreatography (ERCP)

The sphincter of Oddi is cannulated after passing the endoscope into the duodenum via the oesophagus and stomach. A water soluble contrast medium such as Metrizamide (Amipaque) or Megulamine iothalamate (Conray 280) is injected into the common bile duct which is filled retrogradely to reach the intrahepatic biliary system and gall bladder or to the site of obstruction. Gall stones in the common bile duct and gall bladder can be demonstrated as well as strictures due to peancratic carcinoma, primary biliary carcinoma or a post surgical stricture.

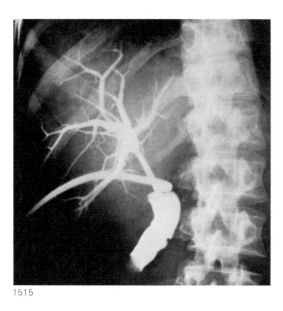

1515

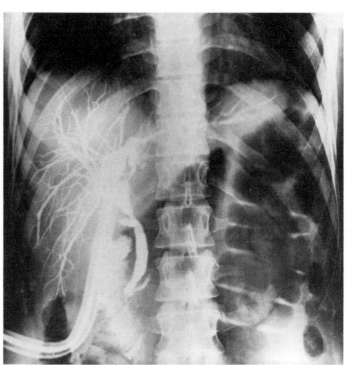

1516

Operative Cholangiography

It is now recognised practice to perform operative cholangiography during cholecystectomy. Just before the gall bladder is removed a syringe and catheter ending in a needle, is filled with a water soluble contrast medium to eliminate air bubbles. The needle is positioned in the cystic duct and a small volume (3–10 mls) of contrast medium is injected to show the common bile duct and common hepatic duct. Three exposures are taken during the procedure and viewed by the surgeon and radiologist to exclude gall stones in the biliary system. The contrast medium should flow freely into the duodenum through the papilla of Vater.

Post-operative (T-tube) Cholangiography

After cholecystectomy the surgeon places a T-tube in the common bile duct which remains in position for two to three weeks to permit healing of the bile duct and maintain patency. Before the T-tube is removed the patient comes to the radiology department for contrast examination of the biliary system via the indwelling T-tube under fluoroscopic control (1515, 1516) The main purpose of this examination is to exclude residual gall stones following a cholecystectomy.

Percutaneous Catheter removal of Gall Stones

Should gall stones have been left behind following cholecystectomy the T-tube remains in position for 6 weeks until a track is produced. Under fluoroscopic control a guided catheter is passed along the residual T-tube track into the biliary system to reach the position of the stone. A "basket guidewire" is passed down the catheter into the bile duct and the "basket" is opened to grab the stone which is then extracted along the residual pathway, thereby avoiding a further operation.

Gall Bladder and Duodenum

When the gall bladder is seen to outline satisfactorily or when its position has been located by the presence of gall stones, a small barium meal may be given to show the relative positions of the gall bladder and duodenum.

Pathological specimens

Radiographs of the gall bladder after its removal are frequently required, sometimes for comparison with the shadows shown in the pre-operative films (1520, 1521).

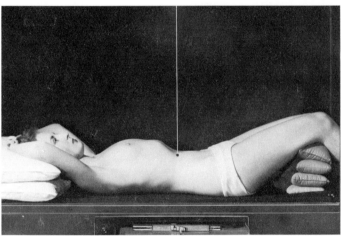

1517

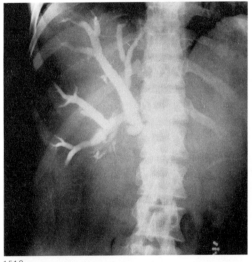

1518

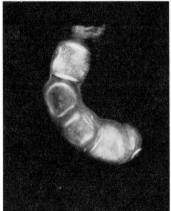

1520

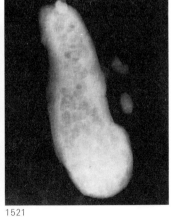

1521

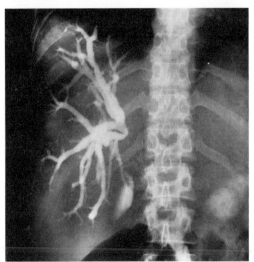

1519

Tomography

Tomography is used routinely during intravenous cholangiography to show the common bile duct. The examination can be carried out in the prone (1522) or supine position. However, the supine oblique position is preferred. To show the common bile duct in the supine position tomographic cuts at 12 to 16 cm from the table top are required depending on the size of the patient. In small patients the duct may be shown at 12 cm but in large patients tomographic cuts at 16 cm may be needed.

Tomography is usually carried out 30 to 40 minutes after the injection of contrast medium or when the common bile duct is well shown on a radiograph of the right hypochondrium. Occasionally tomography of the gall bladder may be used to show small stones when the gall bladder is obscured by overlying gas shadows. Tomographic exposures require an additional 5 kVp for the supine oblique position.

Radiographs (1523, 1524) show how stones can be demonstrated at the lower end of the common bile duct on tomography.

Computed Tomography (C.T.)

Gall stones and dilated bile ducts can be shown on C.T. but is especially useful for acute cholecystitis and empyema of the gall bladder.

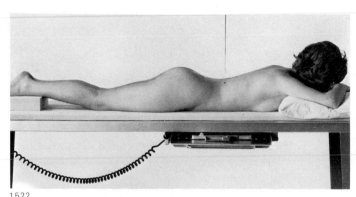

1522

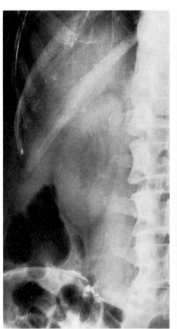 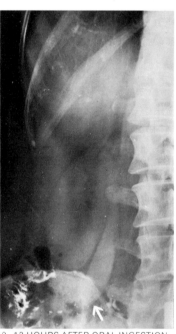 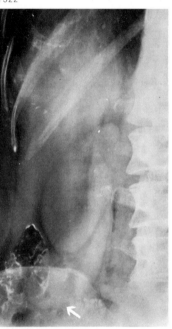

1. PRELIMINARY
1523

2. 12 HOURS AFTER ORAL INGESTION

3. 2 HOURS AFTER INTRAVENOUS INJECTION

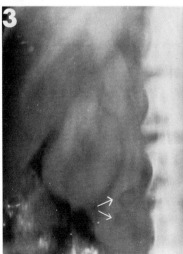 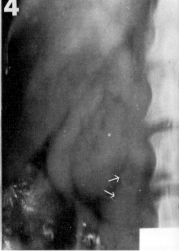 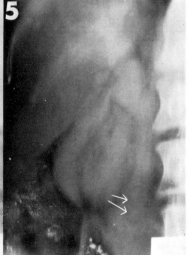

TOMOGRAMS
1524

18

URINARY TRACT

18 SECTION 18

URINARY TRACT

The urinary system consists of the kidneys, ureters, bladder, and urethra. The renal arteries carry blood to the kidneys which is then carried into the arterioles leading to the glomeruli which act as filters. The filtrate passes into the tubules and most of the water and sodium is re-absorbed; the remainder passing down the distal tubules into the calyces, renal pelves and ureters and thence into the bladder. The kidneys have a cortex and medulla.

The cortex is the thin peripheral part of the kidney containing the glomeruli and the medulla lying more centrally contains the renal tubules within the pyramids which have their apices protruding into the minor calyces. The minor calyces join together to form major calyces which in turn become the renal pelvis. (1527)

The hilum of the kidney contains the renal artery, renal vein, renal pelvis and lymphatics embedded in peri-hilar fatty tissue. Surrounding the kidney substance there is a thin, tough membrane called the renal capsule and surrounding this there is a layer of adipose tissue filling in the para-renal space. Kidneys have similar tissue attenuation to surrounding abdominal structures such as liver, spleen, and muscle. The renal outlines are seen, not because of the density of the kidney, but because of the surrounding fatty tissue in the peri-renal space which is bounded by Gerota's capsule. The supra-renal glands also lie within the peri-renal space and bounded by the same peri-renal fascia (Gerota's capsule). Retroperitoneal gas becomes trapped in the peri-renal space showing not only the renal outlines but also the supre-renal glands, and forms the basis of diagnostic retroperitoneal air insufflation for the demonstration of the supra-renals.

The renal pelvis is an expanded area collecting the urine excreted by the kidney and passing it on to the more distal ureter. The ureters lie on the psoas muscles overlying the transverse processes of the lumbar vertebrae and running parallel to the margins of the spine, often over the tips of the transverse processes. At the pelvic brim the ureters cross over the common iliac vessels to lie in front of the sacrum. At the distal end of the sacro-iliac joints the ureters curve around the margin of the pelvic cavity to enter the bladder in the region of the trigone which lies posteriorly and near the base of the bladder. The ureters, extend from the level of the 2nd lumbar vertebra down to the level of the hip joints and are approximately 25 to 30 cm (10–12 ins) long (1526).

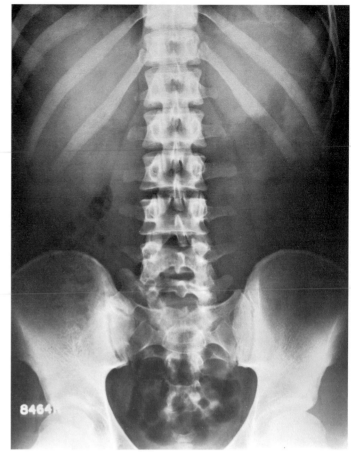

1525

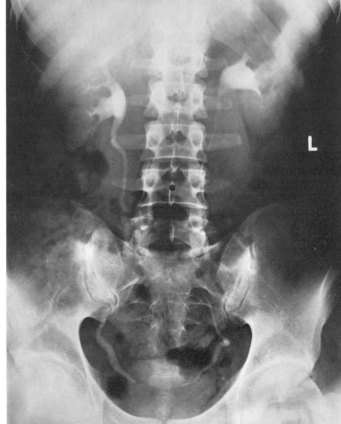

1526

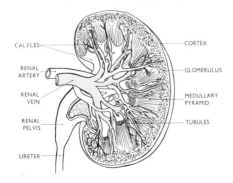

CALYCES — CORTEX
RENAL ARTERY — GLOMERULUS
RENAL VEIN — MEDULLARY PYRAMID
RENAL PELVIS — TUBULES
URETER

1527

The bladder lies behind the symphysis pubis and when full extends well above it to overlie the lower part of the sacrum. In the male the full bladder has a round superior margin, but in the female is often flattened by the impression of the uterus on its superior surface. In the male the prostate lies immediately below the bladder with the urethra passing through it. In the female the vagina lies immediately behind the bladder and the urethra (1531, 1532).

The bladder empties into the urethra through its conical neck and the triangular area between the urethral orifice and the ureteric openings is known as trigone. In the female the urethra is quite short being only some 3 to 4 cm, whereas in the male it is 18 to 20 cm long.

Because the bladder, when full, passes up above the symphysis pubis it is used as a window for ultrasonography of the pelvis, particularly in the early stages of pregnancy. The full bladder is also used to displace small bowel and pelvis in the examination of the terminal ileum.

Radiographs

(1528) is an injected specimen of the renal artery showing the branching pattern around the pyramids of the kidney.

In (1529) there is slight calcification of the bladder wall as occurs in tuberculosis and bilharzia.

(1530) shows the left ureter seen through the contrast in the bladder which is well filled and reaches above the level of the hip joints.

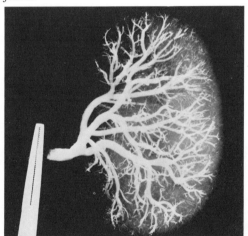

1528

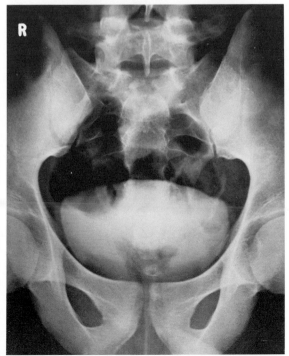

1531/1532

1530

1529

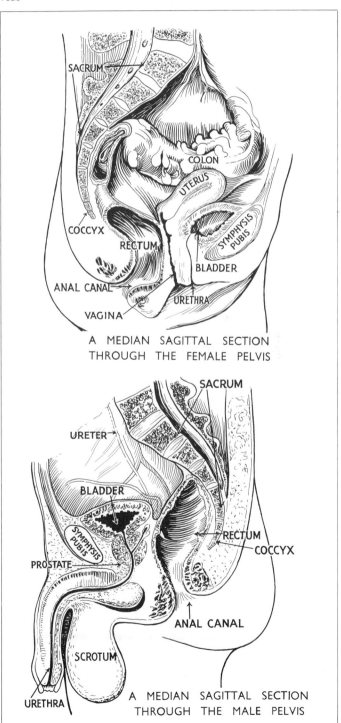

A MEDIAN SAGITTAL SECTION
THROUGH THE FEMALE PELVIS

A MEDIAN SAGITTAL SECTION
THROUGH THE MALE PELVIS

Plain abdominal radiograph

Gas and faeces in the colon frequently obscure the renal areas and is the commonest cause of failure to show the renal outlines. Good bowel preparation is therefore essential for the demonstration of the kidney shadows on a plain radiograph and preparation of the patient must include a laxative.

Renal outlines are visualised because of the adipose tissue in the peri-renal space and are usually better seen in women and adipose subjects than in thin individuals. The spleen lies above the left kidney and often flattens its superior and lateral margin, forming a straight border. The liver lies above and anterior to the right kidney which is against its posterior surface, depressing the right kidney below the level of the left. Thus the upper pole of the left kidney is frequently 2 to 3 cm higher than that of the right. On the plain film of the abdomen, abnormalities of the kidney may be seen because they produce either radiodensities or radiolucencies. Renal and ureteric calculi, (1533, 1534) produce opacities in the renal area or along the line of the ureter. In nephrocalcinosis there is diffuse radiological calcification visible within the renal substance itself. Calcifications can also occur within a renal tumour and in renal tuberculosis.

Gas entering the pelvi-ureteric system will show a pelvi-calicel pattern of radiolucent shadows while gas in the retroperitoneal tissues enters the peri-renal space to outline the kidneys and suprarenals.

Because the kidneys are soft tissue structures they are best shown with relatively low kilovoltage in the region of 60–75 kVp to produce good contrast. After the injection of contrast medium however, the exposure must be increased by 5 to 7 kVp. However, a short exposure time is essential to avoid movement blurring. Radiographs of the renal areas are done on expiration and sufficient time must be allowed for all movement to stop before the exposure is made. However, where there is an opacity overlying a kidney and requires localisation, a film must be taken in deep inspiration. If movement of the opacity exactly coincides with the renal outline then it is renal in origin. However, if it does not move with the kidney oblique views are required to throw the opacity away from the renal outlines.

Calculi, also occur in the bladder and the characteristic feature of bladder calculi is that they move when the position of the patient is changed and is best shown by comparing a frontal view taken in the supine position with a frontal view in the lateral decubitus position.

Transradiencies in the bladder due to gas also occur and may lie within the bladder or in the bladder wall itself, and is particularly associated with diabetes mellitus.

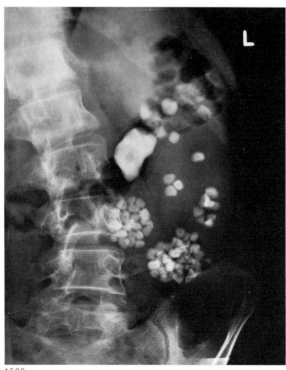

440 1533

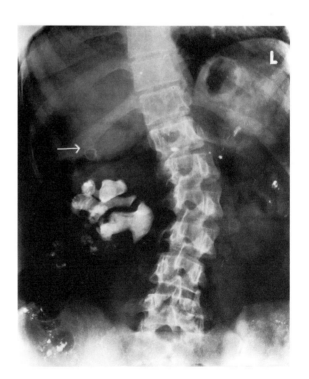

1534

Preparation

The preparation of patients for intravenous urography varies considerably from no preparation at all to a low residue diet and laxatives starting 48 hours before and no fluids for 10 hours prior to the examination. However immediately prior to an intravenous urogram a preliminary film will show whether there is excessive colonic shadowing to require a bowel wash-out before the examination proceeds.

The instructions should be issued to the patient on a written pro forma, which includes the date and time of the appointment. Prior to the examination the patient should have a full explanation of the procedure, especially that an injection will be required. It is however, essential for the radiographer to know that there are certain circumstances when there must be no fluid restriction before an intravenous Urogram and the patient must be well hydrated. Patients with renal failure, high blood urea or multiple myeloma must not have fluid restriction before intravenous contrast medium. It is also most important to know whether the patient has previously had an adverse reaction to a contrast examination.

Ideally all intravenous urograms must be done with equipment which can also perform tomography, particularly when there is overlying colonic shadowing. In children a fizzy drink distends the stomach with gas forming a "window" for the renal areas particularly for the left kidney.

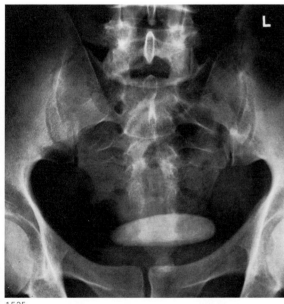

1535

When the appointment for the examination is being given it must be made quite clear to the patient that the 10 day rule is being applied.

In all female patients of child bearing age Urography is done only in the first 10 days of the menstrual cycle unless there is an over-riding clinical indication in which case the 10 day rule must be cancelled by the referring clinician who signs the request form accordingly.

Immediately before the examination starts the patient must have an empty bladder. Although the contrast medium used for urography is now relatively non-toxic occasional reactions do occur. Radiographers and medical staff must be aware contrast medium can provoke an asthmatic attack or produce severe hypotension. Very occasionally sudden respiratory or cardiac collapse may also occur. An emergency resuscitation kit must be at hand during the procedure, including a small ventilator bag and the necessary drugs particularly an intravenous steroid preparation such as hydrocortisone. It is also essential that all radiographic rooms performing contrast examinations must be fitted with an emergency call system.

Positioning

Intravenous Urography (I.V.U.) is almost invariably carried out with the patient horizontal, but occasionally an erect film is required. Routine projections include the antero-posterior and oblique views. Sometimes the prone, postero-anterior or the lateral views are taken. Most examinations are completed within half an hour but where there is ureteric obstruction films may be taken from 6 to 48 hours after the initial contrast injection.

Immobilisation

For urographic examinations the patient must be dressed only in a radiolucent gown provided by the department. However, it is customary to allow women to retain their brassieres and panties and men their underpants. The examination is performed on a radiographic table capable of tomography with the patient lying on a thin plastic sponge mattress which must be free of any opacities that may cause shadowing on the radiograph. Between exposures a blanket must be provided to keep the patient warm and comfortable.

Most urographic examinations will require compression of the lower abdomen to obtain adequate distension of the ureters and pelvi-caliceal system filled with contrast medium. A sphygmomanometer cuff underneath a plastic plate held down by two retaining straps around the patient is effective in the vast majority of cases. The sphygmomanometer bag is positioned immediately above the symphysis pubis. When required it is inflated to a pressure between 90 and 100 mm of mercury and maintained at this level during the examination. Besides compressing the ureters the inflated sphygmomanometer cuff helps in immobilising the patient, (1536). To show the ureters in their full length, the exposure must be made immediately after release of the compression apparatus. However, compression is never used in patients who have abdominal pain or possible ureteric obstruction by a calculus.

18 Urinary tract

Equipment

Most patients requiring a contrast examination of the urinary tract will need a preliminary chest and abdominal radiograph using standard radiographic equipment. However, patients having intravenous urography should be examined on equipment which will allow tomography or zonography.

Retrograde urography is now much less frequently performed because urography has become more detailed and more accurate. When retrograde urography is required the ureteric cather is inserted in the operating theatre, but the radiological examination is usually performed in the X-ray department under fluoroscopic control to avoid over injection of contrast medium which is both painful for the patient and spoils the quality of the examination.

Renal cyst puncture, ante-grade urography, and angiography are usually performed in the special procedures room in the radiology department where fluoroscopy is available and where the examination can be carried out in sterile conditions.

Cysto-urethrography is performed in a conventional fluoroscopic room where spot films can be taken and either rapid sequence 100 mm fluorographic film, Cine or video-tape monitoring is available.

In the last decade the dose of contrast medium for intravenous urography has been increased and now it is common to use between 18 to 22 grams equivalent of iodine e.g. 50 ml Conray "420". The quality of the examination has thereby been greatly improved, resulting in the marked diminution in the number of retrograde pyelograms.

Exposure factors

Relatively low kilovoltages from 60 to 70 kVp is recommended for the preliminary film and should be increased by 5 to 7 kVp during the contrast phase of the examination. However, it is most important to have short exposure times which ideally should be in the order of ·05 to ·08 of a second and can easily be achieved with conventional equipment, using the new rare earth screens. This also results in considerably less radiation to patients.

Focus film distance should be approximately 110 cms (42 ins) to avoid geometric enlargement of the kidney shadows and in addition with 110 cms (42 ins) FFD the whole of the renal tract can be included on a single 43 × 35 cm (17 × 14 ins) film in almost all patients. All exposures are taken on cassettes using intensifying screens and a Potter-Bucky diaphragm.

Respiration

The kidneys are relatively mobile organs which show considerable movement with respiration, abdominal compression and a change in patient position from supine to erect. In elderly patients the kidneys are particularly mobile and the lower pole of the right kidney not infrequently overlies the right iliac crest. All exposures are made during suspended respiration at the end of expiration. However, where an opacity is to be localised to the renal areas a film on inspiration is also taken. The breath holding procedure must be carefully explained to the patient to avoid movement blurring.

Identification of films

Each film taken must clearly show the patient's name, hospital number and date of examination as well as a right or left marker, and the timing of the film following the injection of contrast medium.

A timing device having a clock face with an X-ray opaque moving arm, must be visible on each film taken during an urographic examination. The spacing on the clock face must be at 5 minute intervals up to one hour. The device which should include a right or left letter is placed on the cassette in a standard position preferably in a lower corner away from the renal shadows. The clock is set at zero to coincide with the time of the injection. The preliminary and after micturition films should be clearly labelled as such.

Radiation protection

Careful collimation to the renal areas to avoid unnecessary radiation to the pelvis is most important and in addition a lead rubber sheet may be used over the lower abdomen when the bladder is not being included on the film. In all male patients however, a lead sheet must be used with its upper margin at the lower edge of the symphysis pubis to protect the genitals.

Examples of lead shielding in male children whose age varied from 21 months to 9 years are given in radiographs (1537, 1538 and 1539). Unnecessary radiation can also be avoided by reducing the number of exposures, by careful monitoring of the examination, by good technique to avoid repetition of films, and by the use of modern rare earth film/screen combinations.

Contrast Hyper-sensitivity

Prior to urography a history of possible previous urographic or angiographic examinations must be obtained from each patient and each patient must be questioned specifically as to whether any adverse reactions occurred during the examination. If positive information is obtained the attending radiologist must be informed accordingly and if the procedure is nevertheless continued on clinical grounds the necessary precautions can then be taken.

Ten day rule

Similarly it must be ascertained that all female patients in the child bearing age who are about to have an intravenous urogram or cysto-urethrogram are within the first 10 days of the menstrual cycle or that the 10 day rule has been cancelled by the referring clinician.

Summary of procedures
The following techniques are currently available for examining the urinary tract.

Initial examination
A plain film of the abdomen may be done without preparation to show gross changes but the colonic shadows often obscure a major part of the urinary tract.

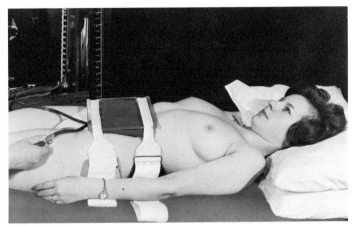

1536

Plain film tomography or zonography
Further information can sometimes be obtained by blurring out the overlying colonic shadows particularly to identify renal opacities without recourse to a bowel wash-out.

Preliminary examination
Immediately before urography a plain film of the abdomen is taken to check that preparation is satisfactory and to localise unusual opacities or transradiencies to the urinary tract.

Intravenous urography
Intravenous urography is the examination of the kidneys, pelvicalyceal systems, ureters, and bladder after the intravenous injection of a water soluble contrast medium.

Intravenous pyelography
This was the term previously used for the examination of the urinary tract but strictly speaking refers only to pelvi-calyceal systems and ureters. The urogram includes visualisation of the renal parenchyma as well as the collecting system.

Retrograde pyelography
After introduction of a catheter into the ureter during cystoscopy, contrast medium is injected retrogradely to show the pelvi-calyceal system and ureters.

Ante-grade pyelography
A percutaneous needle is inserted through the retroperitoneal tissues in the lumbar region to enter the renal pelvis, subsequently a catheter is passed into the renal pelvis and contrast medium is injected. The catheter is also used to drain the obstructed kidney.

Ultrasonography and computed tomography
The kidneys can be visualised by using Ultrasound, especially for cysts and tumours. The kidneys can also be shown on Computed Tomography.

Cystography and cysto-urethrography
The bladder can be examined after catheterisation of the urethra and the injection of contrast medium or contrast medium and air. In a micturating cystogram the bladder and urethra are examined during micturition. This may be combined with pressure and flow studies. Cysto-urethrography includes the examination of the bladder and urethra for stress incontinence in women.

Urethrography
The male urethra may be examined by injecting contrast medium into the tip of the urethra with retrograde filling into the bladder.

Cine radiography/video recording
With an image intensifier this can be used for functional studies, such as ureteric reflux, during micturating cystography.

Tomography and zonography
Tomography or zonography will blur out overlying shadows especially of the colon during urography to show details which would otherwise be obscured.

Seminal vesiculography
This is the introduction of a contrast medium into the vas deferens to show the seminal vesicles.

Renal angiography
This is the examination of the renal arteries by either an injection of contrast medium into the aorta or following selective catheterisation directly into the renal artery.

Renal venography
This demonstrates the renal vein by selective catheterisation and injection of contrast medium.

18

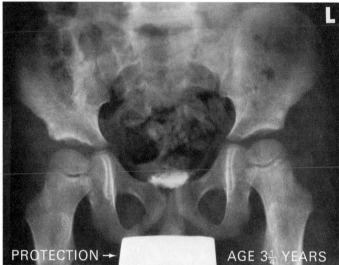

PROTECTION → AGE 3¼ YEARS

1537

Radiographs

In the film of the pelvis (1537) of a 3¼ year old boy taken during a pyelogram there is contrast medium in the bladder. A lead sheet for radiation protection is placed over the scrotum.

In (1538) of a 9 year old child the bladder is filled with contrast medium. The upper part of the lead sheet used for gonad protection is just visible.

The gonad protection lead sheet is clearly visible in (1539) in a 21 month old child. The plain film of the abdomen shows marked faecal retention.

Gas in the transverse colon in (1540) lies across the renal areas. After a colon washout (1541) the renal areas are clearly visible, free of overlying gas shadows. During pyelography, if overlying shadows are present, tomography will blur out overlying gas and faecal shadowing giving a clear view of the kidneys.

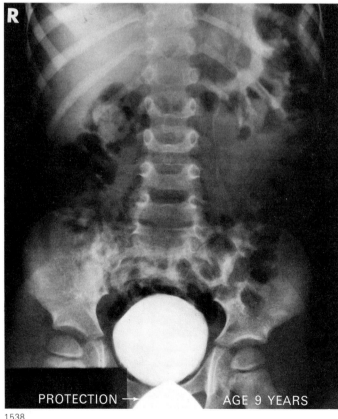

PROTECTION → AGE 9 YEARS

1538

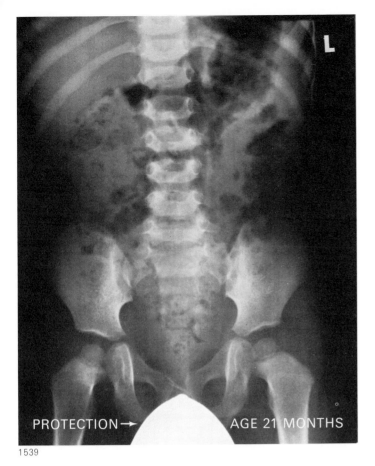

L

PROTECTION→ AGE 21 MONTHS

1539

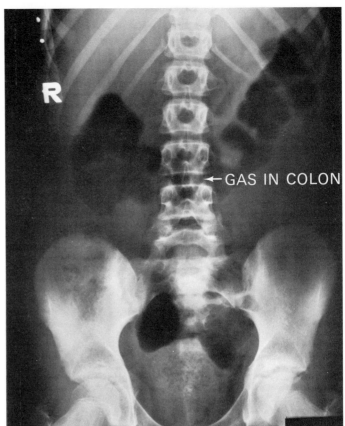

R

←GAS IN COLON

1540

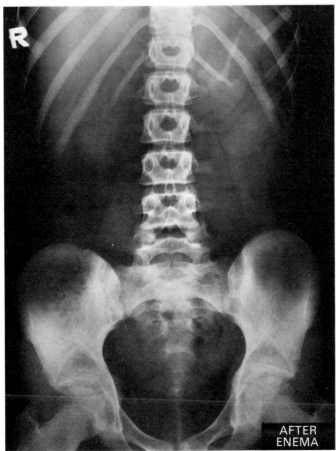

R

AFTER
ENEMA

1541

Initial and preliminary examinations

Preliminary examinations of the abdomen are used for barium meals and barium enemas as well as for intravenous urography. A plain film of the abdomen is especially valuable to show opacities in the kidneys, ureters or bladder or to show transradiencies such as gas in the bladder wall or in the pelvicalyceal systems. Excessive faecal and gas shadowing in the colon will suggest that the patient should have a laxative or bowel wash-out before the intravenous urogram.

The preliminary examination for the urinary system may be done either as a single film or two separate films, one for the pelvis and the other for the upper two-thirds of the abdomen.

Antero-posterior
Single film technique

With the patient supine in the centre of the table and centred to the Potter-Bucky, the knees and shoulders should be slightly raised to straighten out the lumbar arch and bring the kidneys as close to the film as possible. The 43 × 35 cm (17 × 14 ins) cassette is positioned to include the upper pole of the kidneys from the 11th rib to the symphysis pubis.

■ Centre in the midline at the level of the iliac crest. The exposure is made on suspended expiration (1542, 1543, 1544). The line diagram (1544) of a longitudinal section through the abdomen shows the projection of the kidneys, ureters, and bladder on a 43 × 35 cm (17 × 14 ins) film.

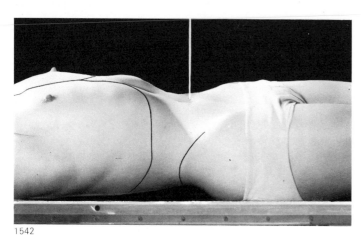
1542

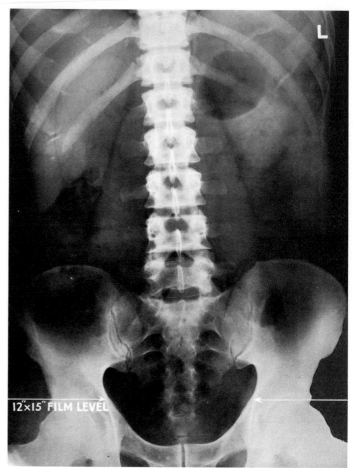
1543

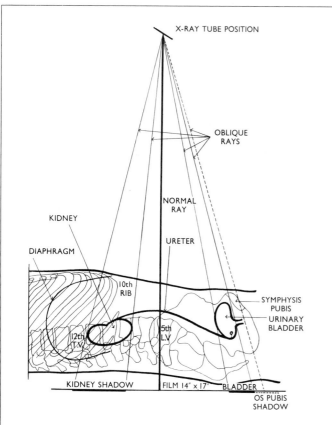
1544

Antero-posterior
Double film technique

With a double film technique the upper two-thirds of the abdomen including the kidneys and ureters is shown on the one film and the bladder and lower ureters on the other. The region of the 5th lumbar vertebra and sacro-iliac joints are overlapped being visible on both films, and helps to identify small ureteric stones which may overly bone.

Kidneys and ureters

For the upper film, with the patient supine a 40 × 30 cm (15 × 12 ins) cassette is placed in position to include the kidneys and the area from the 11th ribs down to the sacro-iliac joints.
■ Centre in the midline at the level of the lower costal margin. Radiograph (1546) shows the area covered by this film.

Bladder

For the lower film the position of the patient and the level of the tube remain unchanged, but the tube is angled 15–25° towards the feet with the central ray passing above the symphysis pubis. The film must be displaced towards the feet to allow for the oblique projection if the whole of the bladder region and the lower two-thirds of the ureters are to be included. The obliquity of the beam increases the FFD slightly (1545, 1546, 1547). When less angulation of the tube is preferred, possible to 10°, the tube is correspondingly moved towards the feet. A 24 × 18 cm (10 × 18 ins) cassette is used for the lower exposure.

The line diagram (1547) shows a longitudinal section of the two-tube projection for the double film technique and should be compared with (1544).

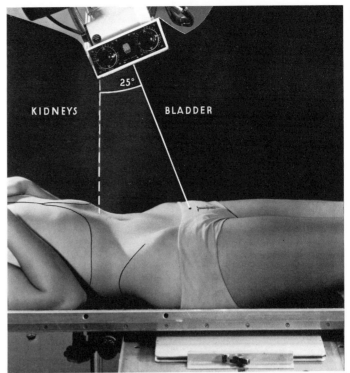

1545

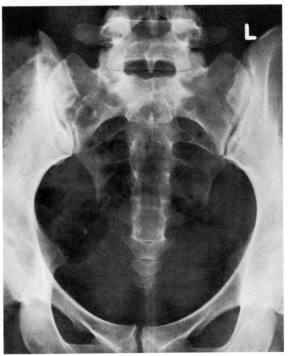

1546

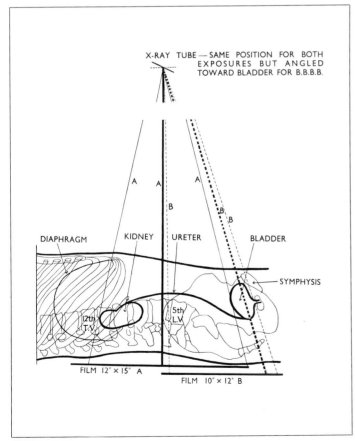

1547

18

447

Kidneys
Differentiation of abnormal shadows
To localise an opacity which overlies the renal area, a second film in inspiration must be done. Opacities overlying the renal area, may in fact be in costal cartilage, lymph nodes, in colon or gall stones in the gall bladder. A constant relationship of an opacity to the kidney on both inspiration and expiration, indicates that it is in the kidney.

Antero-posterior inspiration
Following the initial film a 30 × 24 cm (12 × 10 ins) cassette is placed transversely with its lower margin at the level of the iliac crest.

■ Centre in the midline to the centre of the cassette with a perpendicular central ray.

Increase the kilo-voltage by 5 kVp for a comparable radiographic density (1548a).

Displacement on respiration
On inspiration there is usually considerable downward movement of the kidneys which is well shown when there is contrast medium in the pelvicalyceal systems (1548a, 1548b). In (1548a) the lower pole of the right kidney is at the level of the 4th lumbar vertebra on inspiration, but has moved up to the level of the upper border of the 3rd lumbar vertebra on expiration. Where the lower ribs overlie the upper calyces, a film on inspiration will show them clear of these structures.

Postero-anterior
When there appears to be a hold up of contrast medium at the pelvi-ureteric junction, the ureters can be filled by turning the patient prone (1549) and is the usual method for outlining the ureters when there appears to be a holdup at the pelvi-ureteric junction, but if it fails an erect film will be required.

With the patient prone and central to the couch the ankles are raised over a sandbag. A 30 × 24 cm (12 × 10 ins) cassette is placed in the Potter-Bucky with its lower margin at the level of the iliac crest.

■ Centre in the midline at the level of the lower costal margin and to the centre of the cassette using a perpendicular central ray (1549)

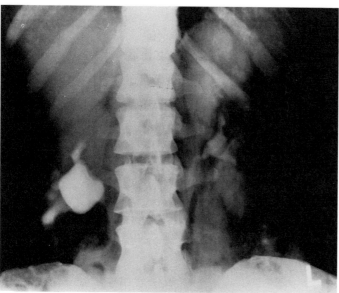

1548a

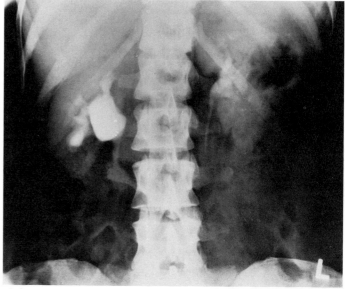

1548b

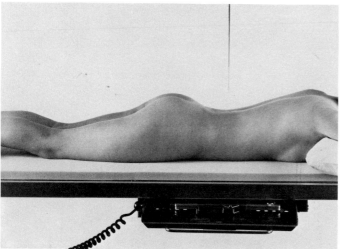

1549

Left and Right antero-posterior oblique

With the patient supine and centred to the centre of the table, raise each side in turn by 30° with a non-opaque support under the buttock and lower thorax.

A 30 × 24 cm (12 × 10 ins) cassette is placed transversely in the Potter-Bucky to include both kidneys with its lower margin at the level of the iliac crest.

■ Centre perpendicular to the film over the midline of the table at the level of the lower costal margin.

The oblique views are used during a urogram to separate superimposed minor calyces filled with contrast medium or if there are overlying colonic shadows which obscure the detail.

Kidneys—lateral

The patient is turned onto the affected side and supported in the lateral position. Position a 30 × 24 cm (12 × 10 ins) cassette transversely with its lower margin at the level of the iliac crests.

■ Centre to the vertebral bodies at the level of the lower costal margin (1551, 1552, 1553).

The kidney shadows tend to overlie the spine with the pelvi-calyceal patterns and ureters becoming visible just anterior to the vertebral bodies.

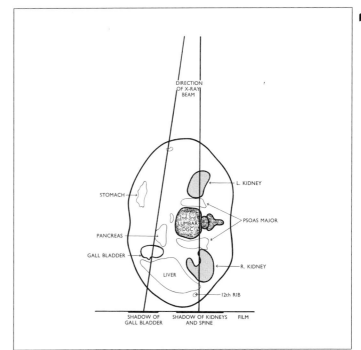

1551

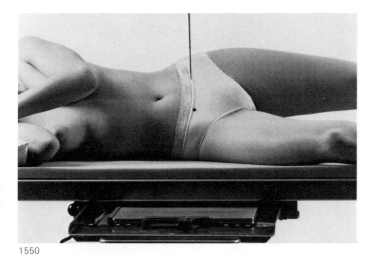

1550

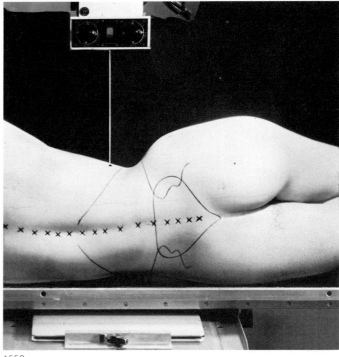

1553

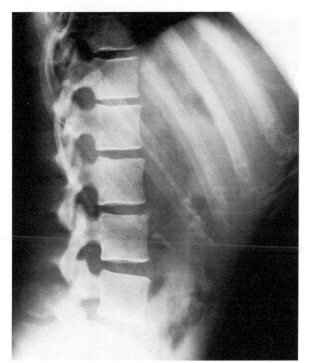

1552

Bladder calculi can move freely within the confines of the bladder and will therefore change their position from supine to oblique or lateral decubitus films. However phleboliths and prostatic calculi are immobile.

Bladder

Turning the patient into the lateral decubitus position, raising the foot of the tilting table, or turning the patient obliquely will alter the position of bladder calculi.

Left and Right antero-posterior oblique

With the patient supine and in the centre of the table raise the left and right sides in turn by 30°. The knee in contact with the table top is flexed and the raised side supported by triangular non-opaque pads.

A 30 × 24 cm (12 × 10 ins) cassette is positioned transversely with its upper margin at the level of the anterior superior iliac spines.

■ Centre to the centre of the cassette with a perpendicular central ray midway between the midline of the patient and the lateral abdominal wall.

Bladder—table tilted

With the patient supine the foot end of the table is raised to 15°. The bladder should be distended with urine and calculi will then tend to fall toward the fundus.

■ Centre in the midline above the symphysis pubis with the tube angle 15° towards the feet (1556, 1557).

A 24 × 18 cm (10 × 8 ins) cassette is placed longitudinally, displaced slightly towards the feet so that the central ray falls on the centre of the cassette.

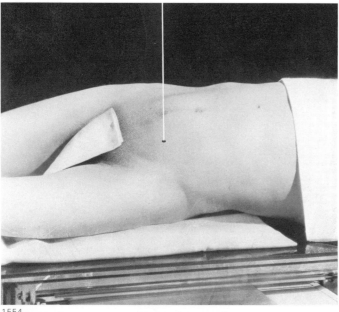

1554

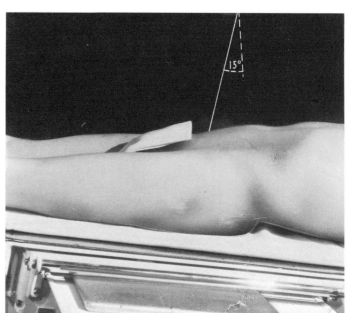

1556

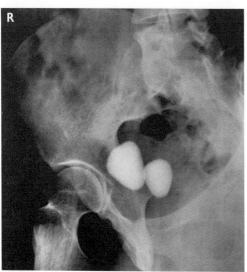

1555

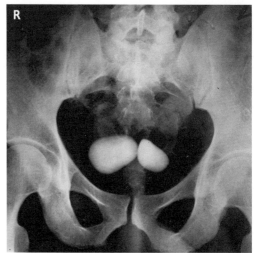

1557

Lateral decubitus

The most convincing radiographic demonstration on a plain film that opacities are intra cystic is obtained with the lateral decibutis film which produces the maximum change in position compared with the supine film.

With the patient lying on the side, and the uppermost limb supported, the pelvis is closely applied to a vertical grid. Calculi in the bladder will fall to the lowest level in the bladder distinguishing between opacities within and outside the bladder (1559).

■ Centre to the bladder with a 10° angulation toward the symphysis pubis using a horizontal ray (1558, 1559)

The prostate

The prostate is a pear shaped gland with its base closely applied to the base of the bladder, surrounding the most proximal part of the male urethra. In middle aged and elderly men it may undergo enlargement due to hypertrophy or carcinoma and cause urinary obstruction. Non-mobile calcifications are also common in the prostate.

On urethrography, prostatic impressions on the urethra can be shown and with prostatic enlargement the urethra is demonstrably narrowed. The prostatic region can be examined either antero-posteriorly or postero-anteriorly.

Antero-posterior (1)

The examination is similar to that used for the bladder with the patient supine and centred to the middle of the table and Potter-Bucky.

■ Centre (a) with the tube directly over the symphysis pubis. Prostatic opacities are shown just above and behind the symphysis pubis (1560, 1562).

■ Centre (b) with the tube angled 15° toward the feet, 2·5 cm (1 ins) above the symphysis pubis. Prostatic opacities are shown above the level of the pubis opening up a gap between (1561).

Radiographs (1560 and 1561) were taken on the same patient with tube straight (1560) and tube angled (1561).

1558

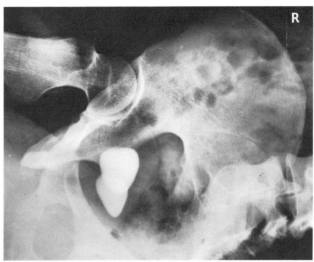

1559

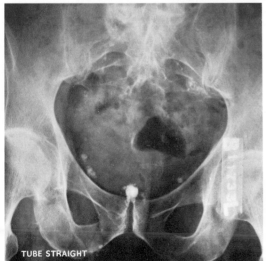

TUBE STRAIGHT

1560

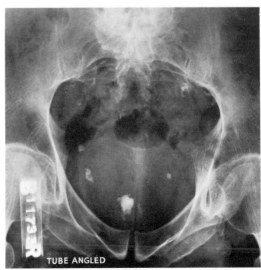

TUBE ANGLED

1561

Prostate
Postero-anterior
With the patient prone place sandbags under the ankles and the thorax can be raised on a pillow.
■ Centre at the tip of the coccyx with the tube angled 10° toward the head.

N.B. By angling the tube the shadow of the coccyx is projected cranially to the prostate (1562, 1563).

For **Exposure Factors** see page 472
As described (page 448) and illustrated (1554, 1556) prostatic calcifications will be stationary and bear a constant relationship to the bony pelvis whereas bladder stones will move with gravity as the position of the patient is changed.

The seminal vesicles
Vesiculography
The seminal vesicles lie behind the angle between the prostate and bladder and retains spermatozoa brought to it by the vas deferens from the seminiferous tubules of the testes. The vas deferens and seminal vesicles are not normally visible but may become calcified in the elderly or after chronic infections such as tuberculosis.

In the investigation of male sterility patency of the vas deferens and the outline of the seminal vesicles are shown by injecting water soluble contrast medium, e.g. Conray "280" into the vas deferens using fluoroscopic control. This examination is called Vesiculography (1564).

A plain film free of overlying gas shadows is used to show a ureteric calculus and appears as an opacity along the line of the ureter. However in the vast majority of cases a stone in the ureter is diagnosed with a pyelogram which shows delayed excretion and retention of contrast medium in the renal parenchyma producing a nephrogram. Late films show

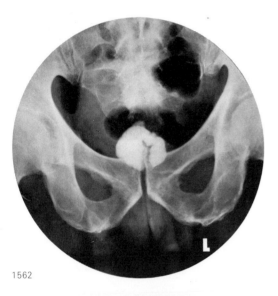
1562

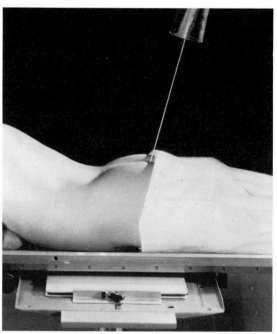
1563

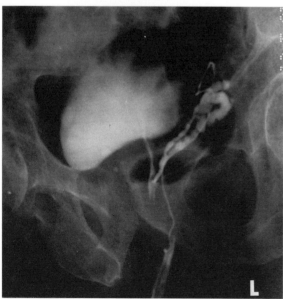
1564

contrast medium in the ureter to the site of obstruction which coincides with the opacity on the plain film.

Occasionally a small opacity may be seen along the line of the ureter and the ureter does not appear to be obstructed. It is then possible to dissociate the opacity from the contrast filled ureter by using a tube shift technique.

Tube shift

After taking the first film an additional film is exposed without moving the patient but with the tube displaced transversely by 10–15 cm (4–6 ins) producing a stereoscopic pair. The second film may clearly show separation of the opacity from the position of the ureter.

Previously this technique was used with a ureteric catheter in position following cystoscopy.

Antero-posterior oblique

With the patient supine the unaffected side is raised and supported on triangular non-opaque pads, turning the patient through approximately 30°.

■ Centre in the line of the ureter midway between the midline of the patient and the lateral abdominal wall to the centre of the Potter-Bucky diaphragm (1567).

For **Exposure Factors** see page 472.

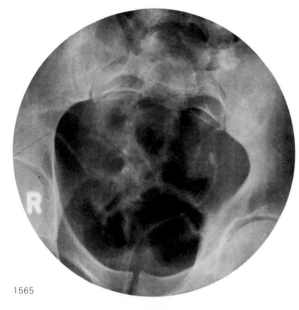

1565

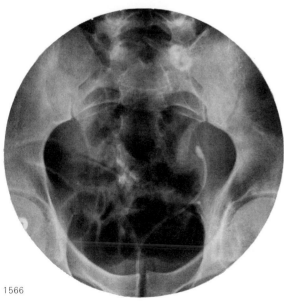

1566

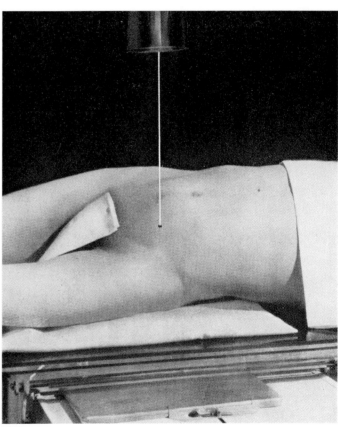

1567

Theatre technique

Radiography of the exposed kidney during operation (1568) requires the strictest asepsis and a meticulous technique to localise small opacities in the kidney.

A non-screen film is used with a backing of lead foil to limit scattered radiation, in a special pack measuring 9 × 12 cm (3½ × 4½ ins). The film pack is sterilised in a formalin vapour steriliser for 2–4 hours and sealed in a plastic envelope.

A rectangular tube applicator 31 cm (12½ ins) long with an aperture of 12 × 14 cm (4½ × 5½ ins) is closed by a linen diaphragm stretched over the applicator and fixed to the sides (1568, 1569). A fine focus tube is essential.

The surgeon raises the kidney in a gauze sling and the applicator depresses the lower border of the incision. The kidney is gently but firmly pressed between the stretched linen diaphragm and the film pack with a metal indicator attached to it (1569). The anaesthetist stops respiration during the exposure and two films are taken so as to exclude artefacts or opacities in the film pack. There must be a darkroom with 90 second development time in the theatre suite for immediate film viewing by the surgeon (1570a).

An operative pyelogram may follow using 10 ml of contrast medium injected directly into the renal pelvis (1570b). More exact localisation of an opacity is achieved using a fine gauze covered metal grid opposed to the kidney on the side nearest the film (1571) and a metal pointer fixed to the grid. Immediate viewing of the film is followed by a local incision of the kidney for removal of the stone and the kidney is then re-examined to ensure that all calculi have been removed (1572b).

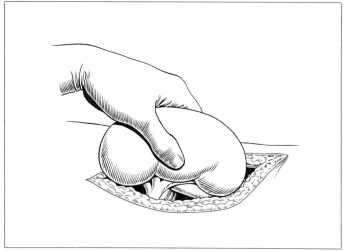

1568a

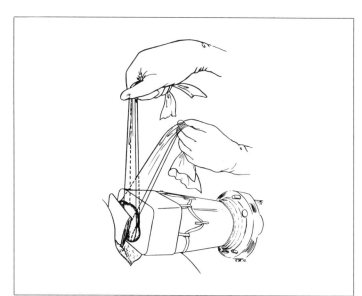

1568b

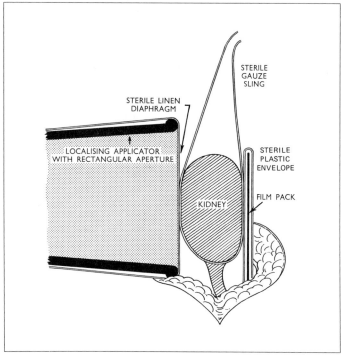

STERILE
GAUZE
SLING

STERILE LINEN
DIAPHRAGM

LOCALISING APPLICATOR
WITH RECTANGULAR APERTURE

STERILE
PLASTIC
ENVELOPE

FILM PACK

KIDNEY

1569

Radiographs

In (1570a) there is a collection of small stones in a major calyx and a separate tiny stone (arrow) in a minor calyx. After injection of contrast medium the relationship of the tiny stone to the minor calyx is shown (1570b).

A small stone has been localised using a metal pointer and grid as shown in (1571).

In (1572) the initial exposure shows two very small renal calculi and in (1573a/b) only one after operation.

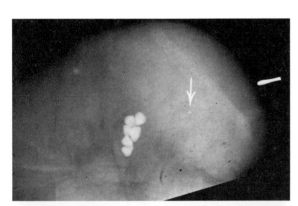

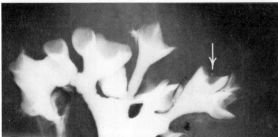

1570a/b

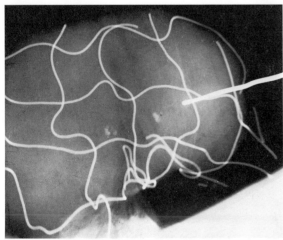

1571

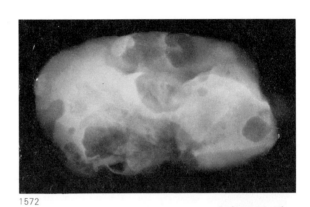

1572

before operation

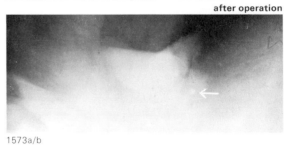

after operation

1573a/b

Urography

The examination of the urinary tract following intravenous injection of contrast medium is called a urogram in preference to a pyelogram because a pyelogram refers only to the pelvicalyceal systems and ureters, whereas a urogram includes the kidneys, pelvicalyceal systems and bladder.

The contrast medium

Water soluble organic iodine compounds of 2,4,6-benzyl rings with extremely low toxicity have now been developed and are produced either as sodium or as meglumine salts. The sodium salts tend to produce more of a local reaction, especially a slight burning sensation along the line of the vein but have a much lower viscosity than the meglumine salts. The usual dose of contrast medium is 18–22 g iodine equivalent given as Conray ('280', '325', '420') sodium and meglumine iothalamate; Urografin or Hypaque (45% or 60%), Sodium diatrizoate or Triosil (25% 45% or 60%) sodium metrizoate.

Preparation

Following the routine use of 18–22 g iodine equivalent as the dose of contrast medium for intravenous urography, patient preparation has been greatly simplified. Nevertheless, at the time the appointment is made a pro forma detailing the preparation and time of appointment is handed to the patient and for females of child bearing age the examination is arranged for the first 10 days of the menstrual cycle. If there has been a previous contrast examination, any adverse reaction must be noted, particularly asthma, skin reactions and possibly hypotension. The patient must be informed that the examination usually takes $\frac{1}{2}$–1 hour but may possibly be longer.

In some centres an aperient is given for 2 nights starting 48 hours before and fluid is restricted for 8 hours prior to renal examination. If considerable overlying faecal shadowing is present on the preliminary film, a cleansing enema is given.

However, there must be no fluid restriction for patients in failure or with myeloma who must on the contrary be well hydrated. For patients with renal failure only the meglumine preparation must be used and not the sodium salts.

Just prior to the injection of contrast all patients are again asked about hypersensitivities and contrast reactions and if a positive history is obtained the radiologist must be informed.

The patient must have an empty bladder before the examination starts.

Radiographic procedure

A preliminary film is taken usually a 43×35 cm (17×14 ins) and clearly labelled "Preliminary" or "Control". If faecal shadows obscure the renal areas the examination must be carried out on a radiographic table with a tomographic attachment or the patient must have a cleansing enema.

The intravenous contrast medium is injected, usually into the antecubital vein at the elbow with the patient in position on the radiographic couch. In the routine examination, the patient remains on the couch until the examination has been completed.

During and immediately after the injection the patient must be observed carefully for any untoward reactions. Not uncommonly there is a transient hot or burning sensation up the arm, possibly even pain in the shoulder. Nausea and vomiting may occur. Skin weals or urticaria and asthma are more serious hypersensitivity reactions and must be reported to the radiologist immediately. Rarely respiratory or cardiovascular collapse may occur requiring immediate resuscitation.

Following the injection of intravenous contrast medium a film is taken immediately which shows the renal parenchyma giving a clear view of the renal outlines to assess the size, shape and position of the kidneys. The first film is often 35×35 cm (14×14 ins) to include the liver and spleen which are also well shown in the parenchymal phase of contrast enhancement.

If faecal shadows overlie the kidneys the "immediate" film of the renal areas should be a tomogram and because of the parenchymal visualisation is called a nephrotomogram.

A full length film on 43×35 cm (17×14 ins) at 5 mins usually shows the ureters filled with contrast medium.

Abdominal compression (1576) with a sphygmomanometer cuff under a plastic plate held in position with straps, is applied to the lower abdomen to obstruct the ureters and distend the pelvicalyceal systems. A pressure of 90–110 mm Hg in the sphygmomanometer cuff is required which is inflated slowly. Abdominal compression must not be used when the patient has abdominal pain or ureteric obstruction.

Films are taken at 10 and 15 mins after injection with compression applied and the films are viewed. Oblique films may then be needed. The 10 and 15 minute and oblique films are 30×25 cm (12×10 ins) with the lower margin of the cassette at the level of the iliac crests and the tube centred to the centre of the cassette.

If the films taken with compression show the pelvicalyceal patterns satisfactorily, abdominal compression is released and a further full length film 43×35 cm (17×14 ins) is taken to show the urinary tract including the ureters and bladder.

The patient then goes to the toilet to pass urine and followed by a post micturition film of the bladder region on a 25×20 cm (8×10 ins) film.

Variations on the timing of films

For hypertension (high blood pressure) a rapid sequence of films at 2, 4 and 6 minutes after injection and before compression was previously used to show the pyelographic signs of renal artery stenosis but in recent years has been replaced by functional renal isotope studies which is a much more accurate procedure.

Delayed films at 4–6 hours and even up to 24–28 hours may be needed where there is ureteric obstruction or slow excretion due to renal failure. No abdominal compression is used in these cases.

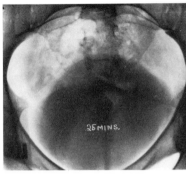

1574b

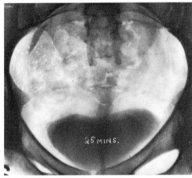

1575b

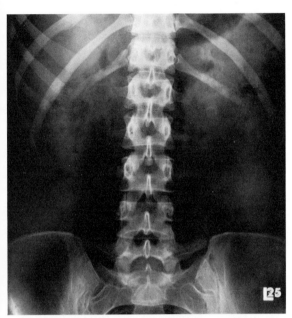

1574a

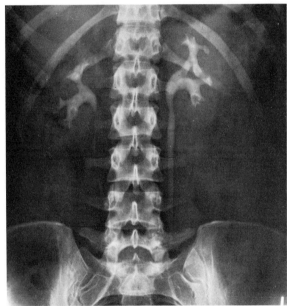

1575a

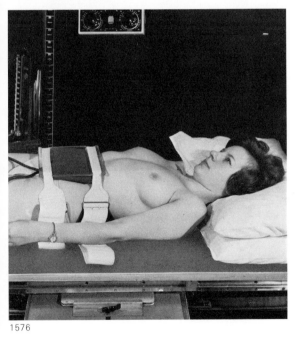

1576

Prone or Erect Film
An obstructed ureter causes delayed contrast excretion which often pools in the renal pelvis in the supine position. The ureter may then be shown down to the site of obstruction on a film taken after turning the patient prone.

Nephrotomography or Zonography
Tomography or zonography with sections taken 10–12 cm (4–6 ins) from the table top, immediately after the intravenous contrast medium, clearly shows the renal parenchyma and renal outlines and is used to differentiate cysts and tumours. Tomography is done with a longer tube swing and produces thinner sections than zonography for which only a short tube swing is needed and produces thicker sections.

Radiographs
A typical series of films of an intravenous urogram (1577–1579) of a normal adult were taken at 5, 15 and 25 mins (1577a,b,c) after injection with abdominal compression and show progressive filling of pelvicalyceal systems and ureters. (1578) was taken after release of compression and (1579) after micturition.

A similar series of a child (1580–1584) starts with the preliminary film (1580) and films at 5, 12 and 20 mins after injection with abdominal compression (1581, 1582) while (1583) was at 30 mins after injection when abdominal compression had been released and (1584) after micturition at 85 mins.

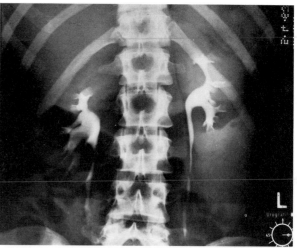

1577b

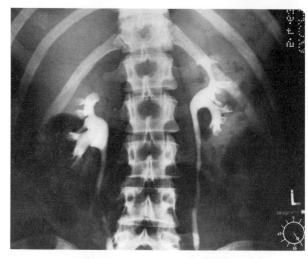

1577c

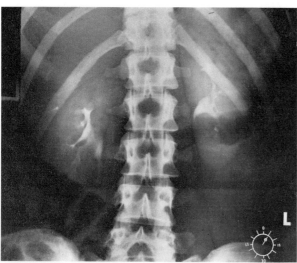

1577a

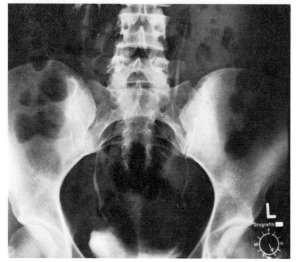

1578

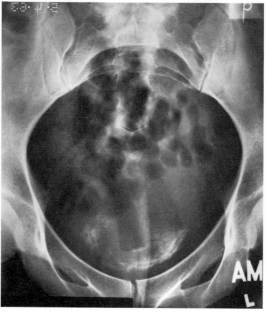

1579

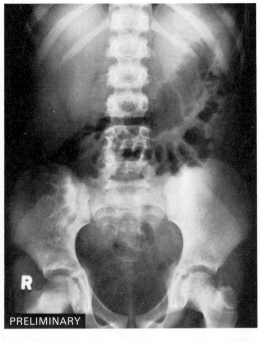

PRELIMINARY

1580

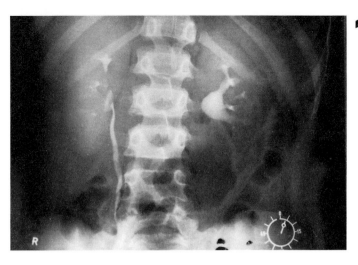

1581

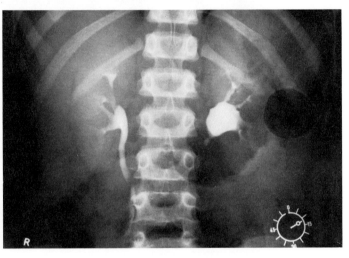

1582a

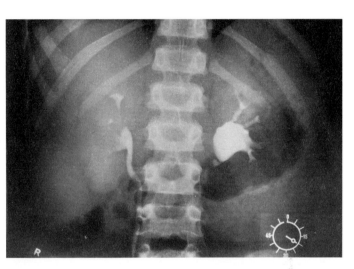

1582b

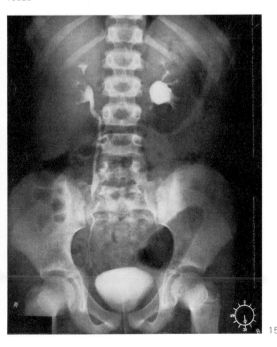

1583

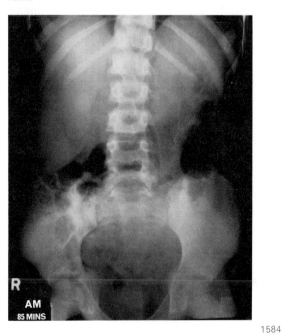

AM
85 MINS

1584

Radiographs

Long-standing obstruction to a ureter produces hydronephrosis in which there is dilatation of the pelvicalyceal patterns (1585). A prone film is often required to show the ureter down to the site of obstruction which may be anywhere along the length of the ureter to the bladder (1586, 1587). In (1587) the irregularity of the left margin of the bladder wall is due to a carcinoma and in (1588) the pelvicalyceal patterns are shown on a lateral projection.

In the full length film (1589) taken supine the pelvicalyceal systems are filled with contrast which largely drains away in the erect position (1590). A lateral view is shown in (1591) and a film in the sitting position in (1592).

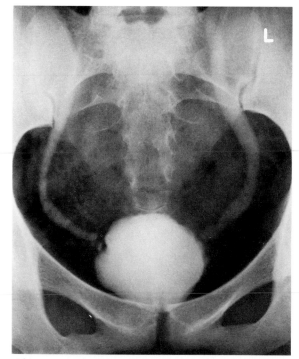

1586

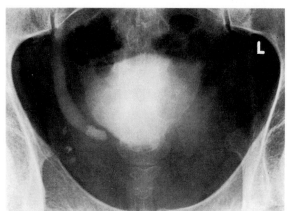

1587

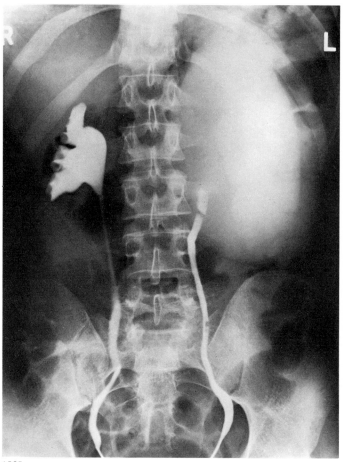

1585

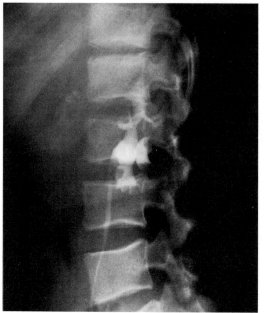

1588

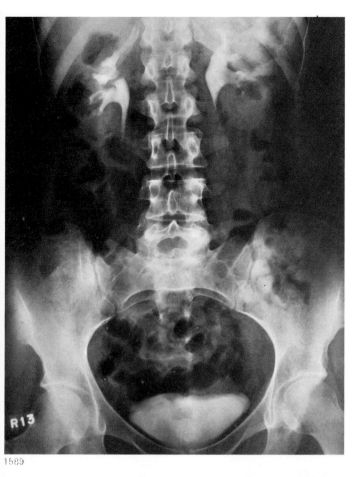

1589

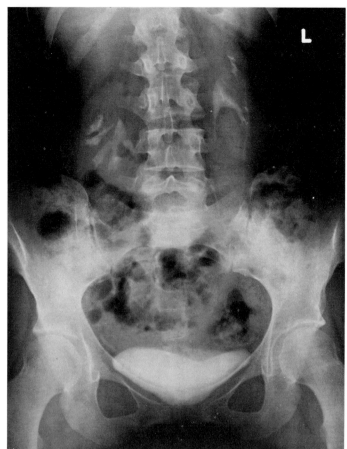

1590

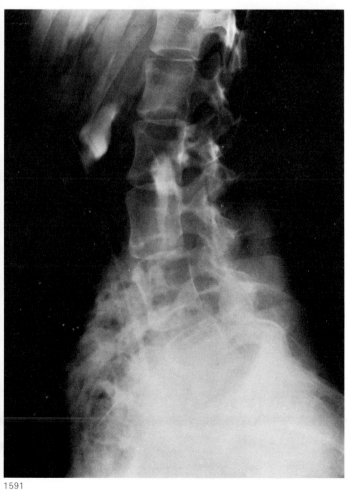

1591

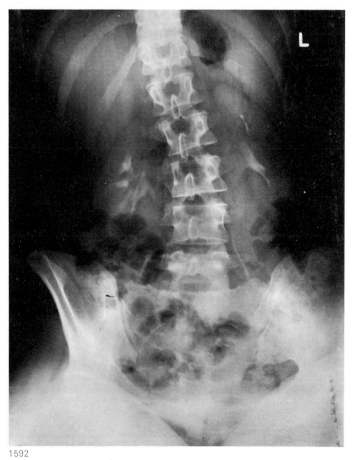

1592

Oblique projections

Minor calyces are not infrequently superimposed on the frontal view, overlying colonic shadows may obscure part of the kidney or more detail of a mass lesion may be required necessitating oblique views.

With abdominal compression being maintained turn the patient 30° towards the right and left sides in turn, using non-opaque triangular pads to support the patient in position.

Radiographs

In (1593) and (1594) a frontal view (a) is compared with the oblique view (b) to show calyces free of overlying colonic gas.

Children—Gas distention of the Stomach

In children a fizzy drink will distend the stomach producing a gas "window" through which the pelvicalyceal systems can be seen (1596a/b) often better on the left than the right (1595a/b).

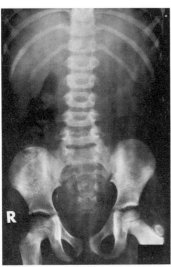

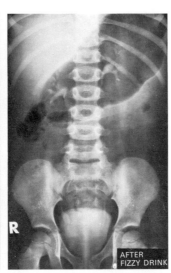

1595a/b

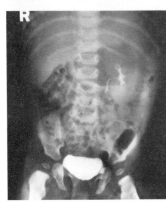

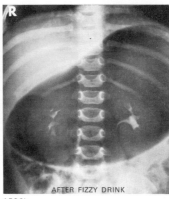

1596a   1596b

Radiographs

In (1595) a full length film of a child of 3½ years is shown with gas distension of the stomach. The left pelvicalyceal system is seen through gas in the body of the stomach and the right pelvicalyceal system through the gas in the antrum. In (1596b) there is marked gas distension showing both pelvicalyceal systems in a child of 15 months.

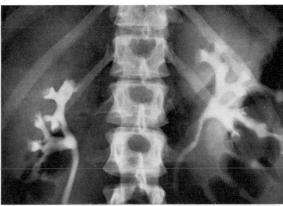

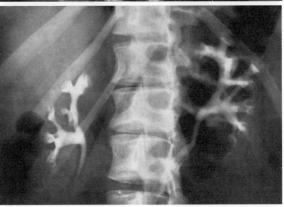

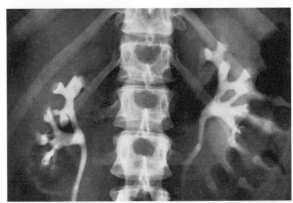

1593a/b

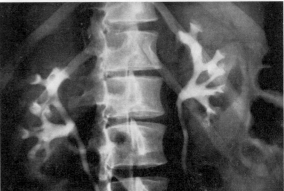

1594

Tomography and Zonography

Not too infrequently especially in patients confined to bed, gas and faeces obscure the renal areas. Tomography which produces thinner sections of 2–5 mm and zonography thicker sections of 10–20 mm can show the kidneys and pelvicalyceal systems by diffusing the overlying shadows (1597a/b). It is now standard practice to perform all intravenous urograms with equipment having a tomographic attachment.

Radiographs

In 1597(a) the pelvicalyceal systems are obscured by bowel gas but shown in 1597(b) after tomography.

In (1598) there is delayed excretion on the left side; due to a stone at the lower end of the ureter in (1599). In the retrograde pyelogram (1600) a ureteric catheter has been introduced into the left ureter and shows dilatation of the minor calyces.

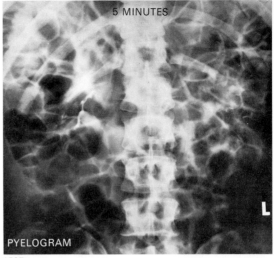

1597a

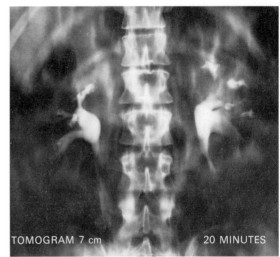

1597b

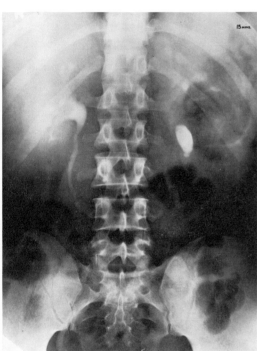

1598

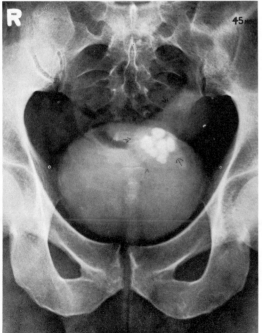

1599

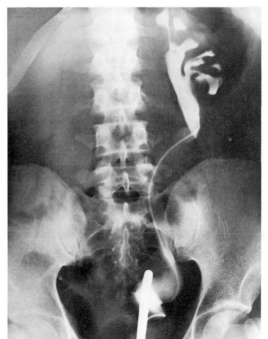

1600

The renal arteries and aorta are demonstrated by injection of contrast medium through a catheter or direct needle puncture of the aorta by the translumbar route (1601–1604).

The catheter is usually introduced by a percutaneous technique into the femoral artery and threaded up into the aorta under fluoroscopic control. An injection of contrast medium into the aorta shows the aorta and renal arteries from their origin into the kidneys and is known as a free flush aortogram. If the catheter tip is positioned in a renal artery and the contrast medium injected directly into it the examination produced is a selective renal arteriogram. These examinations are now almost exclusively done with the patient on a moving table top with fluoroscopic control for positioning the catheter and an automatic serial changer for a sequence of films at 1–2 second intervals up to 15 seconds.

The free flush injection of contrast medium into the aorta is delivered with a pressure pump which is set to trigger the serial changer but the selective injection into the renal artery is often done by hand, the serial changer being started by the radiographer after a signal from the radiologist.

The contrast medium used is similar to that for intravenous urography (p. 454); 30–40 ml being used for the free flush arteriogram and 8–10 ml for the selective renal arteriogram.

Radiographic technique

For a catheter arteriogram a preliminary film is taken with the patient supine, positioned over the serial changer and the diaphragm accurately collimated to the renal areas. The previous pyelogram should act as a guide for the expected position of the kidneys. The position of the light beam diaphragm is marked on the patient's skin and the central ray is centred to the centre of the serial changer. The preliminary film is viewed for radiographic quality and to exclude interfering opacities such as barium from a previous examination.

Radiographic technique

The procedure is fully explained to the patient who signs a consent form. It is especially important for the patient to know that the injection of contrast medium will cause a hot feeling in the loin which travels down the legs. Premedication with diazepam (Valium) is commonly used.

The patient then lies on the fluoroscopic table which should have image intensification. The radiologist inserts a radiopaque catheter under local anaesthesia into the femoral artery using the Seldinger percutaneous technique. The tip of the catheter is positioned using a small test injection of contrast medium which is observed on fluoroscopy or video. The catheter is strapped to the groin and the patient positioned over the serial changer, making the necessary radiographic adjustments based on the results of the preliminary film.

With the exposure factors and film sequence set, the contrast

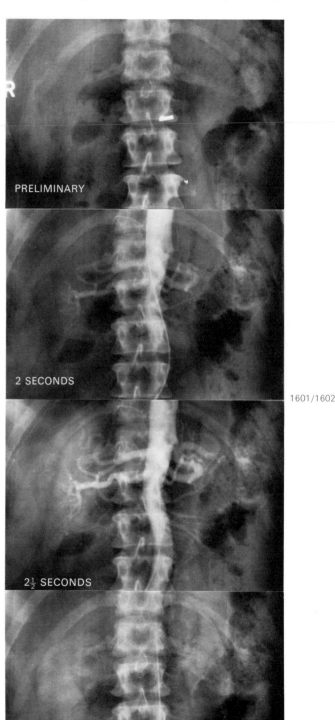

1601/1602

1603/1604

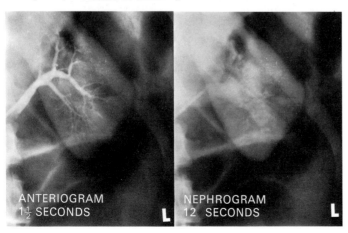

1605a/1605b

loaded pressure pump is attached to the catheter and the patient is warned of the effects of the injection. The examination is done in suspended expiration. The pressure pump is then triggered which in turn sets off the serial changer and exposures.

For selective arteriography the radiographic procedure is similar but the light beam diaphragm is collimated to each kidney in turn and often the contrast medium is injected by hand. The serial exposures are started by the radiographer after a signal from the radiologist.

In selective renal venography the radiopaque catheter is inserted into the femoral vein and the end of the catheter placed in the renal vein.

Magnification or Macro Angiography

If a fine focus high output tube of 0·3–0·1 mm is available magnification arteriography is obtained by increasing the subject film distance using an air gap.

Intramuscular Injection

In the vast majority of children the contrast medium can be injected intravenously. However very rarely it needs to be given intramuscularly (1606) and hyalase is then added to aid absorption of the contrast medium.

Radiographs

In (1606–1609) the intramuscular contrast medium is slowly disappearing as the pyelogram proceeds.

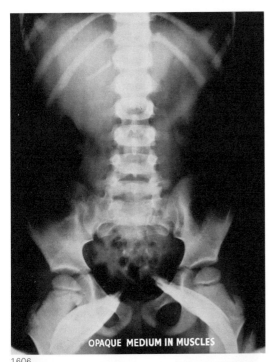

1606

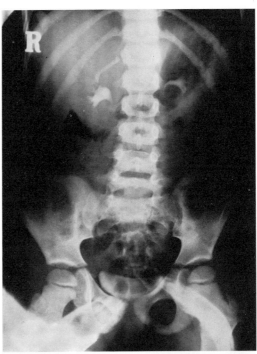

1607

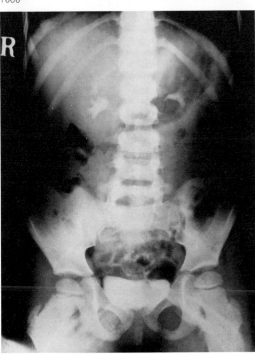

1608

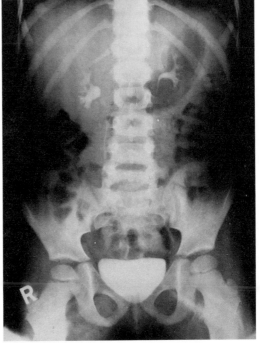

1609

Retrograde or Ascending Pyelography

With the use of high dose contrast medium urography, tomography and abdominal compression, retrograde pyelography is now used relatively infrequently. The only definite indication is for the completely non-visualised kidney.

A retrograde catheter is passed into the ureter during cystoscopy done under a general anaesthetic. The patient is then moved to a fluoroscopy unit with the catheter still in position. Under fluoroscopy a 30% urographic contrast medium (p. 454) is injected slowly up the catheter to outline the pelvicalyceal system (1610, 1611). Care is taken not to inject more than the required amount of contrast medium because pyelosinus backflow occurs which obscures the detail of the minor calyces and also causes loin pain.

Films are taken on the fluoroscopy unit and for greater detail an overcouch film may be required at the end of the examination.

Radiographs

In (1610) the tip of the ureteric catheter is at L3/4 in the left ureter and after contrast medium has been injected the pelvicalyceal system is deomonstrated while in (1611) a bilateral retrograde or ascending pyelogram shows both pelvicalyceal systems.

In (1612) a left retrograde pyelogram shows a bifid or duplication of the renal pelvis and calyces which were poorly demonstrated on the intravenous pyelogram (1653). An adequately performed urogram would make the retrograde examination unnecessary.

Ante-grade Pyelography

Where there is complete obstruction of a ureter usually from a tumour the pelvicalyceal system and proximal ureter can be shown by percutaneous translumbar injection and subsequent insertion of a catheter to drain the urine and reestablish kidney function. Subsequently a ureteric prosthesis can similarly be inserted down the ureter through the tumour or stricture to drain into the bladder.

With the patient prone, using fluoroscopy control the tip of a translumbar needle is inserted into the renal pelvis and contrast medium injected. A guide wire with a curved flexible tip is passed down the needle and into the renal pelvis. The needle is removed leaving the guide wire in position and an opaque catheter threaded over the guide wire which is then removed leaving the catheter in the renal pelvis.

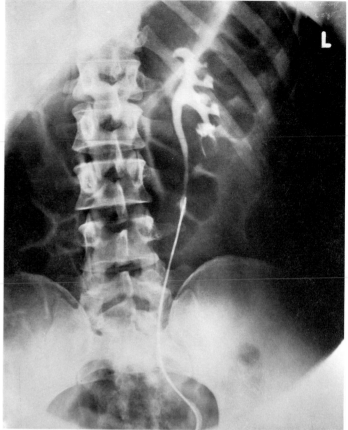

1610

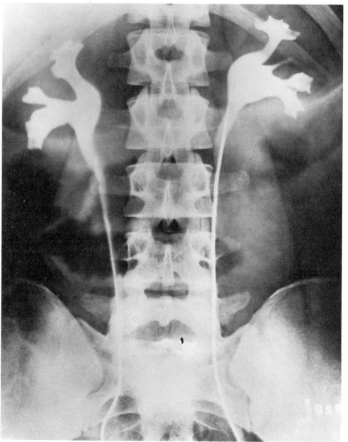

1611

Fluroscopy of the Pelvicalyceal System

Very occasionally peristaltic activity in the pelvicalyceal system is recorded either on video tape, cinefluorography or serial exposures (1614) during the course of a urogram when the pelvicalyceal system has been opacified.

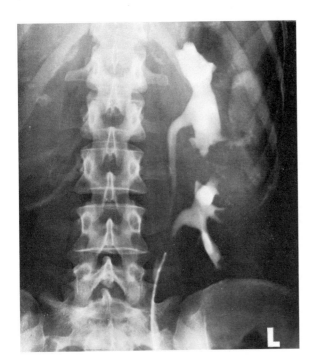

1612

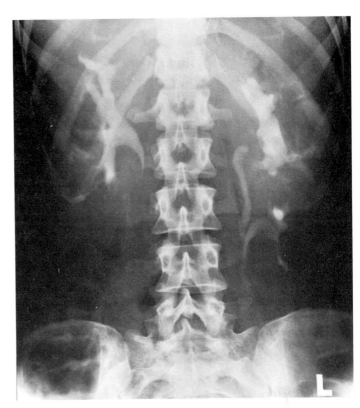

1613

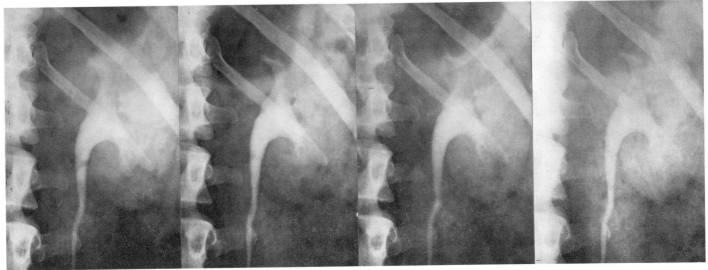

1614

Cystography

There are a number of radiographic methods for examining the bladder, the commonest being part of an intravenous urogram. The bladder is also examined as part of a functional study to show the urethra, cystourethrogram.

The bladder can in addition be examined using the single or double contrast methods as a static examination for bladder tumours. These static examinations however, have largely been abandoned because the extramural part of the tumour is not shown, being replaced by ultrasonography and computed tomography which give a clear view of both the inner and outer margins of the bladder wall (1625).

The Static Cystogram

The bladder is catheterised using strict asepsis emptied of urine and 300 ml of a 10% solution of a urographic contrast medium such as urografin or conray is injected and the catheter withdrawn. An antero-posterior, true lateral and two oblique projections are taken using a high kVp to obtain adequate penetration of the contrast filled bladder.

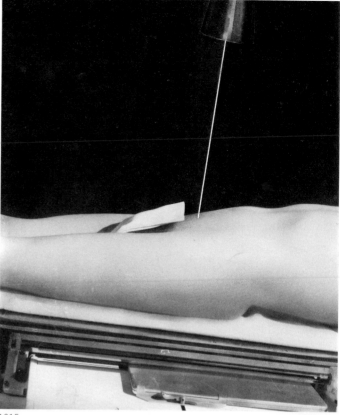

1615

Antero-posterior

With the patient supine, in the centre of the couch and the foot end raised 10° to fill the bladder, a 30 × 25 cm (12 × 10 ins) cassette is placed longitudinally with its upper border at the level of the anterior-superior iliac spines. Raising the foot end of the couch helps to fill the fundus of the bladder.

■ Centre in the midline just below the level of the anterior-superior iliac spine with the tube angled 15° towards the feet.

The difference in appearance of the bladder with the table horizontal and tilted is shown in (1586, 1587).

Left and right antero-posterior obliques

With the patient supine the left and right sides are raised in turn through 30° and triangular non-opaque foam pads are used for support. The legs are flexed at the hips and knees with the knees in contact and supported on the table with a foam pad.

■ Centre with the central ray perpendicular just below the anterior-superior iliac spine on the raised side, examining each side in turn. The film must be carefully labelled as to the side in contact with the table (1617, 1618, 1619).

N.B. If the bladder is overfilled with contrast medium and underpenetrated then only the silhouette will be visible 1617, 1618) but with less contrast and more penetration a better view of the bladder is obtained (1620, 1621, 1622). However, for a really adequate view of the bladder ultrasonography or computed tomography must be used (1625).

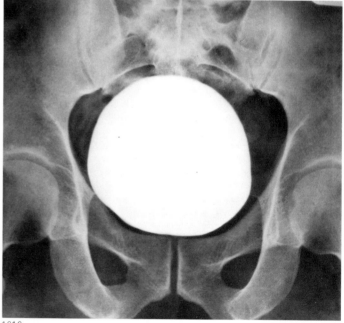

1616

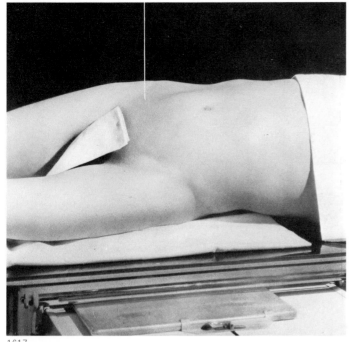

1617

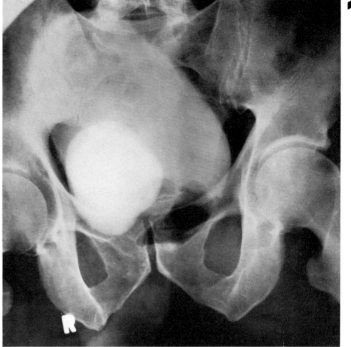

1620

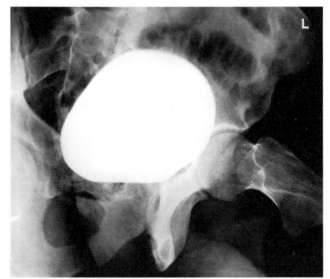

1618

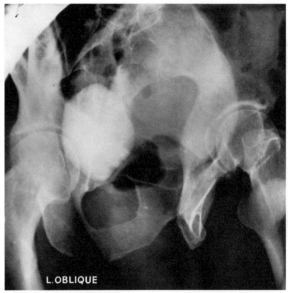

L.OBLIQUE

1621

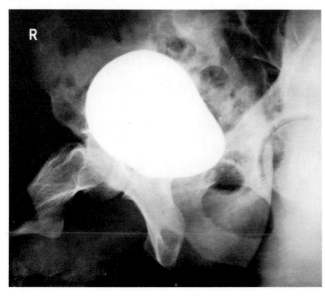

1619

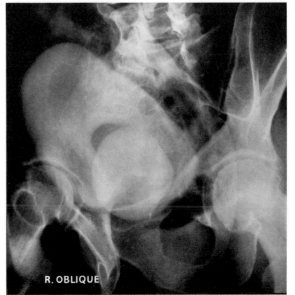

R. OBLIQUE

1622

Radiographs

In (1623) there is a large right sided bladder diverticulum, in (1624) bladder calculi with an indwelling catheter in a patient with a traumatic paraplegia and (1625) shows the bladder using computed tomography.

Lithotomy position

An additional projection of the bladder can be taken in the lithotomy position with the tube centred on the upper margin of the symphysis pubis (1627). With the patient supine, the hips are acutely flexed and the legs supported on rests attached to the couch or end of the urography table (1626a and b).

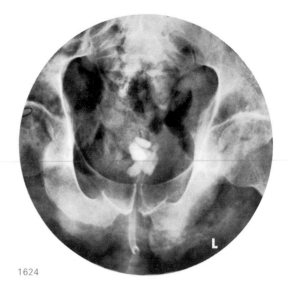

1624

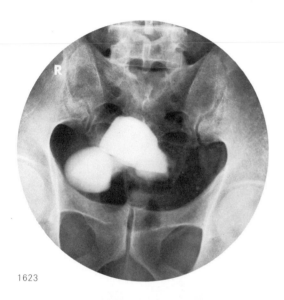

1623

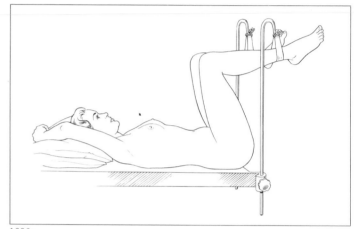

1626a

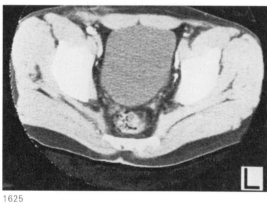

1625

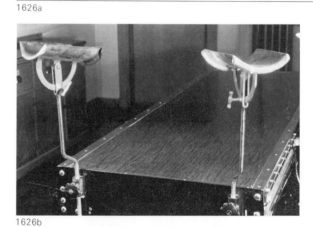

1626b

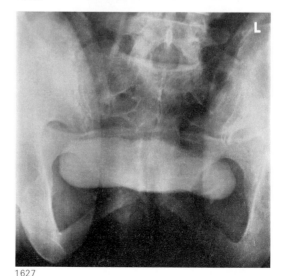

1627

470

Cysto-urethrography

The examination of the bladder and urethra by micturating cystourethrography follows catheterisation.

Immediately after the patient has urinated the urethra is catherised and the bladder emptied using strict sterility. The "residual urine" thus removed from the bladder is noted.

(1) Voiding or micturating cystourethrography for ureteric reflux or urethral valves is most commonly performed in children. The bladder is filled with a 25% solution of a urographic contrast medium such as sodium diatrizoate (Hypaque). The catheter is removed and spontaneous micturation is viewed fluoroscopically with image intensification and television monitoring. Ureteric reflux is recorded on spot films, cinefluorography or on videotape.

(2) Cystourethrography is also performed for stress incontinence in women to assess prolapse at the base of the bladder and to measure the angle between the urethra and bladder.

Three hundred millilitres of contrast medium is injected into the bladder and thereafter the patient is seated on a lavatory chair (1628) in a true lateral position. The descent of the bladder base and urethral leak on straining and coughing is recorded on spot films, videotape or cinefluorography. As with cysto-urethrography for reflux the examination is performed under fluoroscopy control with image intensification and television monitoring.

Films are taken in the relaxed position, on straining, during micturition and possibly after corrective surgery (1629–1632).

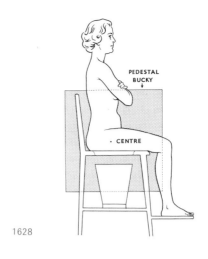

1628

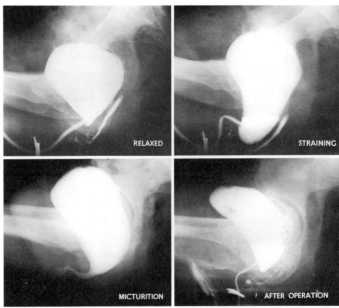

1629/1630 (top)   1631/1632 (above)

Urethrography

The male urethra is demonstrated by injecting contrast medium retrogradely from the end of the penis. Previously a viscous 50% contrast medium (Umbradil viscous) was used together with a clamp to seal off the tip of the penis. Presently a gravity pressure method with a non-irritant water soluble contrast agent such as methyl-glucamine acetrizoate 50% is most commonly used.

Spot films are taken during fluoroscopy with image intensification and television monitoring.

In the frontal view (1633) there is foreshortening of the urethra, whereas in the oblique views (1634, 1635) the full length of the urethra becomes visible. In the lateral view the overlying bone and soft tissue obscure the urethra necessitating a marked increase in exposure and is therefore not recommended.

After filling the bladder with contrast medium a micturating cysto-urethrogram can be performed to show the urethra (1636, 1637, 1638) and is particularly valuable for demonstrating congenital urethral valves.

Rarely a urinary calculus becomes impacted in the urethra and can be shown on plain films.

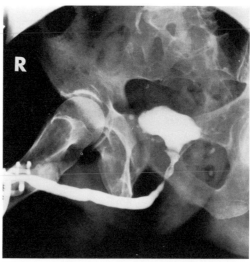

1634

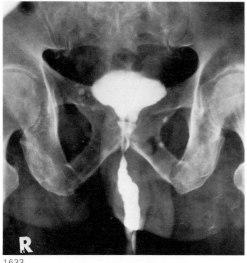

1633

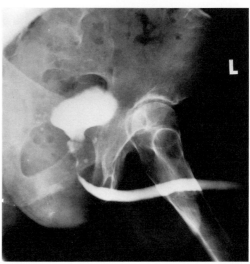

1635

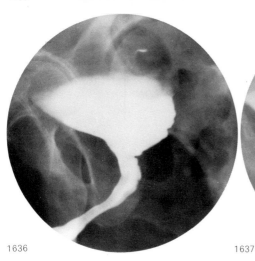

1636

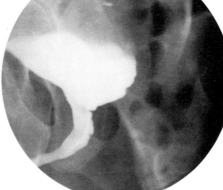

1637

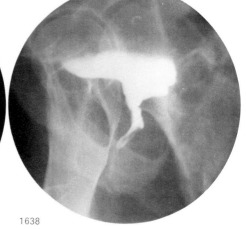

1638

Antero-posterior

The patient is seated on the end of a radiographic couch over a Potter-Bucky diaphragm with a back support. The legs are separated and flexed over the end of the couch.

■ Centre over the symphysis pubis with the tube angle 10° toward the head (1639).

Postero-anterior

The patient is prone with the legs separated and lying on a radiographic table with a Potter-Bucky diaphragm.

■ Centre to the symphysis pubis with the tube angled 10° towards the head (1640).

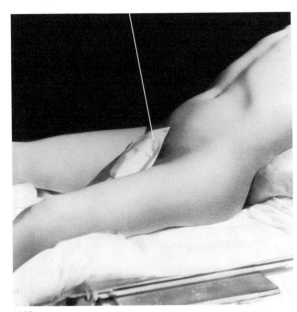

1639

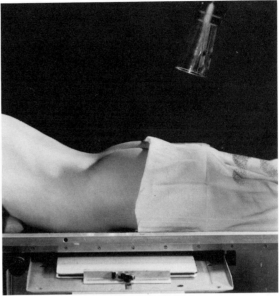

1640

A summary of exposure conditions for the urinary tract suitable for an adult of average physique

Region	Position	kVp	mAS	FFD	Film ILFORD	Screen ILFORD	Grid
Urinary Tract	Antero-posterior	70	50	100 cm (40″)	RAPID R	FT	Grid
	Postero-anterior	70	55	100 cm (40″)	RAPID R	FT	Grid
	Lateral	90	80	100 cm (40″)	RAPID R	FT	Grid
Ureters-Pelvic	Antero-posterior	70	50	100 cm (40″)	RAPID R	FT	Grid
	Oblique	80	50	100 cm (40″)	RAPID R	FT	Grid
Bladder	Antero-posterior						
	Antero-posterior lateral decubitus	90	40	100 cm (40″)	RAPID R	FT	Grid
Cystography	Antero-posterior	100	20	100 cm (40″)	RAPID R	FT	Grid
	Oblique	100	20	100 cm (40″)	RAPID R	FT	Grid
	Lateral	110	50	100 cm (40″)	RAPID R	FT	Grid
	Lithotomy	100	30	100 cm (40″)	RAPID R	FT	Grid
Cystourethrography	Lateral	90	50	100 cm (40″)	RAPID R	FT	Grid
Urethra	Antero-posterior	70	20	100 cm (40″)	RAPID R	FT	Grid
	Oblique	70	25	100 cm (40″)	RAPID R	FT	Grid
Prostate	Antero-posterior	75	30	100 cm (40″)	RAPID R	FT	Grid
	Postero-anterior						

477